In loving memory of
John Rutledge Boring, Jr., June Gibson Daniels,
Hubert Wayne Eley, Sr., William Dana Flanders, Jr.,
and Bernard George Greenberg

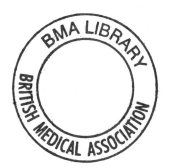

Contents

Preface

The authors of Medical Epidemiology are pleased to introduce the fourth edition of this book. Much has transpired in the field of epidemiology since the publication of the previous edition of this book just a few years ago. In September and October of 2001, several letters containing powders with spores of *Bacillus anthracis* were mailed in the United States, resulting in 22 cases of anthrax and five deaths. This episode emphasized the potential threat to human health that can arise when biological agents are used as weapons by terrorists. It also underscored the role that epidemiology can play in investigating and controlling such exposures.

Not much more than a year later, the world witnessed the dramatic emergence of a novel coronavirus, resulting in an epidemic new illness, Severe Acute Respiratory Syndrome (SARS). The rapid spread of this infection around the globe was aided by the highly contagious nature of this disease and the frequency of international travel. Through global cooperation, epidemiology once again proved to be critical in identifying and controlling an emerging infectious disease.

Accordingly, this new edition of *Medical Epidemiology* appears at a time when there is great focus on the role of epidemiology in studying both natural and man-made influences on human health. Moreover, the fast pace of external events reminds us of the importance of presenting the most current information possible. As with previous editions, we have updated information on patterns of disease occurrence and presented new self-assessment questions at the end of each chapter.

Although this book has been extensively revised, it remains faithful to the original intent of the authors—to provide a text that would serve the basic needs of medical students, as well as students of other health disciplines, such as public health, nursing, pharmacy, and dentistry. It is written concisely and can be used as a course textbook or as a stand-alone study guide.

OBJECTIVES

The aim of this book is to provide the reader with an overview of the principles and concepts of epidemiology. In so doing, it attempts to illustrate the complementary relationship between population-based science and the care of patients. Specific topic areas include:

- Measuring disease frequency
- Describing patterns of disease occurrence
- Investigating outbreaks of disease
- Assessing the utility of diagnostic tests
- Testing the effectiveness of treatments
- Identifying the causes of diseases
- Predicting the outcome of illness
- Decision-making about treatment strategies
- Summarizing evidence on clinical questions

Upon completion of this book, the reader should be able to calculate and interpret basic epidemiologic measures, recognize the various epidemiologic study designs with their respective advantages and limitations, understand the concepts of variability and bias, and characterize the means by which clinical evidence can be systematically summarized for decision-making.

APPROACH AND FEATURES

From the first edition of this book to the present version, the authors have taken the viewpoint that epidemiology should be both an understandable and interesting topic for students of the health professions. In order to introduce the topic in that manner, the following elements are emphasized:

- Conceptual topics are explained in nontechnical language.
- Liberal use is made of illustrations to facilitate comprehension and retention of material.
- The most current information available is presented on disease patterns and risk factors.
- Key concepts are highlighted for emphasis, with summaries at the beginning and end of each chapter.
- The relationship between population-based science and patient care is demonstrated through patient profiles.
- A full range of clinical areas of application is shown, including infectious diseases, cancer, Alzheimer's disease, and perinatal disorders.
- Critical formulas and equations are provided without undue emphasis on the mathematical applications of epidemiology.
- Questions are provided in standardized test format at the end of each chapter to help the student assess their knowledge and prepare for examinations.
- An updated glossary is provided to help the student master the vocabulary of epidemiology.

   If the response to the first three editions of this book is any indication, this approach is appealing to students of the health professions. The authors hope that the present edition continues to satisfy the demand for an engaging introductory text in epidemiology.

Charleston, South Carolina   Raymond S. Greenberg, MD, PhD
September, 2004

Acknowledgments

The fourth edition of this book was made possible through the dedicated efforts of many individuals, including Janet Foltin, Karen Edmonson, Regina Y. Brown, and Charissa Baker.

The comments and suggestions of several anonymous reviewers were helpful in refining the original style and contents of this book. In addition, Dr. Beth Dawson and Dr. Paul Levy provided valuable advice in the initial developmental process. The didactic approach used in this book was developed largely through the experience of teaching epidemiology to medical students at Emory University and the University of Cincinnati. We have learned a great deal from these students, and we hope that their suggestions are adequately represented in the pages that follow.

The authors have had the good fortune to study under and to work with a number of outstanding epidemiologists. In writing an introductory text, we were inevitably drawn back to the teachers who first attracted us to the field. The influences of former mentors can be found throughout this book. Of particular note are the teachings of Dr. Philip Cole at the School of Public Health of the University of Alabama-Birmingham, Dr. Kenneth Rothman at Boston University, Dr. David Kleinbaum, formerly of the University of North Carolina and now of Emory University, and Dean Michel Ibrahim at the School of Public Health of the University of North Carolina.

The support and encouragement of our respective institutions were essential for the completion of this project. We thank Dr. Jeffrey Houpt, former Dean of the Emory University School of Medicine, for promoting strong educational and research linkages with the faculty of the Rollins School of Public Health. Dr. Charles Hatcher, Jr., former Vice President for Health Affairs at Emory University, provided the resources and environment necessary for epidemiology and public health to develop at that institution. We also thank former Emory University President James T. Laney for his vision of the role of public health in serving human needs.

Ms. Essie Mills spent many long hours in the original preparation of the manuscript. For her extraordinary tolerance in dealing with countless revisions, erratic work schedules, and urgent deadlines, the authors will remain forever in her debt. We are especially grateful to Ms. Judy Holz for her outstanding efforts in revising the third and fourth editions of this text.

This book could not have been completed without the understanding and support of our wives and families. Time and again, precious hours at home were preempted by writing tasks, and we are grateful for the sacrifices that were made by our loved ones.

Charleston, South Carolina   Raymond S. Greenberg, MD, PhD
September, 2004

Introduction to Epidemiology

KEY CONCEPTS

1. Epidemiology is the study of the distribution and determinants of diseases within human populations. Research in this field is based primarily upon observing people directly in their natural environments.

2. Epidemiology can be used for descriptive purposes, such as surveillance of the occurrence (incidence) of a particular illness.

3. Epidemiology can be used for analytic purposes, such as studying risk factors for disease development.

4. Epidemiologic methods can be used to assess the performance of diagnostic tests.

5. Epidemiology can be used to study the progression or natural history of a disease.

6. Epidemiologic methods can be used to study prognostic factors, which are determinants of the progression of a disease.

7. Epidemiology can be used to evaluate treatments for a disease.

PATIENT PROFILE

A 29-year-old previously healthy man was referred to the University of California at Los Angeles (UCLA) Medical Center with a history of fever, fatigue, lymph node enlargement, and weight loss of almost 25 lb over the preceding 8 months. He had a temperature of 39.5°C, appeared physically wasted, and had swollen lymph nodes. Laboratory evaluation revealed a depressed level of peripheral blood lymphocytes. The patient suffered from simultaneous infections involving Candida albicans *in his upper digestive tract, cytomegalovirus in his urinary tract, and* Pneumocystis carinii *in his lungs. Although antibiotic therapy was administered, the patient remained severely ill.*

INTRODUCTION

Epidemiology is a fundamental medical science that focuses on the distribution and determinants of disease frequency in human populations. Specifically, epidemiologists examine patterns of illness in the population and then try to determine why certain groups or individuals develop a particular disease whereas others do not.

Knowledge about who is likely to develop a particular disease and under what circumstances they are likely to develop it is central to the daily practice of medicine and to efforts to improve the health of the public. To prevent an illness, health care providers must be able both to identify persons who because of personal characteristics or their environment are at high risk, and to intervene to reduce that risk. This type of knowledge emerges in many cases from epidemiologic research.

This book serves as an introduction to epidemiologic methods and the ways in which these methods can be used to answer key medical and public health questions. This chapter begins by considering a particular disease, as described in the Patient Profile. Focusing attention on one disease enables us to demonstrate the important contribution of epidemiology to current knowledge about this condition. Although the emphasis is on a single disease, it should be recognized that epidemiologic methods can be applied to a wide spectrum of conditions, ranging from acute illnesses, such as outbreaks of food-borne infections, to long-term debilitating conditions, such as Alzheimer's disease.

The man in the Patient Profile was referred to the UCLA Medical Center in June 1981. At the time, there was no obvious explanation as to why a healthy young man would suddenly develop concurrent infections in three different organ systems involving three different microorganisms. More surprising was the nature of the infections that were present. Opportunistic infections, such as those caused by the parasite *P carinii,* are infectious illnesses that tend to occur only in persons with lowered resistance, such as that which results from impaired immune responses. However, the young man described in the Patient Profile did not have any obvious underlying causes of immune dysfunction. For example, he did not have cancer or severe malnutrition and he did not use immunosuppressants. Why then was his body overwhelmed by the infections? This question was given a heightened sense of urgency by the severity of the patient's illness.

This patient was not the first to be referred to the UCLA Medical Center with this clinical presentation. Within the preceding 6 months three other previously healthy young men with recent histories of weight loss, fever, and lymph node enlargement had been examined. All had *P carinii* pneumonia and *C albicans* infections.

Why were four patients with similar symptoms appearing at about the same time in the same location? Suspecting that the illnesses in these four patients might be related, the UCLA physicians notified public health officials and prepared a descriptive report of their findings for publication.

Was this new appearance of a rare and life-threatening form of pneumonia confined to the UCLA Medical Center, or was it being observed by physicians elsewhere? If the experience at UCLA was unique, the entire episode might be regarded as a medical curiosity—unusual, but not a reason for great public health concern. On the other hand, if patients similar to those at UCLA were appearing in clinics or medical offices elsewhere, this episode could not be so easily dismissed. Within a matter of weeks, public health authorities received reports of outbreaks of *P carinii* pneumonia among previously healthy young men in San Francisco and New York City.

In the United States, the federal agency that is responsible for monitoring unusual patterns of disease occurrence is the Centers for Disease Control and Prevention (CDC). Recognizing the potential for the widespread emergence of this new, unexplained, and debilitating condition, the CDC established a special task force to collect more detailed information on the affected persons. In addition, the CDC issued a formal request to report such patients to all state health departments. Between June and November 1981, 76 instances of *P carinii* pneumonia were identified in persons who did not have known predisposing illnesses and were not taking immunosuppressants. A few months later, the disease that afflicted these patients was named the acquired immune deficiency syndrome (AIDS).

PERSON, PLACE, & TIME

The physicians at UCLA played a crucial role in establishing the presence of a new disease in their community. The first few affected patients identified with any outbreak of disease are referred to as **sentinel cases.** The story of the first few AIDS patients is particularly dramatic because of the severity of the illness and the extent and speed with which the disease spread to others. A sudden and great increase in the occurrence of a disease within a population is referred to as an **epidemic.** It quickly became apparent, however, that the emergence of AIDS was not confined to a few communities. A rapidly emerging outbreak of disease that affects a wide range of geographically distributed populations is described as a **pandemic.** In 1981, no one could have predicted that through 2002 almost 900,000 persons in the United States would be diagnosed with AIDS and over 500,000 deaths from AIDS would be reported nationally. By 1996, AIDS was the eighth most common cause of death in the United States and the third most common cause of death for persons between the ages of 25 and 44 years. With the introduction of effective combination drug therapy, the death rate from AIDS has declined in the United States and in other industrialized nations. In developing nations a much more devastating picture is emerging; for instance, of the estimated 3,000,000 deaths annually from AIDS worldwide, about three-fourths occur in sub-Saharan Africa.

Looking back to 1981, when AIDS had not yet been recognized as a clinical entity, it is instructive to consider the features of the sentinel cases that suggested a possible connection. All the patients with AIDS who presented to the UCLA clinicians suffered from the same rare opportunistic infections. Had the infections involved more conventional human pathogens—or less severe symptoms—the entire episode might have gone unnoticed for some time.

Beyond their clinical similarities, the sentinel cases shared other features as summarized in Table 1–1. All four patients were previously healthy homosexual men in their early 30s (personal characteristics) who resided in Los Angeles (place) and first became ill in the 9 months ending in June 1981 (time). These three dimensions—**person, place,** and **time**—are the features traditionally used to characterize patterns of disease occurrence, as discussed in Chapter 3.

THE EPIDEMIOLOGIC APPROACH

Epidemiology is the study of the distribution and determinants of disease frequency in human populations. Interest in frequency or occurrence of disease derives largely from a basic tenet of epidemiology, namely that disease does not develop at random. In essence, all persons are not equally likely to develop a particular disease. The level of risk for different individuals typically is a function of their personal characteristics and environment.

As applied to the outbreak of AIDS, for instance, it is highly unlikely that of the first four cases seen in Los Angeles all would have occurred in homosexual males if the disease was striking at random. The repeated occurrence of AIDS in homosexual men suggested that this segment of the population had an increased risk of developing the disease. Other high-risk groups for AIDS, including hemophiliacs and injecting drug users, were soon identified. On the surface, these three groups seemed to have little in common. On closer examination, however, it became evident that an increased risk of exposure to the blood of other persons was the factor they all shared.

Contemporary medical research is devoted largely to investigating the biologic elements of disease development. For example, in the study of AIDS, a microbiologist tends to focus on the infectious agent, the human immunodeficiency virus (HIV). An immunologist might concentrate on the primary target of HIV infection, the CD4$^+$ T lymphocyte, which coordinates a number of immune functions. The epidemiologist, on the other hand, views a disease from both a biologic and a social perspective. It is not enough to know that HIV is transmitted primarily through contaminated blood. The epidemiologist must be able to understand the circumstances of HIV transmission among humans. Here, the influence of social factors is undeniable. The spread of AIDS in human populations cannot be fully appreciated without recognizing the role of certain behaviors, such as sexual practices or injecting drug use.

The desire to study social factors that impinge on health has definite implications for how epidemiologic research is conducted. In most instances, this research involves observations of phenomena that occur naturally within human populations. Such an approach is unique among the medical sciences. Two features distinguish the epidemiologic approach from other biomedical sciences: (1) the focus on human populations and (2) a heavy reliance on nonexperimental observations.

At first, the focus on human populations may not seem distinctive. Ultimately, all medical research is motivated by a desire to prevent or control human illnesses. However, the process leading to that goal may take various routes. Laboratory scientists, for example, often rely on experiments that involve nonhuman animals, cells in tissue culture, or biochemical assays. Although these studies offer important advantages to the investigator, such as precise control over the experimental conditions, certain limitations must also be recognized. Obviously, a laboratory environment may not accurately reflect the actual conditions of exposure in the external world. Of equal importance is the recognition that animals of different species may have dissimilar responses to experimental manipulations. It cannot be assumed that biologic effects detected in rodents, for instance, will necessarily apply to humans.

Epidemiologists avoid these concerns by attempting to study people directly in their natural environments. With this approach, it is not necessary to make assumptions about similarity of effects either across species or across doses and routes of exposure. The epidemiologist actually observes the patterns of exposure and disease development as they naturally occur within human populations. Without such information, it would not be possible to reach a definitive conclusion about the extent of disease related to a particular agent.

As with any scientific method, the epidemiologic approach has inherent constraints. In observational research, which comprises much of epidemiology, the investigator merely watches the phenomena under study (ie, the epidemiologist has no control over the events

Table 1–1. Characteristics of sentinel cases of AIDS in Los Angeles,1981.

Characteristics of Sentinel Cases	Personal Attributes
Age	Early 30s
Gender	Male
Prior health	Good
Sexual preference	Homosexual
Place of occurrence	Los Angeles
Time of occurrence	October 19, 1980 to June 19, 1981

that occur). It is often difficult, therefore, to separate the causal contributions of the exposure of interest from the causal contributions of other background influences in the population. Even direct measurement of the degree of exposure may not be possible in some settings, thereby forcing the epidemiologist to rely on indirect estimates.

The epidemiologist's perspective of the relationship between exposure to risk factors and the development of disease in human populations may appear rather crude in comparison to exacting research performed at the molecular level. Indeed, epidemiology is not particularly useful for characterizing the precise biologic mechanisms of disease development. The epidemiologist frequently sees only how different levels of exposure across groups of the population affect the comparative likelihood that those groups will develop disease. Typically, the epidemiologist can identify the personal, social, and environmental circumstances under which a disease tends to occur, without being able to explain the exact processes that give rise to the disease.

Medical progress often is best advanced when the sciences that focus on subcellular and molecular basic research work in tandem with the population-oriented science of epidemiology. For example, as bench scientists were struggling to characterize the molecular properties of HIV, epidemiologists already determined that AIDS is a contagious disease that is spread through certain interpersonal behaviors. As the painstaking search continues for improved treatment, or even a cure or vaccine, public health professionals have recommended measures to prevent the spread of HIV by reducing the frequency of high-risk practices, such as casual, unprotected sex and sharing needles among injecting drug users.

THE APPLICATIONS OF EPIDEMIOLOGY

Epidemiologic methods can be used for a number of distinct purposes. In the following sections, these areas of application are specified, with corresponding illustrations drawn from the literature on AIDS.

Disease Surveillance

Perhaps the most basic question that can be asked about a disease is "What is the frequency with which the disease occurs?" To answer this question, it is necessary to know the number of persons who acquire the disease (cases) over a specified period of time, and the size of the unaffected population. Measures of frequency of occurrence of a disease, described in Chapter 2, are used to characterize the patterns of the occurrence of the disease, described

in Chapter 3, and the medical surveillance of the disease, discussed in Chapter 4. Typically, the criteria used to define the occurrence of a disease depend on current knowledge about the disease; such criteria may become more refined as the causes of a disease are delineated and new diagnostic tests are introduced. For example, in 1982, the CDC created an initial, relatively simple surveillance definition for AIDS: "A disease, at least moderately indicative of a defect in cell-mediated immunity, occurring in a person with no known cause for diminished resistance to that disease."

A more specific definition became possible once the causative agent, HIV, was identified and tests for the detection of antibodies to the virus were developed. In 1987, the CDC surveillance definition was expanded to incorporate clinical conditions that are indicative of AIDS. A 1993 revision further expanded the surveillance definition to include three additional indicator conditions (pulmonary tuberculosis, recurrent pneumonia, or invasive cervical cancer), or the presence of a severely depressed $CD4^+$ T-lymphocyte count. In 2000, the CDC integrated monitoring of both HIV infection and AIDS.

Such changes in diagnostic criteria can have a profound effect on the apparent frequency of a disease. The expanded definition of AIDS introduced in 1987 led to an increase in the number of reported AIDS patients by about 50% during the next 2 years. The 1993 revision more than doubled the number of persons who met the surveillance definition. Most of the latter increase was attributable to persons made eligible on the basis of reduced $CD4^+$ T-lymphocyte counts and HIV infection. Accordingly, analysis of trends in disease occurrence over time must account for the possible effects of any temporal changes in diagnostic criteria.

The identification of patients with a disease can occur through various mechanisms, most commonly by physician and laboratory reporting. In the United States, a number of diseases, including AIDS, must be reported to public health authorities. Monitoring the patterns of occurrence of a disease within a population is referred to as **surveillance.** There are many potential benefits from the collection of surveillance data. This type of information (1) can help to identify the new outbreak of an illness, such as AIDS, (2) can provide clues, by considering the population groups that are most affected by the illness, to possible causes of the condition, (3) can be used to suggest strategies to control or prevent the spread of disease, (4) can be used to measure the impact of disease prevention and control efforts, and finally, (5) can provide information on the burden of illness, data that are necessary for determining health and medical service needs.

The course of the AIDS pandemic in the United States is depicted in Figure 1–1. To diminish the im-

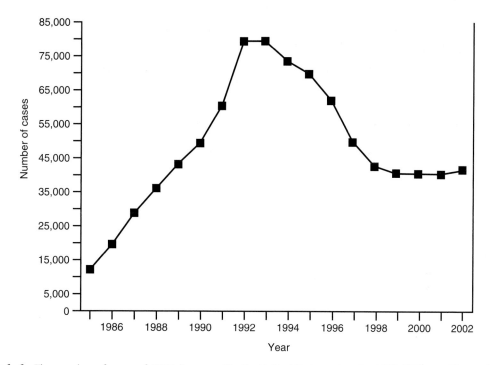

Figure 1–1. The number of cases of AIDS diagnosed in the United States using the 1993 CDC surveillance defini-tion, after adjustments for reporting delays, 1985–2002. (Modified and reproduced from CDC: HIV/AIDS Surveillance Report 2002;**14**:1.)

pact of changes of the surveillance definition over time, a single definition, the 1993 CDC version, was used throughout. From 1985 through 1992 there was an un-relenting rise in the number of newly reported cases. From 1993 through 1998 there was a progressive fall in the number of newly reported cases. Between 1999 and 2001 the level of AIDS cases was unchanged, with a slight increase in 2002. It should be noted that the in-formation in Figure 1–1 relates to the **number** of newly diagnosed cases per year. Changes in the counts of new cases can be affected by a number of factors, including among others, changes in the following:

1. Frequency with which the disease occurs
2. Definition of the disease
3. Size of the population from which the cases de-velop
4. Completeness of the reporting of the cases.

With respect to point 2, the same surveillance defin-ition was used consistently for all years in Figure 1–1,

minimizing any confounding influence of a change in definition of the disease over time. With regard to point 3, growth in the size of the population of the United States could not explain more than a trivial amount of the rise in the cases seen between 1985 and 1992. The national population grew at only about 1% per year, whereas the average annual increase in re-ported persons with AIDS exceeded 30%. Moreover, the declines in AIDS cases observed between 1993 and 1998 occurred while the population of the United States continued to grow. Concerning point 4, the overall completeness of reporting of AIDS cases is esti-mated to be about 85% in the United States. Although there is some internal variation by geographic subregion and patient population, it is unlikely that these patterns could have given rise to more than a small part of the trend observed in Figure 1–1. Since items 2 through 4 do not appear to account for the marked changes in the annual numbers of reported AIDS cases, it is reasonable to conclude that the observed trends reflect true changes in the occurrence of the disease.

For surveillance purposes, the size of the source population from which cases arise usually is estimated from census data. The frequency of disease occurrence is then expressed as the number of new cases developing within a specified time among a standard number of unaffected individuals. For example, during 2002 over 42,000 cases of AIDS were reported in the United States; the U.S. population in 2002 was about 288,000,000. Dividing the number of reported cases by the size of the population yields 0.00015 cases per person during that year. For ease and consistency of expression of such figures, epidemiologists typically express such frequencies of disease occurrence for a population of a specified size, say 100,000 persons. By multiplying 0.00015 by 100,000, the number 15 is obtained. That is to say, within a standard population of 100,000 persons in the United States, 15 persons would have been reported as developing AIDS during 2002. This measure of the rapidity of disease occurrence is referred to as an **incidence rate.** More information on incidence rates is presented in Chapter 2.

To characterize patterns of disease occurrence, incidence rates may be determined for groups defined by geographic area. For example, Figure 1–2 in annual incidence rates for AIDS are presented by place of residence in the United States. During 1997, the incidence rate for the District of Columbia was the highest observed, with 162.4 reported cases for every 100,000 residents. At the other extreme, North Dakota experienced the lowest annual incidence rate (0.5 cases per 100,000 residents). In other words, AIDS occurred in the District of Columbia about 325 times (162.4/0.5 = 325) more frequently than in North Dakota. Why are persons in the District of Columbia so frequently diagnosed with AIDS; conversely, why are persons in North Dakota so infrequently affected?

Answers to such questions typically do not derive from surveillance information alone. Surveillance data usually are limited to general characteristics of affected persons, such as their age, race, sex, and place of residence. Although variations in incidence rates according to these demographic features can lead to the identifica-

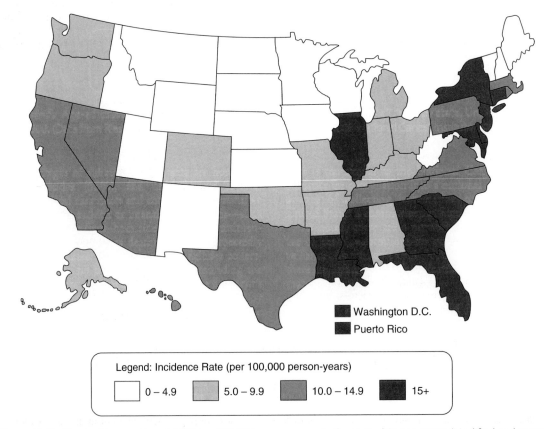

Figure 1–2. The incidence rates of AIDS per 100,000 person-years in the United States, 2002. (Modified and reproduced from CDC: HIV/AIDS Surveillance Report 2002;**14**:27–28.)

tion of high-risk groups, explanations for these patterns generally require more in-depth investigation into personal characteristics, behaviors, and environments.

Searching for Causes

To study personal and environmental characteristics, epidemiologists often rely on interviews, review of records, and laboratory examinations. Through such sources of information, a profile of characteristics that accompany the disease can be generated. Associations between these characteristics and the occurrence of disease can arise by coincidence, by noncausal linkages to other features, or by cause-and-effect relationships.

The epidemiologist is primarily interested in the last category, ie, determinants of disease development, also known as **risk factors.** Identification of risk factors can provide a better understanding of the pathways leading to disease acquisition, and consequently, better strategies for prevention.

Again, returning to the AIDS example, early epidemiologic studies played an important role in determining the cause of this disease. Within the first 5 months after recognition of this syndrome, the CDC had received reports on 70 patients with AIDS in four urban centers. Of these individuals, 50 homosexual

male patients with AIDS were interviewed; also interviewed were 120 unaffected homosexual male comparison subjects. Persons who are affected with a disease are referred to by epidemiologists as **cases,** and unaffected comparison persons are called **controls.** Comparison of the responses from cases and controls revealed that the AIDS patients had a higher number of sexual partners. This type of investigation is referred to as a **case–control study;** the basic design of such a study is illustrated in Figure 1–3.

In essence, this study is an attempt to look backward in time to identify characteristics that may have contributed to the development of the disease. The increased number of sexual partners—as well as a greater frequency of syphilis among cases—suggested that AIDS resulted from a sexually transmitted infectious agent, later discovered to be the HIV virus. Case–control studies are described in Chapter 9.

Comparison of historical exposures reported by cases and controls can provide suggestive evidence of a cause-and-effect relationship. This type of information, however, may be distorted or **biased** by the fact that the ability of cases and controls to recall earlier exposures differs. Such bias could be avoided by using a **cohort study** design, in which exposure is assessed among unaffected persons, and subjects are then observed for sub-

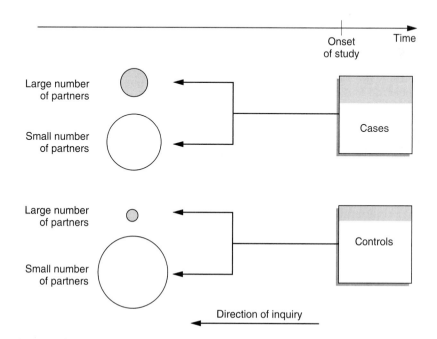

Figure 1–3. Schematic diagram of a case–control study of the association between the number of male sexual partners of homosexual men and the risk of AIDS. Shaded areas represent subjects with a large number of sexual partners, and unshaded areas represent subjects with a small number of sexual partners.

sequent development of illness. To collect such data, a cohort of 2507 homosexual men without antibodies to HIV (seronegative) was questioned about their sexual practices, and then followed for development of antibodies to HIV (seroconversion). Within 6 months, 95 men (3.8%) seroconverted, and the likelihood or **risk** of developing HIV antibodies was found to be related to receptive anal intercourse. The basic design of this cohort study is illustrated schematically in Figure 1–4. Cohort studies are discussed in Chapter 8.

The proportion of new AIDS cases related to sexual transmission between homosexual men has declined over time in the United States. In 2002, slightly more than half of all reported AIDS cases occurred among men who have sex with men. Use of injected drugs accounted for almost one-fourth of cases, and heterosexual contact was responsible for almost one-sixth of all cases. The diminished role of homosexual contact as a contributing factor in the occurrence of AIDS in the United States reflected avoidance of high-risk behaviors, although there is evidence that high-risk behaviors continue in some communities.

HIV transmission through heterosexual intercourse continues to increase in the United States and is the leading mode of transmission worldwide. The practice of safe sex can prevent the transmission of AIDS among

heterosexuals, as demonstrated clearly in a cohort study by de Vincenzi (1994). That European study included heterosexual couples in which only one partner was HIV seropositive at the outset. Couples were followed for an average of almost 2 years to determine the relationship between certain sexual practices and the risk of HIV transmission to the uninfected partner. Condom use was found to be an effective barrier to HIV transmission. Among 124 couples who consistently used condoms there were no episodes of seroconversion of uninfected partners. However, among 121 couples whose condom use was inconsistent, there were 12 instances of seroconversions of initially uninfected partners.

Diagnostic Testing

The purpose of diagnostic testing is to obtain objective evidence of the presence or absence of a particular condition. This evidence can be obtained to detect disease at its earliest stages among asymptomatic persons in the general population, a process referred to as **screening.** In other circumstances, diagnostic tests are used to confirm a diagnosis among persons with existing signs or symptoms of illness. Ideally, a diagnostic test would correctly distin-

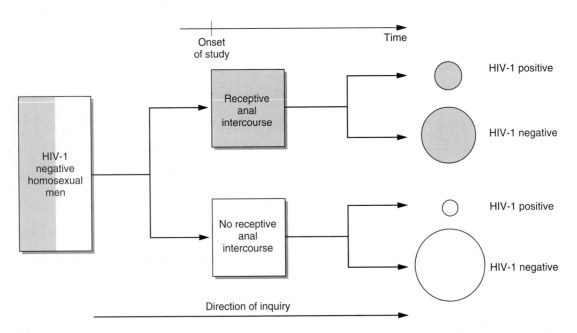

Figure 1–4. Schematic diagram of a cohort study of the association between receptive anal intercourse and risk of being HIV positive. Shaded areas indicate subjects who practice receptive anal intercourse, and unshaded areas represent subjects who do not.

guish affected persons from unaffected persons; unfortunately, as is true of most diagnostic tests, assays for HIV infection are not perfect.

Occasionally, a positive test result will incorrectly suggest that infection is present in an unaffected person. This type of outcome is referred to as a **false positive,** because the positive test result was in error. Obviously, a false-positive finding for HIV infection could be devastating to the tested individual, so every effort must be made to keep such errors to a minimum. A test with a very low percentage of false-positive results is said to have **high specificity** (Figure 1–5).

Another type of error occurs when a test incorrectly suggests that infection is not present (negative test result) in an affected person. This type of outcome is referred to as a **false negative,** because the negative test result was in error. A false-negative finding for HIV infection could provide inappropriate reassurance to an infected person, thereby delaying the start of treatment and possibly increasing the risk of spread to other persons. A test with a very low percentage of false-negative results is described as having **high sensitivity** (Figure 1–6). More detail on measures of test accuracy is presented in Chapter 6.

A number of different tests for the presence of HIV infection are available. The screening approach used most widely is to attempt to detect antibodies to the virus. This strategy is based on two assumptions: (1) HIV-infected

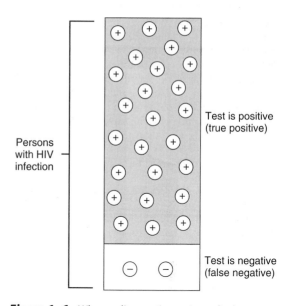

Figure 1–6. When a diagnostic test is applied to persons with HIV infection, it is highly sensitive if the true positive test results (shaded area) greatly outnumber the erroneous negative test results (unshaded area).

persons have detectable antibodies, and (2) persons with detectable antibodies to the virus are infected with HIV. In practice, these assumptions appear to be reasonably valid among patients beyond the first few months of infection. The time required to mount an antibody response sufficient for detection (seroconversion) varies across patients, but the vast majority seroconvert in less than 6 months following initial HIV infection.

The performance of an enzyme-linked immunosorbent assay (ELISA) test for antibodies to HIV was first reported in 1985. Among 74 patients who met the CDC clinical surveillance definition for AIDS and had unequivocal ELISA test results, 72 (97%) had detectable antibodies. In other words, a false-negative outcome was observed for only 2 patients (3%). Among 261 healthy blood donors with unequivocal ELISA test results, 257 (98%) had no detectable antibodies (ie, a false-positive outcome was found for 4 persons [2%]). Thus, the ELISA test was judged to be both sensitive and specific, and it has become the most widely employed screening test for HIV infection.

A number of different ELISA kits are commercially available. When false-negative ELISA results occur among high-risk individuals, the most likely explanation is that the test was performed prior to the development of detectable antibody levels in the immediate postinfection period. False-positive ELISA test results have been observed among patients with medical con-

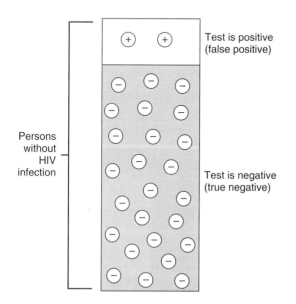

Figure 1–5. When a diagnostic test is applied to persons without HIV infection, it is highly specific if the true negative test results (shaded area) greatly outnumber erroneous positive test results (unshaded area).

ditions unrelated to HIV, such as autoimmune disorders, hematologic malignancies, and infections with viruses other than HIV, among patients recently vaccinated against hepatitis B or influenza, and among patients who have received immune globulin. Technical or human errors in performing the ELISA test also can produce false-positive results.

Considering the potential for error, it is recommended that a positive ELISA test be repeated in duplicate. If either of the follow-up tests is positive, a supplementary test should be performed. The most widely used confirmatory test is the Western blot. This type of test is not recommended for screening purposes, because Western blot can produce a substantial proportion of equivocal results among persons who are negative to all other HIV tests.

The presence of infection with HIV also can be detected through other approaches, such as the detection of viral genetic material in plasma.

Determining the Natural History

After being informed of a new diagnosis, patients most frequently ask "What will happen to me?" This question cannot be answered with absolute certainty because of variations in outcome across individual patients. Usually the best guidance for predictions is the experience of other patients who are similar to the patient in question. Even when the ultimate outcome can be predicted with some confidence, the actual sequence of events can vary widely among patients.

Consider, for example, a patient newly diagnosed as being HIV positive. In this instance, with the advent of new treatments it is reasonable to question whether the full syndrome of AIDS will develop, and if it does how long it will take to occur. In attempting to address these questions, the physician might consult published research on the progression of HIV-related illness. Usually these data are collected on large groups of patients. By noting the timing of critical events for each patient (eg, date of determination of HIV infection, development of clinical symptoms of illness, demonstrable changes in immune function, diagnosis of AIDS, and subsequent clinical events), the progression of the disease can be divided into phases.

When these events are summarized for many patients, precise and accurate estimates of the typical sequence of events—the **natural history** of the illness—can be constructed. Some authors restrict the use of the descriptor "natural" to situations in which medical treatment is unavailable or ineffective. Others use the term more broadly, to indicate the typical course of an illness, regardless of whether it can be treated effectively.

There are several ways to characterize the natural history of an illness. One straightforward measure is the **case fatality,** which represents the percentage of patients with a disease who die within a specified observation period. For example, among the 11,740 reported adolescent and adult patients diagnosed with AIDS in 1985 in the United States, 10,946 are known to have died before 1998. In other words, the case fatality was

$$\frac{10{,}946}{11{,}740} \times 100\% = 93.2\%$$

The approach to determining the case fatality is illustrated schematically in Figure 1–7.

Another method of characterizing the natural history of a disease is to estimate the typical duration from diagnosis to death (**survival time**). As an illustration, a study was conducted in a rural part of Uganda, a country with a high prevalence of HIV infection. In this setting, in which economic and other conditions limited treatment to simple and affordable drugs, the natural history of HIV infection was characterized. The study involved persons who were seropositive for HIV and a comparison group of seronegative individuals. All subjects were identified in 1990 and were evaluated clinically every 3 months until death or the end of calendar year 1995, whichever came first. For the initial 3 years after seroconversion, there was no difference in survival between the HIV-positive persons and the persons without infection. However, by 5 years following seroconversion only 83% of the HIV-positive persons were still alive, compared with 94% of the seronegative persons.

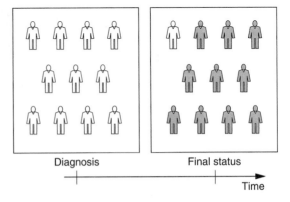

Diagnosis   Final status

Time

Figure 1–7. Schematic diagram of the concept of case fatality. Shaded figures represent patients who are deceased and unshaded figures represent patients who are alive.

A number of factors can affect the apparent natural history of HIV-related illnesses. HIV infection may exist for a prolonged period of time prior to the development of symptoms that lead to a clinical diagnosis of AIDS. Recognition of the presence of infection during this preclinical phase clearly depends on the availability of an effective screening test, the sensitivity of the test to detect early infection, and the extent to which the screening test is applied in the population. The expectation, therefore, is that in the earliest years of the AIDS epidemic, prior to the development and widespread application of screening tests for HIV, the diagnosis was made at comparatively advanced stages of infection, when symptoms already were evident.

Comparisons of the survival experience of patients with AIDS both regionally and internationally also might be distorted by differences in the extent to which screening for HIV and CD4+ T-lymphocyte counts are employed in the different locations.

Changes over time in the criteria used to diagnose AIDS could also alter the apparent survival experience of patients with this disease. For example, analysis of patients with HIV registered in Italy between July 1987 and December 1991 revealed that when the 1987 CDC case definition for AIDS was applied, half of the patients survived for 24 months more or longer. The length of survival that is met or exceeded by 50% of the study population is referred to as the **median survival time.** When the broadened 1993 CDC case definition

was retrospectively applied to this same population, not only did a larger number of patients meet the definition, but the median survival time was found to exceed 57 months. In other words, the population of patients who met the 1993 case definition tended to have a more favorable outcome than the subset that met the earlier definition.

In estimating the natural history of HIV infection, an increasingly important issue is the impact of more effective treatments on the progression of illness. The benefits of improved clinical treatment are not confined to persons in advanced stages of disease. As shown schematically in Figure 1–8, the introduction of effective therapy can delay the onset of AIDS after infection with HIV, as well as extend the duration of survival after a diagnosis of AIDS. Several studies in industrialized countries have demonstrated that the rate of progression from HIV infection to a diagnosis of AIDS was reduced by about 75% after the introduction of highly active antiretroviral therapy (HAART). Similarly, the rate of progression from AIDS to death declined by about two-thirds after the introduction of HAART.

Searching for Prognostic Factors

Analysis of survival can be employed to identify groups of patients with unusually favorable (or unfavorable) clinical outcomes. Characteristics that relate to the likelihood of survival are referred

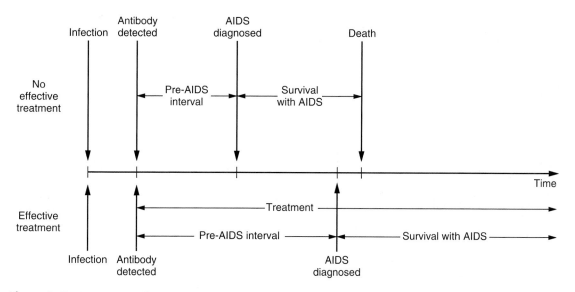

Figure 1–8. Comparison of the clinical progression of HIV infection prior to effective treatment and after the introduction of effective treatment. Aggressive early treatment delays the onset of AIDS and prolongs survival after the diagnosis of AIDS.

to as **prognostic factors.** The approach to identifying prognostic factors can be illustrated by a study conducted by Mellors and colleagues (1997). Using data collected from the Multicenter AIDS Cohort Study of homosexual men in the United States, the investigators evaluated factors related to the progression from initial infection with HIV to two clinical end points: (1) the development of AIDS and (2) AIDS-related death. A total of 1604 men were enrolled in the study, which included a follow-up period on average of almost 10 years. Over this time period, 998 of the participants developed AIDS and 855 died of AIDS. The design of this study is depicted schematically in Figure 1–9. Figure 1–9 shows that the study design is similar to that of the cohort study (Figure 1–4), except that the focus is on predicting survival rather than on determining risk factors for the onset of disease.

In the study by Mellors and associates, a number of potential prognostic factors were assessed, including, among others, oral candidiasis or fever, markers of immune stimulation, various lymphocyte counts including CD4+ T-lymphocytes, and an assay of the plasma concentration of HIV-1 RNA (ribonucleic acid—the genetic material of the virus). The HIV-1 RNA assay provides a precise measurement of the load of the virus circulating in a patient's blood. As might be expected, some association was seen between the initial levels of the individual prognostic factors. For example, patients with higher viral loads at the start of the study were more likely to have fever or oral candidiasis and reduced levels of CD4+ T-lymphocytes. Viral load also was seen as the single best predictor of the subsequent decline over time in CD4+ T-lymphocyte levels, as well as in the progression to AIDS and death. Specifically, when study subjects were grouped into five ordered categories based on plasma viral load, the 6-year probability of AIDS-related death ranged from 1% among those with the lightest load, to 70% among those with the heaviest load. By combining information on HIV-1 RNA concentrations with CD4+ T-lymphocyte levels, even more effective determination of the likelihood of disease progression could be made (Table 1–2).

Testing New Treatments

In the United States, all new medications must be tested and proved effective before they can be introduced into routine clinical care. The standard approach used to evaluate treatment effectiveness is the **randomized controlled clinical trial.** The term "controlled" means that patients (experimental subjects) who receive the new medication are compared with patients (control subjects) who receive either an inactive substance (placebo) or a standard treatment if one

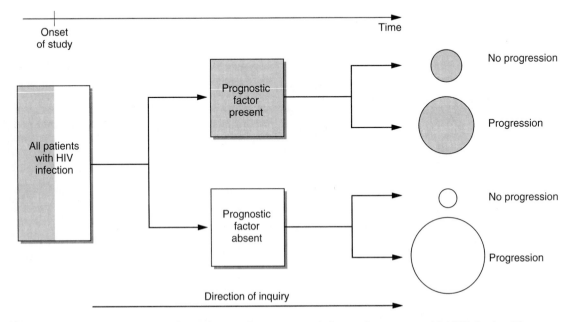

Figure 1–9. Schematic diagram of a study to evaluate prognostic factors for persons with HIV infection. The shaded areas represent patients with the favorable prognostic factor of interest and the unshaded areas represent patients without the prognostic factor of interest.

Table 1–2. Independent prognostic factors for AIDS.

Factor	Poor Prognosis Level
Age	37 years or older
Initial presentation	Multiple diagnoses
Single diagnosis other than Kaposi's sarcoma or *P carinii* pneumonia	Thrush
CD4+ T lymphocytes	Low
HIV-1 RNA level	High

exists. "Randomized" refers to a method of assignment of subjects to either the experimental or control group that is determined by chance rather than patient preference or physician selection. This type of allocation system is desirable because it tends to result in study groups that are comparable with respect to important prognostic factors. Randomized controlled clinical trials are discussed in Chapter 7.

The principles of randomized controlled clinical trials can be demonstrated by a study that has contributed to a revolution in the treatment of HIV-infected persons. That study, published by Hammer and colleagues in 1997, compared a standard therapy with a new ex-perimental treatment regimen. The standard therapy employed two drugs (zidovudine and lamivudine), both of which are inhibitors of the HIV reverse transcriptase. By interfering with the conversion of viral genetic material to a form that can be incorporated into the host, these drugs limit the replication of HIV within host cells. The experimental treatment involved these two drugs plus another one (indinavir), which is an inhibitor of the HIV protease. Protease inhibitors interfere with the process of assembling viral components after replication of HIV genetic material. The experimental therapy, therefore, involved a simultaneous attack on two separate and distinct steps in the process of HIV reproduction. Prior studies had demonstrated that this combined therapy was capable of reducing viral plasma load and raising CD4+ T-lymphocyte levels. Since favorable responses were seen in these prognostic factors, it was reasonable to anticipate that this combination therapy might diminish the rate of progression of HIV-related disease.

Hammer and colleagues undertook a randomized controlled clinical trial in which a standard two-drug reverse transciptase regimen was compared with a three-drug combined reverse transcriptase/protease inhibition experimental treatment. The basic design of the trial is depicted in Figure 1–10. Participants were recruited from 40 different clinical centers throughout the United

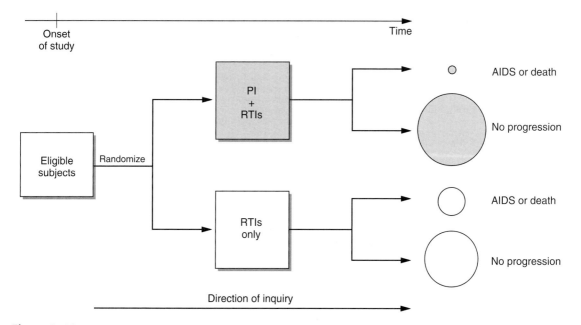

Figure 1–10. Schematic diagram of a randomized controlled clinical trial of reverse transcriptase inhibitors (RTIs), with or without a protease inhibitor (PI), for the treatment of HIV infection. The shaded area indicates patients randomized to receive combined treatment with RTIs and a PI.

States. The subjects were required to have documentation of HIV infection and a CD4$^+$ T-lymphocyte level diminished below a predetermined level. To minimize effects of prior therapy, eligible subjects were limited to those who had not been treated previously with a protease inhibitor. A total of 1156 patients were randomized between January 1996 and January 1997, with 579 assigned to the standard therapy group and the remaining 577 assigned to the experimental therapy group. The clinical characteristics of the two groups were similar at the onset of treatment. After an average of about 38 weeks of observation, the trial was terminated because of a dramatic difference in risk of disease progression between the two groups. Within the experimental treatment group of the study, 33 patients (6%) progressed to AIDS or died. In contrast, within the standard treatment group, 63 patients (11%) progressed to AIDS or died.

The results of this trial and other similar studies clearly demonstrated the short-term therapeutic benefit of combined treatment with reverse transcriptase inhibitors and protease inhibitors. The ethical imperative to terminate this study early because of the substantial advantage of combination therapy left unresolved the question of whether this effect is sustainable over longer periods of time. Even without data on the long-term benefits, the striking results of the studies of combined reverse transcriptase and protease inhibition changed the whole approach to clinical management of HIV infection. As the search for even more effective treatments continues, randomized controlled clinical trials will serve as the definitive approach to establishing therapeutic superiority.

SUMMARY

In this chapter, we have seen how epidemiologic research has contributed to basic knowledge about AIDS:

1. The techniques of surveillance were used to determine the patterns of HIV infection and occurrence of AIDS by person, place, and time.
2. Comparisons of affected and unaffected persons led to the identification of risk factors and ultimately to the suspicion that an infectious agent was responsible for the disease.
3. Evaluation of tests for antibodies to HIV allowed improved diagnosis and prevention of spread by contaminated blood products.
4. Studies of natural history helped to define the clinical course of the illness.
5. Prognostic factors were determined through comparison of patients with favorable and unfavorable outcomes.

6. Finally, improvement in treatment was demonstrated through randomized controlled clinical trials.

The story of HIV and AIDS is particularly dramatic because it involves a devastating disease that emerged rapidly in the population and developed with minimal advance warning. It is an unfinished story because new cases are still occurring with considerable frequency, and a cure has not yet been identified. Epidemiology will continue to play an important role in monitoring progress in the prevention and treatment of HIV-related illness and AIDS.

Epidemiologic research has been pivotal in gaining insight into many different diseases. From infectious illnesses to heart disease to cancer to congenital malformations, epidemiology has provided insights into patterns of disease occurrence and underlying causal factors. Ultimately, this information can be used to help control the impact of diseases either through preventive measures or improved clinical management.

STUDY QUESTIONS

An outbreak of illness from West Nile virus (WNV) infection took place in the northeastern United States between July and October, 2001 (CDC: Serosurveys for West Nile virus infection—New York and Connecticut counties, 2000. MMWR 2001; 50:37.)

Questions 1–10: For each numbered situation below, select the most appropriate term from the following lettered options. Each option can be used once, more than once, or not at all.

   A. *Epidemic*
   B. *Sentinel case*
   C. *Incidence rate*
   D. *Risk*
   E. *False-positive*
   F. *False-negative*
   G. *Risk factor*
   H. *Prognostic factor*
   I. *Natural history*
   J. *Case fatality*
   K. *Median survival*
   L. *Randomized controlled clinical trial*
   M. *Cohort study*
   N. *Case–control study*

1. Persons with fever/headache were ten times more likely than others to have serum evidence of WNV infection. Fever/headache is best described as

2. Among Staten Island residents, 2.5 per 100,000 persons developed severe WNV neurologic disease during this time period. This measure is best described as

3. West Nile virus had occurred for the first time in the United States the preceding year. This unusual pattern of occurrence is best described as

4. A person who has the symptoms consistent with severe WNV neurologic disease, but does not have definitive serologic evidence of infection

5. Two of 21 patients with severe WNV neurologic disease died. This is best described by

6. The first person with severe WNV neurologic disease became ill the week of July 15. This individual is best described as

7. Clinical outcome of severe WNV neurologic disease was substantially worse for elderly patients. Advanced age is best described as

8. A study of antiviral agents is conducted for the treatment of severe WNV neurologic disease in which treatment assignments to individual patients are made by chance

9. A study is conducted comparing prior use of mosquito repellent by persons with and without severe WNV neurologic disease. This is best described as

10. A study is conducted in which the rates of subsequent WNV infection are compared in communities with and without mosquito abatement programs. This is best described as

FURTHER READING

Overview of Epidemiology

Szabo RM: Principles of epidemiology for the orthopedic surgeon. J Bone Joint Surg 1998;**80:**111.

Overview of AIDS

Sabin CA: The changing clinical epidemiology of AIDS in the highly active antiretroviral therapy era. AIDS 2002;**16**(suppl 4):S61–S68.

REFERENCES

Patient Profile

Gottlieb MS et al: *Pneumocystis carinii* pneumonia and mucosal candidiasis in previously healthy homosexual men. N Engl J Med 1981;**305:**1425.

Person, Place, and Time

CDC: HIV/AIDS Surveillance Report 1997;**9**(No. 2):1.

Disease Surveillance

CDC: 1993 revised classification system for HIV infection and expanded surveillance case definition for AIDS among adolescents and adults. MMWR 1992;**41**(No. RR-17):1.

CDC: HIV/AIDS Surveillance Report. 2002;**14:**1–40.

Fleming PL et al: Declines in AIDS incidence and deaths in the USA: A signal change in the epidemic. AIDS 1998;**12**(Suppl A):555.

Searching for Causes

de Vincenzi I, for the European Study Group on Heterosexual Transmission of HIV: A longitudinal study of human immunodeficiency virus transmission by heterosexual partners. N Engl J Med 1994;**331:**341.

Jaffe HW et al: National case-control study of Kaposi's sarcoma and *Pneumocystis carinii* pneumonia in homosexual men: Part 1, epidemiologic results. Ann Intern Med 1983;**99:**145.

Kingsley LA et al: Risk factors for seroconversion to human immunodeficiency virus among male homosexuals. Lancet 1987;**1:**345.

Lemp GF et al: Seroprevalence of HIV and risk behaviors among young homosexual and bisexual men. JAMA 1994;**272:**449.

Diagnostic Testing

Phair JP, Wolinsky S: Diagnosis of infection with the human immunodeficiency virus. Clin Infect Dis 1992;**15:**13.

Proffitt MR, Yen-Lieberman B: Laboratory diagnosis of human immunodeficiency virus infection. Infect Dis Clin North Am 1993;**7:**203.

Weiss SH et al: Screening test for HTLV-III (AIDS agent) antibodies. JAMA 1985;**253:**221.

Determining the Natural History

CDC: HIV/AIDS Surveillance Report 1997;**9**(No. 2):19.

Morgan D et al: An HIV-1 natural history cohort and survival times in rural Uganda. AIDS 1997;**11:**633.

Vella S et al: Differential survival of patients with AIDS according to the 1987 and 1993 CDC case definitions. JAMA 1994;**271:**1197.

Searching for Prognostic Factors

Mellors JW et al: Plasma viral load and CD4+ lymphocytes as prognostic markers of HIV-1 infection. Ann Intern Med 1997;**126:**946.

Testing New Treatments

Hammer SM et al: A controlled trial of two nucleoside analogues plus indinavir in persons with human immunodeficiency virus infection and CD4 cell counts of 200 per cubic millimeter or less. N Engl J Med 1997;**337**:725.

e-PIDEMIOLOGY

Overview of Epidemiology

http://bmj.com/epidem/epid.1.html
http://www.pitt.edu/~super1/lecture/lec0151/index.htm
http://www.pitt.edu/~super1/lecture/lec0841/index.htm
http://www.pitt.edu/~super1/lecture/lec7261/index.htm
http://hivinsite.ucsf.edu/InSite?page=kb-01-03

Disease Surveillance

http://www.cdc.gov/hiv/stats.htm
http://www.unaids.org/en/resources/epidemiology.asp

Searching for Causes

http://www.niaid.nih.gov/factsheets/evidhiv.htm

Diagnostic Testing

http://www.cdc.gov/mmwr/pdf/rr/rr5019.pdf

Searching for Prognostic Factors

http://hivinsite.ucsf.edu/InSite?page=kb-03-02-04#53X

Testing New Treatments

http://www.aidsinfo.nih.gov/guidelines/adult/AA_111003.pdf
http://www.cdc.gov/hiv/treatment.htm
http://www.pitt.edu/~super1/lecture/lec10331/index.htm

Epidemiologic Measures

2

KEY CONCEPTS

1. A variety of measures are employed in epidemiology, each of which has a specific definition and use.

2. When characterizing the likelihood of developing a disease within a specified period of time, the appropriate measure is risk.

3. Prevalence is used to describe the proportion of a population that is affected by a disease.

4. When measuring the rate of new occurrences of a disease, incidence is the appropriate measure.

5. Case fatality is used to describe the natural history of a disease and corresponds to the proportion of affected persons who die from that illness. Conversely, survival is the likelihood of escaping death from that illness.

PATIENT PROFILE

A 60-year-old previously healthy female research chemist recently developed shortness of breath and nosebleeds. On physical examination, the patient was pale and her pulse was elevated at 110 beats per minute. Her hematocrit was 20% (low), indicating anemia, her white blood cell count was 20,000/μL (elevated), her platelet count was 15,000/μL (low), and examination of her peripheral blood smear revealed atypical myeloblasts. The patient was hospitalized for suspected acute myelogenous leukemia. The diagnosis was confirmed by examination of a bone marrow aspirate and biopsy. Chemotherapy was started and about 3 weeks later, the patient's temperature rose abruptly to 39°C, and her neutrophil count dropped to 100/μL (abnormally low). Although no source of infection was apparent, cultures were obtained of her blood and urine, and antibiotics were administered to cover a wide range of potential infections. These cultures confirmed the presence of Staphylococcus aureus in the blood.

CLINICAL BACKGROUND

Acute myelogenous leukemia (AML), also known as acute nonlymphocytic leukemia, is a heterogeneous group of disorders involving uncontrolled proliferation of primitive blood-forming cells. AML accounts for almost one third of all leukemias, with over 9000 patients newly diagnosed in the United States each year. This disease tends to occur in later life, with a median age at onset of 65 years. Males are at a slightly higher risk than females.

Although for most patients the cause of AML is unknown, a number of risk factors have been identified, including exposure to ionizing radiation, benzene, certain drugs, and perhaps cigarette smoke. This disease also occurs with unusual frequency among patients with certain congenital disorders—such as Down syndrome.

Patients with AML may present with a variety of symptoms, including weakness, fatigue, unexplained weight loss, infection, and bleeding. On physical examination, these patients often are pale, have multiple bruises, and have fevers, with evidence of localized infections. In some instances, enlargement of the lymph nodes, spleen, or liver may be found. Examination of blood specimens reveals anemia, low platelet counts, and markedly elevated leukocyte counts, with immature granulocytes abnormally appearing in the circulating blood. The bone marrow of these patients tends to be packed densely with cells, including a high proportion of immature cells.

The clinical management of AML involves an attempt to induce remission with chemotherapy. The likelihood of achieving remission is reduced for patients who are older, are obese, have impaired renal function, or have preexisting medical conditions, particularly prior disorders of the bone marrow. Remissions may be induced in two thirds or more of patients, with remission failures most commonly attributable to infection or hemorrhage leading to death. Even among patients in remission, about 75% will eventually relapse, and only one fifth of patients can be expected to live 5 years beyond the time of diagnosis.

The complications of infection and bleeding among these patients are directly related to chemotherapy-induced suppression of the bone marrow, with consequent reductions in the circulating levels of neutrophils and platelets. Very low neutrophil counts increase susceptibility to a wide variety of infections, with clinical or microbiologic evidence of infection in about 30–40% of patients. Among the most common types of infection are those involving in-dwelling catheters, the urinary tract, and the soft tissues. The leading bacterial pathogens are *S aureus, Staphylococcus epidermidis, Viridans streptococci, Escherichia coli, Enterobacter, Pseudomonas,* and *Klebsiella* species. *Candida albicans* and other fungi can also cause infections among these patients. Treatment with broad-spectrum antibiotics has reduced the risk of life-threatening infections in these individuals. An evolving area of therapy is the use of so-called **growth factors** to stimulate the patient's ability to produce replacement neutrophils. The use of these growth factors can lower the rate of infection and the need for antibiotics, but it is unclear whether the ultimate prognosis of the disease is affected.

In about half of the instances of fever among neutropenic patients, an infection cannot be documented either clinically or microbiologically. These episodes, therefore, are referred to as **unexplained fever.** Even in the absence of an identified specific infectious agent, fever is an ominous sign in a neutropenic patient and is associated with a high risk of adverse outcomes, including death. It has become standard practice to treat febrile neutropenic patients with combinations of antibiotics that are effective against a wide range of infectious agents. The selection of a regimen of antibiotic treatment on the basis of likely infectious agents, in the absence of documentation of those agents, is referred to as **empiric** treatment. Evidence about the likely pathogens is derived from experience in managing other febrile neutropenic patients in whom responsible infectious agents were identified.

INTRODUCTION

The importance of risk assessment is evident in the Patient Profile. Antibiotics were administered to the patient even before an infectious cause of fever was identified. In this situation, the attending physician concluded that the potential risk of complications from delayed antibiotic treatment outweighed the likelihood of harm from treatment administered before the cause of the fever was determined. Virtually every treatment decision involves a counterbalancing of risks and benefits. In this chapter, emphasis will be placed on how epidemiologic measures can be used to assess outcomes and thereby guide decision making.

MEASURES OF DISEASE OCCURRENCE

In this chapter, three basic measures to assess the frequency of health events are introduced. These measures, which play key roles in medicine, epidemiology, and public health, are **risk** (the likelihood that an individual will contract a disease), **prevalence** (the amount of disease already present in a population), and **incidence rate** (how fast new occurrences of disease arise). In addition, these measures can be used to assess the prognosis and mortality of patients with disease.

Risk

Risk, or cumulative incidence, is a measure of the occurrence of new cases of the disease of interest in the population. More precisely, *risk is the proportion of unaffected individuals who, on average, will contract the disease of interest over a specified period of time.* Risk is estimated by observing a particular population for a defined period of time-the risk period. The estimated risk (R) is a proportion; the numerator is the number of newly affected persons (A), called *cases* by epidemiologists, and the denominator is the size (N) of the unaffected population under observation:

$$R = \frac{\text{New cases}}{\text{Persons at risk}} = \frac{A}{N}$$

All members of the population, or cohort, are free of disease at the start of observation. Risk, which has no units, lies between 0 (when no new occurrences arise) and 1 (when, at the other extreme, the entire population becomes affected during the risk period). Alternatively, risk can be expressed as a percentage by multiplying the proportion by 100.

In Figure 2–1 a hypothetical study of six subjects illustrates the calculation of risk. This study began in 1995 and concluded in 2004. Individual subjects entered the study at various times, were all free of the disease of interest at the time of enrollment, and were followed up for at least 2 years. For example, Patient A was enrolled in 1995, was diagnosed with the disease just prior to 1997, and was followed up until death in 2002. Patient B was enrolled in 1997, was followed up

until 1999 without developing the disease, and then discontinued participation in the study. Patient C was enrolled in 1999, was diagnosed with the disease just prior to 2002, and survived through the end of the observation period in 2004. Patients D, E, and F entered the study in 1997, 2002, and 1998, respectively; each patient was followed through 2004 without developing the disease.

Of the six subjects under observation ($N = 6$), only one ($A = 1$) developed the disease within 2 years of entry into the study. The 2-year risk of disease, therefore, is estimated by

$$R = \frac{A}{N} = \frac{1}{6} = 0.17 - 17\%$$

These same data are also summarized in Figure 2–2, where the time scale on the horizontal axis represents the duration of observation for each subject. In other words, observation of a particular individual begins at time zero and continues until that person dies or is lost from the study or until the study is concluded. The for-

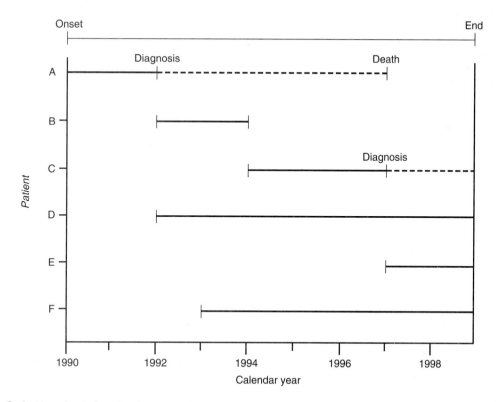

Figure 2–1. Hypothetical study of a group of six subjects between 1995 and 2004. The solid horizontal lines indicate time observed while the subjects are at risk for developing the disease of interest. The dashed horizontal lines indicate time observed after the subjects are diagnosed.

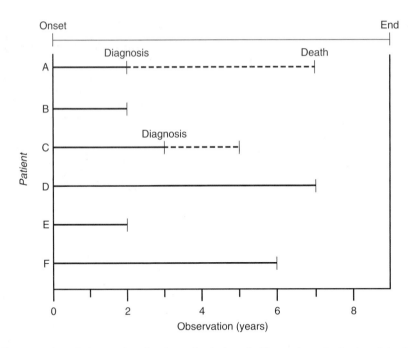

Figure 2–2. Restructuring of observations in a hypothetical study. Times along the horizontal axis reflect years of observation for each subject, rather than calendar years.

mat used in Figure 2–2 is sometimes preferred as a matter of convenience, because it may be easier to visualize the actual lengths of observation for individual subjects. The following example further illustrates the use of risks and how they are estimated.

Example 1. In deciding whether to treat the patient in the Patient Profile with antibiotics prior to determining the cause of the fever, the clinician had to address this key question: How likely is it that the patient has a bacterial infection? The answer can be based on experience with similar patients. For example, to estimate a cancer patient's risk of acquiring an infection in the hospital (a nosocomial infection), a study was conducted of 5031 patients admitted to a comprehensive cancer center. The investigators carefully defined a nosocomial infection as an infection that (1) is documented by cultures, (2) was not incubating at admission, (3) occurred at least 48 hours after admission, and (4) occurred no more than 48 hours following discharge (somewhat longer for surgical wound infections). Of the 5031 patients, 596 developed an infection that met these criteria. The risk was

$$R = \frac{596}{5031} = 0.12 = 12\%$$

In this example, the risk period for each patient began 48 hours after hospitalization and ended 48 hours after discharge. This equation indicates that about 12% of cancer patients similar to those studied will develop a nosocomial infection during or soon after hospitalization. The risk is greater than would be expected for the average hospitalized patient, suggesting that cancer patients are at an unusually high risk of developing a hospital-acquired infection.

A broad range of hospitalized cancer patients were involved in this study. The woman in the Patient Profile, however, had a fever and a low granulocyte count. A more refined estimate of the likelihood of infection could be derived from a study of patients with similar conditions. In one such study, 1022 cancer patients with fever and granulocytopenia were studied according to a defined protocol. Of these patients, 530 had a clinically or microbiologically documented bacterial infection. Thus, the risk of infection in granulocytopenic, febrile cancer patients is estimated to be

$$R = \frac{530}{1022} = 0.52 = 52\%$$

This result suggests that patients similar to the one described in the Patient Profile have a very high risk of a bacterial infection, thus supporting the decision to treat the patient with antibiotics even before an infection is diagnosed.

Prevalence

Prevalence indicates the number of existing cases of the disease of interest in a population. Specifically, the point prevalence (P) is the proportion of a population that has the disease of interest at a particular time, eg, on a given day. This value is estimated by dividing the number of existing affected individuals, or cases (C), by the number of persons in the population (N):

$$P = \frac{C}{N}$$

Prevalence, like risk, ranges between 0 and 1 and has no units. The calculation of prevalence can be illustrated using the data summarized in Figure 2–1. For example, to calculate the prevalence of the disease of interest in 2001, it is necessary to know (1) the number of persons under observation in 2001 and (2) the number of individuals affected at that time. First, four persons are under observation in 2001 (Patients A, C, D, and F) ($N = 4$). Second, at that time one of these persons (Patient A) is affected ($C = 1$). Thus, the prevalence in 2001 is

$$P = \frac{C}{N} = \frac{1}{4} = 0.25 = 25\%$$

Example 2. An important question in deciding whether to administer antibiotics to the patient described in the Patient Profile is the type of infection involved. As indicated earlier, individuals with low neutrophil counts are susceptible to a wide variety of bacterial infections. Therefore, broad-spectrum antibiotics are used empirically in these patients until the specific infecting organism is identified.

These bacteria often can be cultured from persons without symptomatic illness. For example, the prevalence of skin colonization with *S aureus* was estimated among 96 people attending an outpatient clinic for the first time. Patients with skin infections were excluded from the study. *S aureus* was cultured from specimens from 62 patients. The prevalence of colonization with *S aureus* in this group was

$$P = \frac{62}{96} = 0.65 = 65\%$$

From this equation, it is estimated that in a group of patients similar to the patients studied, the prevalence of skin colonization with *S aureus* is about 65%.

Incidence Rate

The incidence rate (IR), like risk, reflects occurrence of new cases of the disease of interest. Thus, *incidence rate measures the rapidity with which newly diagnosed cases of the disease of interest develop.* The incidence rate is estimated by observing a population, counting the number of new cases of disease in that population (A), and measuring the net time, called person-time (PT), that individuals in the population at risk for developing disease are observed. A subject at risk of disease followed for 1 year contributes 1 person-year of observation. The incidence rate is

$$IR = \frac{A}{PT}$$

To illustrate calculation of person-time and incidence rate, consider the small hypothetical cohort illustrated schematically in Figure 2–2. Patient A developed the disease 2 years after entry into the study. Because subjects contribute person-time only while eligible to develop the disease, the person-time for Patient A was 2 years. Similarly, Patients B, C, D, E, and F contributed 2, 3, 7, 2, and 6 years, respectively. Patients A and C developed disease. Thus, A (the number of new cases of disease in the population) = 2, the total PT = 2 + 2 + 3 + 7 + 2 + 6 = 22 person-years, and the incidence rate is

$$IR = \frac{A}{PT} = \frac{2}{22} = 0.09 \text{ cases / person-year}$$

Note that the total person-years of observation is obtained simply by addition of the years contributed by each subject. Alternatively, this rate can be expressed as 9 cases/100 person-years by multiplying the numerator and denominator by 100. Although these two expressions are equivalent, the latter might be preferred since it does not require use of decimal points.

Example 3. Returning to the study cited in Example 1, the incidence rate of nosocomial infections can be calculated from additional data reported in that investigation. The 5031 patients remained under observation for a total of 127,859 patient-days (or an average length of stay of 127,859/5031 = 25.4 days). Since 596 patients developed an infection that met the definition for a hospital-acquired infection, the incidence rate can be estimated as

$$IR = \frac{596}{127,859} = 0.0047 \text{ cases / patient-day}$$
$$= 4.7 \text{ cases / 1000 patient-days}$$

This means that among patients similar to those studied, on average, about 0.47% of patients would be expected to develop a nosocomial infection per day.

Calculation of incidence rates for a large population, such as that in a city, by separately enumerating the person-years at risk for each individual, as described above, would require a tremendous amount of work. Fortunately, person-time for a large population can often be calculated by multiplying the average size of the population at risk by the length of time the population is observed:

$$PT = \text{(Average size of population at risk)} \times \text{(Length of observation)}$$

In many instances, relatively few people in the population develop the disease, and the population undergoes no major demographic shifts during the time period of observation. In such situations, the average size of the population at risk can be estimated by the size of the entire population, using census or other data. The person-time of a large, stable population can often be estimated by

$$PT = \text{(Size of entire population)} \times \text{(Length of observation)}$$

Example 4 illustrates calculation of incidence rates using this alternative approach to estimating person-time.

Example 4. In the United States, the National Cancer Institute maintains a network of registries that collect information on all new occurrences of cancer within populations residing in specific geographic areas. Collectively, these registries cover about 14% of the population of the United States, and between 1996 and 2000, 2957 females were newly diagnosed with acute myelocytic leukemia in these areas. An estimated 19,185,836 females lived in these combined areas on average during this 5-year period. Thus, the number of woman-years of observation for this population was 19,185,836 women × 5 years = 95,929,180 woman-years. Therefore, the average annual incidence rate of acute myelocytic leukemia among females was 3.1 cases for every 100,000 woman-years of observation in these specific study areas.

DIFFERENCES BETWEEN RISK, PREVALENCE, & INCIDENCE

As summarized in Table 2–1, risk, prevalence, and incidence rates differ in at least three important ways. First, the measures have different units. Incidence rates are expressed as units of newly diagnosed patients per unit of person-time, whereas risk and prevalence have no units. Second, these measures reflect different aspects of disease. Incidence rates and risk describe occurrence of new disease, whereas prevalence reflects already existing disease. Third, these measures are calculated differently. As shown in Figure 2–1, in 2001 the prevalence was 25%, the 2-year risk was 17%, and the incidence rate was 9 cases per 100 person-years. These differences indicate that the three measures cannot be compared directly with one another.

In view of these inherent differences, the measures have different applications. Risk is most useful if interest centers on the proportion of a population that will become ill over a specified period of time. Risk also can be used to estimate the probability that a particular individual within a population will become ill over a specified period of time. Incidence rates are preferred if interest centers on the rapidity with which new cases arise in a population (the time period may be long or unspecified). Prevalence is preferred if interest centers on the number of existing cases within a population or the proportion of cases of a given type. Example 5 illustrates some of the differences among these measures.

Example 5. The use of an antibiotic, norfloxacin, was studied for prevention of gram-negative bacterial infections in patients with acute leukemia who had treatment-related low neutrophil counts. All 35 patients who received norfloxacin developed fever. The 35 patients were observed for a total of 220.5 person-days before first developing fever; each day, on average, about 28% of the patients had a fever. Thus, the risk of developing a fever was 35/35 = 1 in this group of patients, the incidence rate was 35/220.5 = 0.16 cases/person-day = 16 cases/100 person-days, and the average prevalence was 28%.

A risk of 1 suggests that treatment with norfloxacin does not ultimately prevent infectious fevers or reduce the risk of developing fever. On the other hand, the in-

Table 2–1. Characteristics of risk, prevalence, and incidence rate.

Characteristic	Risk	Prevalence	Incidence Rate
What is measured	Probability of disease	Percentage of population with disease	Rapidity of disease occurrence
Units	None	None	Cases/person-time
Time of disease diagnosis	Newly diagnosed	Existing	Newly diagnosed
Synonyms	Cumulative incidence	—	Incidence density

cidence rate in the norfloxacin-treated group was lower than that in a group of similar patients who did not receive norfloxacin, suggesting that treatment slowed or delayed the onset of fever. Furthermore, prevalence of fever was lower in the norfloxacin-treated group, which indicates that patients treated with norfloxacin are less likely to be febrile on an average day.

SURVIVAL

Survival is the probability of remaining alive for a specific length of time. For a chronic disease such as cancer, 1-year survival and 5-year survival rates are often used as indicators of the severity of disease and the prognosis. For example, the 5-year survival for acute myelocytic leukemia is about 0.19, indicating that only 19% of patients with acute myelocytic leukemia survive at least 5 years after diagnosis.

In simple situations, survival (*S*) is estimated as

$$S = \frac{A-D}{A}$$

where *D* is the number of deaths observed in a specified period of time and *A* is the number of newly diagnosed patients under observation. Survival for at least 2 years after diagnosis can be determined from the data in Fig-

ure 2–3. Observation of each patient begins at diagnosis (time = 0), and continues until one of the following outcomes occurs: death, survival for 5 years, or follow-up ceases (the subject is "censored"). A patient is censored when follow-up ends prior to death or completion of a full period of observation. Follow-up could end for one of several reasons: (1) the patient decides to discontinue participation, (2) the patient is "lost" to follow-up, or (3) the study ends. Five of the six people under observation (*N* = 6) in Figure 2–3 survive at least 2 years. Thus, the 2-year survival is

$$S = \frac{5}{6} = 0.83 = 83\%$$

Calculation of survival indicates the probability of surviving a specified length of time and is inversely related to the risk of death. Survival estimates provide a useful way to summarize prognosis, as illustrated in Example 6.

Example 6. The patient described in the Patient Profile has acute myelogenous leukemia. Data collected by the National Cancer Institute for patients diagnosed with this disease in the United States between 1992 and 1999 indicate that only about 19% of patients survived for at least 5 years from the time of diagnosis. For per-

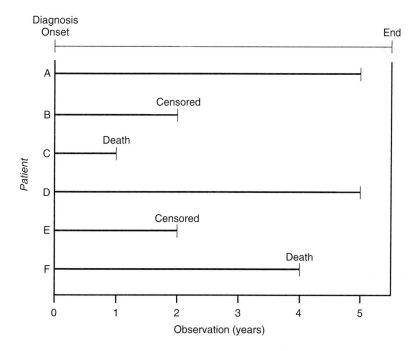

Figure 2–3. Survival experience of a hypothetical group of six patients. The time of observation for each subject, beginning with diagnosis, is measured in years.

sons who were *under 65 years of age* at diagnosis, the 5-year survival rate (31%) was higher than for persons who were *65 years or older* at diagnosis (4%). Nevertheless, it can be concluded from these data that, regardless of age, patients with acute myelogenous leukemia as a group have an extremely poor prognosis. The group experience also serves as the best indicator of prognosis for individual patients with this diagnosis. For example, a patient with acute myelogenous leukemia who is under 65 years of age would be expected to have a 1-in-3 chance of surviving at least 5 years from the time of diagnosis. For a patient 65 years or older with the same diagnosis, the chance of surviving at least 5 years from diagnosis is reduced to 1 in 25.

Life Table & Other Survival Analyses

When studying survival and risk, problems may arise if the investigator cannot follow some subjects for the entire risk period, either because the subjects move away or miss a follow-up appointment. In Figure 2–3, for example, observation of Patients B and E stopped after 2 years (censored). In determining the survival for a 5-year period, observation of Patients B and E is incomplete; we have less than 5 years of observation on these individuals. It is known only that these individuals survived for at least 2 years, not if they survived a full 5 years. It might seem, therefore, that these patients do not contribute any useful information toward the estimation of a 5-year survival probability. In the absence of information about what happened to these patients over the full observation period, we might consider two extreme scenarios. In the first scenario, both Patients B and E survive the full 5 years. The overall 5-year survival estimate in this situation would be

$$S = \frac{4}{6} = 0.67 = 67\%$$

In the second scenario, neither Patient B nor E survives for the full 5 years. The overall 5-year survival estimate in this situation would be

$$S = \frac{2}{6} = 0.33 = 33\%$$

Clearly, these two extreme assumptions lead to very different estimates of the 5-year probability of survival. Since the observations are incomplete, we do not know which, if either, of these two extreme situations is closer to the correct answer. In this case, the inability to estimate survival probabilities indicates the need for analytic methods to handle censored observations.

Statisticians have developed special techniques, called *survival analyses,* to account for such incomplete observations. Two particularly useful methods of survival analysis are life table analysis and Kaplan-Meier analysis. Life table and Kaplan-Meier analyses allow calculation of risk even if some of the observations are incomplete. Descriptions of these and other methods of survival analysis can be found in Dawson and Trapp (2004), *Basic and Clinical Biostatistics.*

The results of a survival analysis can be presented graphically, as shown in Figure 2–4. The information

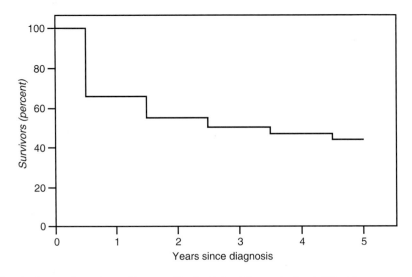

Figure 2–4. Survival curve for patients diagnosed in the United States during 1995 with any type of leukemia.
(Adapted from Ries LAG et al: *SEER Cancer Statistics Review,* 1975–2000. National Cancer Institute, 2003.)

portrayed in this graph relates to the survival experience of patients diagnosed in the United States during 1995 with any type of leukemia. The horizontal axis plots time in years since diagnosis (0 = time of diagnosis) and the vertical axis plots the percentage of patients who are alive. The survival curve begins at the time of diagnosis, when 100% of patients are alive. During the first year following diagnosis, 32% of the patients die (or equivalently, 100% − 32% = 68% survive). During the next year, another 10% of patients die (cumulative survival = 68% − 10% = 58%). The process of attrition to death continues each year through the end of the 5-year observation period.

The survival curve can be used to determine basic summary measures about the prognosis of leukemia in adults, for example, the percentage of patients who survive to some fixed period of time following diagnosis. Typically, cancer prognosis is assessed by determining the percentage of patients who survive for at least 5 years after diagnosis. The approach to estimating this percentage is depicted in Figure 2–5. Beginning on the horizontal axis at 5 years, a line is drawn to the survival curve (Step A). From the point of intersection with the survival curve, a line is drawn across to the vertical axis (Step B). The percentage of survivors (47%) is then read from the vertical axis.

Another summary measure of prognosis is the **median survival time,** which is the time following diagnosis at which one half of the patients remain alive. The approach to estimating the median survival time is shown in Figure 2–6. Beginning on the vertical axis at the 50% (median) survival level, a line is drawn across to the survival curve (Step A). From the point of intersection with the survival curve, a line is drawn down to the horizontal axis (Step B). The median survival time in this example is estimated to be between 3.5 and 4.5 years, with a best estimate around 4 years. That is to say on average, patients with leukemia diagnosed in the United States during 1995 tended to survive about 4 years from the time of diagnosis. For any individual patient out of this population, 4 years serves as an estimate of the likely survival time. As noted in Chapter 1, additional prognostic factors often can be identified that help to refine the predictions for groups of patients or individuals with those characteristics.

Case Fatality

The propensity of a disease to cause the death of affected patients is referred to as the **case fatality.** The terms *rate* and *ratio* are sometimes associated with case fatality, although mathematically this is not appropriate since case fatality is a proportion. Case fatality (*CF*) is estimated by

$$CF = \frac{\text{Number of deaths}}{\text{Number of diagnosed patients}} = \frac{D}{A}$$

The resulting estimate can be left as a proportion or multiplied by 100 to convert it to a percentage. Note

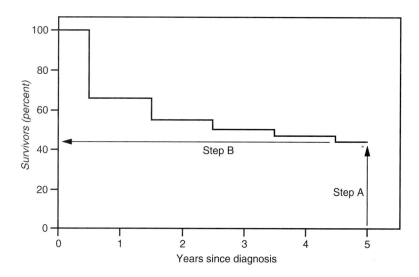

Figure 2–5. Approach to estimating the survival 5 years after diagnosis for patients diagnosed in the United States during 1995 with any type of leukemia. (Adapted from Ries LAG et al: *SEER Cancer Statistics Review,* 1975–2000. National Cancer Institute, 2003.)

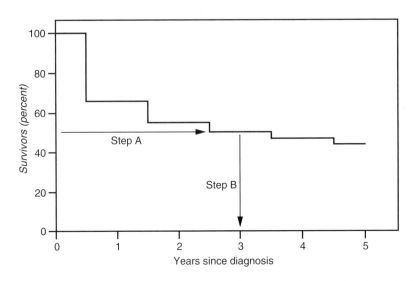

Figure 2–6. Approach to estimating the median survival time for patients diagnosed in the United States during 1995 with any type of leukemia. (Adapted from Ries LAG et al: *SEER Cancer Statistics Review, 1975–2000.* National Cancer Institute, 2003.)

that this equation is analogous in structure to the equation previously described for risk, or cumulative incidence. The difference between these two measures is the phase of illness to which they are applied. Risk of disease refers to the initial development of the condition, and case fatality refers to the likelihood of death among persons in whom the disease is diagnosed. Case fatality can be thought of as the risk of death among those who have been just diagnosed with the disease. Both measures require specification of some time period over which events are counted.

The relationship between risk and case fatality is depicted schematically in Figure 2–7. The initial population at risk of disease consists of 15 women ($N = 15$), five of whom develop the condition of interest ($A = 5$). Risk, or cumulative incidence, therefore, is

$$R = \frac{A}{N} = \frac{5}{15} = 0.33 = 33\%$$

Only two ($D = 2$) of the affected women ($A = 5$) subsequently die from the condition. The case fatality, therefore, is

$$CF = \frac{D}{A} = \frac{2}{5} = 0.40 = 40\%$$

The case fatality can range from 0, when no patients die from the disease, to 1 (or 100%), when all patients die from the disease. Since the case fatality represents the proportion of persons affected with a disease who

die from it, the case fatality may be thought of as the complement to survival. In other words, for a given period of observation, the case fatality and survival should sum to 100%. Returning to Figure 2–7, survival is

$$S = \frac{(A-D)}{A} = \frac{(5-2)}{5} = \frac{3}{5} = 0.60 = 60\%$$

Thus, the case fatality ($CF = 40\%$) and the survival ($S = 60\%$) total 100%.

SUMMARY

Five of the basic descriptive measures used in epidemiology have been introduced in this chapter. Although other indicators of disease frequency and prognosis exist, the following five measures are central to the descriptive function of epidemiology.

1. Risk, or cumulative incidence, is the proportion of unaffected persons within a population that develops the disease of interest in a specified period of time.

2. Prevalence is the proportion of a population affected by the disease of interest at a particular time.

3. Incidence rate measures the rapidity with which unaffected persons within a population develop a particular disease.

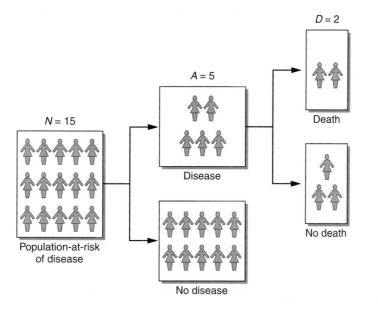

Figure 2–7. Schematic diagram of the natural history of an illness, indicating the population at risk of disease (*N*), incident cases (*A*), and deaths from the disease (*D*).

4. Survival is the proportion of persons affected by the disease of interest that lives for at least a specified period of time.

5. Case fatality is the proportion of persons within a population affected by a particular disease that dies from the disease within a specified period of time.

Survival and case fatality represent mutually exclusive outcomes. Together they must account for all individuals affected with the disease who have known vital status.

Application of these measures to the questions raised by the Patient Profile results in the following conclusions:

1. Hospitalized cancer patients have a substantial risk (*R* = 0.12, or 12%) of developing an infection during hospitalization.

2. The agents (eg, *S aureus*) that cause infections in the bloodstream of cancer patients are commonly cultured from the skin of healthy persons (prevalence [*P*] = 0.65, or 65%).

3. The incidence rate of infection among hospitalized cancer patients is appreciable (*IR* = 4.7 cases per 1000 patient-days), but the corresponding incidence rate among patients with impaired immune systems is more than 30 times greater (*IR* = 160 cases per 1000 patient-days).

4. The 5-year survival for adult patients with acute myelogenous leukemia is extremely low (*S* = 0.19, or 19%).

5. Based on the survival data, it can be concluded that 81% of patients with acute myelogenous leukemia die from this disease or its complications within 5 years of diagnosis.

With this information in mind, the physician in the Patient Profile can conclude that the patient is at an unusually high risk for a life-threatening nosocomial bacterial infection. Rapid initiation of broad-spectrum antibiotic therapy is warranted, even before the results of culture specimens are known. When the results of pretreatment cultures and antibiotic susceptibilities become available, the antibiotic regimen can be modified, if necessary. By appropriate use and interpretation of standard epidemiologic measures such as risk and incidence rate, the physician can make informed and potentially life-saving treatment decisions.

STUDY QUESTIONS

Questions 1–7: For each numbered situation below, select the most appropriate measure from the following lettered options. Each lettered option can be used once, more than once, or not at all.

A. *Five-year survival*

B. *Prevalence*

C. *Incidence rate*

D. *Risk*

E. *Case fatality*

F. *Median survival*

1. *Which is the best measure to estimate the proportion of the U.S. population that is overweight?*

2. *Which is the best measure to estimate how fast new cases of acute myelogenous leukemia develop among workers exposed to benzene?*

3. *Which is the best measure to estimate the proportion of patients with breast cancer who will be alive 5 years after diagnosis?*

4. *Which is the best measure to estimate the typical length of life of patients with breast cancer after diagnosis?*

5. *Which is the best measure to estimate the proportion of professional football players who will suffer a knee injury during a season?*

6. *Which is the best measure to assess the risk of death among persons with West Nile Virus infection?*

7. *Which is the best measure to estimate how quickly people develop hypertension, after age 21?*

Questions 8–0: A study about risk of myocardial infarction among cigarette smokers was conducted for five years, between 1998 and 2003. The results of observations on six patients are depicted schematically in Figure 2–8.

8. *The prevalence of myocardial infarction in mid-2002 was*

   A. *1/6 = 0.17*

   B. *2/6 = 0.33*

   C. *1/4 = 0.25*

   D. *2/4 = 0.50*

   E. *2/3 = 0.67*

9. *Among these patients, the risk of developing a myocardial infarction by the end of the first year of follow-up is*

   A. *1/6 = 0.17*

   B. *1/5 = 0.20*

   C. *2/6 = 0.33*

   D. *2/5 = 0.40*

   E. *3/5 = 0.60*

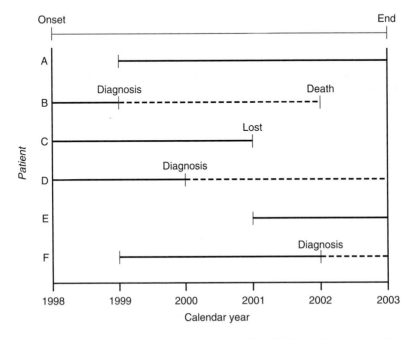

Figure 2–8. Observations on six elderly cigarette smokers (A–F). Solid lines indicate times observed while subjects were at risk of developing myocardial infarctions; dashed lines indicate times observed after myocardial infarctions.

10. The incidence rate of myocardial infarction over the observation period was:
    A. $3/6 = 0.50$ cases/person year
    B. $3/10 = 0.30$ cases/person year
    C. $2/15 = 0.13$ cases/person year
    D. $3/15 = 0.20$ cases/person year
    E. $3/5 = 0.60$ cases/person year

Questions 11–12: A survival curve for patients with multiple myeloma is shown in Figure 2–9.

11. From this curve, the median survival is estimated to be between
    A. 0 and 1 year
    B. 1 and 2 years
    C. 2 and 3 years
    D. 3 and 4 years
    E. 4 and 5 years

12. From this curve, the proportion of patients surviving 1-year is estimated to be closest to
    A. 40%
    B. 50%
    C. 60%
    D. 70%
    E. 80%

Questions 13–15: For each measure below, select the most appropriate answer from the following lettered options. Each option can be used once, more than once, or not at all.
    A. 0.0001
    B. 0.0001 cases/person-year
    C. 0.001
    D. 0.001 cases/person-year
    E. .010
    F. .010 cases/person-year
    G. .10
    H. .10 cases/person-year
    I. 1.0
    J. 1.0 cases/person-year

13. Estimate the prevalence of melanoma in a retirement community of 10,000 among whom 10 are found to have melanoma during an initial screening and 1 new case is found at a subsequent screening exam 1 year later.

14. Estimate the approximate 1-year risk of developing melanoma in the population described in question 13, assuming no entries or losses of subjects and no deaths from other causes.

15. For the population described in question 13, estimate the approximate incidence rate of developing melanoma, assuming no entries or losses of subjects and no deaths from other causes.

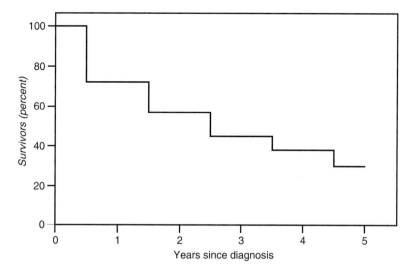

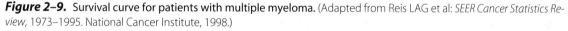

Figure 2–9. Survival curve for patients with multiple myeloma. (Adapted from Reis LAG et al: *SEER Cancer Statistics Review,* 1973–1995. National Cancer Institute, 1998.)

FURTHER READING

Flanders WD, O'Brien TR: Inappropriate comparisons of incidence and prevalence in epidemiologic research. Am J Public Health 1989;**79:**1301.

Tapia Granados JA: On the terminology and dimensions of incidence. J Clin Epidemiol 1997;**50:**891.

REFERENCES

Clinical Background

Estey EH: Therapeutic options for acute myelogenous leukemia. Cancer 2001;**92:**1059.

Koll BS, Brown AE: The changing epidemiology of infections at cancer hospitals. Clin Infect Dis 1993;**17**(Suppl 2):S322.

Ohno R: Granulocyte colony-stimulating factor, granulocyte-macrophage colony stimulating factor and macrophage colony stimulating factor in the treatment of acute myeloid leukemia and acute lymphoblastic leukemia. Leukemia Res 1998;**22:** 1143.

Rolston KV: Expanding the options for risk-based therapy in febrile neutropenia. Diagn Microbiol Infect Dis 1998;**31:** 411.

Scheinberg DA, et al: Acute leukemias. In: DeVita VT, Hellman S, Rosenberg SA (editors): Principles & Practice of Oncology, 6th ed. Lippincott, Williams & Wilkins, 2001.

Stone RM: The difficult problem of acute myeloid leukemia in the older adult. CA Cancer J Clin 2002;**52:**363.

Risk

European Organization for Research and Treatment of Cancer International Antimicrobial Therapy Cooperative: Ceftazidime combined with a short or long course of amikacin for empirical therapy of gram-negative bacteremia in cancer patients with granulocytopenia. N Engl J Med 1987;**317:**1692.

Rotstein C et al: Nosocomial infection rates at an oncology center. Infect Control Hosp Epidemiol 1988;**9:**13.

Prevalence

Schimpff SC: Empiric antibiotic therapy for granulocytopenic cancer patients. Am J Med 1986;**80:**13.

Incidence Rate

Ries LAG et al: *SEER Cancer Statistics Review, 1975–2000.* National Cancer Institute, 2003.

Differences Between Risk, Prevalence, and Incidence

Karp JE et al: Oral norfloxacin for prevention of gram-negative bacterial infections in patients with acute leukemia and granulocytopenia. Ann Intern Med 1987;**106:**1.

Survival

Clark TG et al: Survival analysis part I: basic concepts and first analyses. Br J Cancer 2003;**89:**232.

Ries LAG et al: *SEER Cancer Statistics Review, 1975–2000.* National Cancer Institute, 2003.

Life Table and Other Survival Analyses

Dawson B, Trapp RG: *Basic and Clinical Biostatistics,* 4th ed. Appleton & Lange, 2004.

Evans C et al: High-dose cytosine arabinoside and L-asparaginase therapy for poor-risk adult acute non-lymphocytic leukemia. Cancer 1990;**66:**2624.

e-PIDEMIOLOGY

Rates

http://bmj.com/epidem/epid.2.html#pgfId=1003279

http://www.pitt.edu/~super1/lecture/lec0441/index.htm

http://www.pitt.edu/~super1/lecture/lec0891/index.htm

Measures of Disease Occurrence

http://www.pitt.edu/~super1/lecture/lec0441/index.htm

Clinical Background

http://www.meds.com/pdq/myeloid_pro.html

http://www.meds.com/leukemia/trends/mon_pt1.html

http://www.meds.com/leukemia/trends/mon_pt4.html#tef_1

Incidence Rate

http://seer.cancer.gov/csr/1975_2000

Survival

http://seer.cancer.gov/csr/1975_2000

Patterns of Occurrence

KEY CONCEPTS

① *The distribution of a disease within a population can be characterized by three basic questions: Who develops the disease? Where does the disease occur? When does the disease occur?*

② *A rapid and dramatic increase in the occurrence of a disease is referred to as an epidemic.*

③ *Studies of migrant populations can be used to help distinguish whether a disease is more environmentally or genetically determined.*

PATIENT PROFILE

A 34-year-old female domestic worker who had recently emigrated from Southeast Asia to the United States came to the emergency room with a 6-week history of cough, fever, night sweats, weakness, fatigue, and shortness of breath. Previously she had been in good health. She had experienced two uncomplicated pregnancies and deliveries, followed by a tubal sterilization. Cavitary lesions were visible on the patient's chest x-ray. A smear of a sputum specimen revealed acid-fast bacilli. Mycobacterium tuberculosis subsequently grew from cultures of the sputum, and these organisms were susceptible to all drugs tested. The patient was placed on an initial antibiotic regimen involving four drugs administered daily under direct observation by the health care provider. After 2 weeks of daily therapy, the patient improved clinically and she was maintained on directly observed, four-drug therapy daily for the next 6 weeks. The patient remained asymptomatic, and there was no evidence of bacilli in her sputum. Her treatment regimen was reduced to two drugs administered three times

each week, and she remained under direct observation for an additional 18 weeks.

The patient resided with her husband and two young children in an apartment building. Tuberculin skin tests were administered to each of the family members at the time of the patient's initial diagnosis, and results were positive for the patient's husband and 3-year-old daughter. Although no evidence of clinically active tuberculosis was found in either the spouse or daughter, preventive therapy was administered to all three family members. Skin testing of 54 other residents of the apartment building revealed one other infected adult, who lacked evidence of active disease and received preventive antibiotic therapy. None of the tuberculin skin tests administered to the patient's contacts at work were positive.

CLINICAL BACKGROUND

Tuberculosis is caused by mycobacteria transmitted on small airborne particles that are created when an individual with pulmonary tuberculosis coughs or sneezes.

Air currents circulate these particles throughout an entire room or building. When a susceptible person inhales these particles, tubercle bacilli may become established in the lungs and spread throughout the body. Usually the host's immune system contains this initial infection within a short period of time. A small proportion (10%) of patients will develop active clinical illness months or years later, when the mycobacteria begin to replicate and cause symptoms.

As shown in Table 3–1, environmental as well as personal factors affect the likelihood of tuberculosis transmission. Each of the environmental features listed tends to increase the concentration of mycobacteria in the air. Transmission also is promoted by (1) characteristics of the infected individual that contribute to greater release of mycobacteria and (2) characteristics of the susceptible person that diminish the immune response.

Public health officials in the United States have established the elimination of tuberculosis in this country as a national priority. An effective plan for the control of tuberculosis requires that persons who are infectious with active tuberculosis be identified early, isolated from susceptible persons, and treated with adequate antibiotic therapy. Control strategies also include screening for the presence of asymptomatic infection within groups at high risk of tuberculosis, followed by antibiotic therapy to prevent the development of active disease. On the basis of epidemiologic data, a number of groups with an elevated risk of developing tuberculosis have been identified (Table 3–2).

The Patient Profile illustrates many important points about tuberculosis. Because the patient had recently emigrated from an area with an elevated prevalence of tuberculosis, she was a member of a high-risk group. The presence of symptoms, in conjunction with cavitary lung lesions and tubercle bacilli in the sputum, indicated that the patient was highly infectious. Although the infectious state may end after several weeks of appropriate antibiotic treatment, relapse may occur unless therapy is sustained for at least 6 months.

The emergence of antibiotic-resistant tuberculosis has complicated the clinical management of this disease. Drug-resistant strains of tubercle bacilli arise from spontaneous chromosomal mutations; different mutations affect susceptibility to different drugs. Under conditions in which therapy is inadequate, because too few drugs are prescribed, the dosages are inadequate, or patient adherence to the prescribed regimen is poor, resistance to multiple antibiotic agents can arise. Recent surveillance data in the United States indicate that about 1 in 13 patients with tuberculosis has a strain resistant to one of the leading antibiotics, isoniazid. Foreign-born persons with tuberculosis are about twice as likely as those born in the United States to have antibiotic-resistant strains of the organism. Even more vexing is the challenge of multidrug-resistant tuberculosis, in which the organism is resistant to two or more antibiotics. Multidrug-resistant tuberculosis is particularly difficult to treat, often requiring an extended duration of therapy and the use of alternative antibiotics that are expensive and have higher risks of adverse effects.

Because of the rise in incidence of multidrug-resistant forms of tuberculosis, treatment recommendations for the disease have been modified as follows:

- In vitro testing of isolated tubercle bacilli for drug resistance and reporting of these results to the health department
- The use of a four-antibiotic regimen for initial treatment of tuberculosis infections
- Direct observation of initial therapy by a health care provider.

Directly observed therapy, involving ingestion of antibiotics by the patient in the presence of the health care provider or another designated person, is intended to ensure adherence to the prescribed antibiotic regimen. Surveillance data in the United States indicate that over half of tuberculosis therapy is now administered totally through directly observed therapy, with

Table 3–1. Factors that increase the probability of tuberculosis transmission.

Environment	Infectious Individuals	Susceptible Individuals
1. Close contact of infections and susceptible people in small, enclosed spaces	1. Pulmonary or laryngeal disease (particularly with bacilli in sputum or cavitary lesions in the lung)	1. Compromised immune system
2. Poor ventilation	2. Cough or other cause of forceful expiration; uncovered mouth when coughing	2. Presence of certain predisposing medical conditions (eg, silicosis, cancer)
3. Recirculation of contaminated air	3. Less than 2–3 weeks of appropriate antimicrobial therapy	3. Lack of adequate nutrition
		4. Injection drug use or heavy alcohol intake

Table 3–2. Populations at high risk for developing tuberculosis.

Individuals Who Have Daily Contact with a Patient with Tuberculosis	Individuals with Predisposing Medical Conditions	Other Individuals
1. Family members and close personal contacts	1. Persons with the human immunodeficiency virus (HIV)	1. Foreign-born persons from countries where the prevalence of tuberculosis is high
2. Health care workers	2. Persons with silicosis, hematological disorders, cancer, chronic renal failure, or diabetes mellitus	2. Residents of long-term facilities (eg, correctional institutions, nursing homes, and mental institutions)
	3. Medically underserved low-income populations	3. Alcohol and injection drug users

another one fourth of patients receiving a combination of directly observed and self-administered treatment.

Once a patient is diagnosed with clinically active tuberculosis, the patient's close personal contacts should be tested for tuberculosis. The husband and two children of the woman in the Patient Profile were considered close contacts. Because asymptomatic infection was demonstrated in the husband and one child, preventive therapy was administered. The other child showed no signs of infection. Guidelines for preventive therapy dictate that children who are close contacts and have a negative skin test should receive antibiotics until a skin test repeated 12 weeks later is also negative. Residents of the patient's apartment building and her contacts at work also were considered to be at high risk and were investigated for infection. The single infected resident was treated with preventive antibiotics, in accordance with established guidelines.

DESCRIPTIVE EPIDEMIOLOGY

Broadly speaking, epidemiologic work can be divided into two main categories:

1. **Descriptive epidemiology,** which includes activities related to characterizing the distribution of diseases within a population; and
2. **Analytic epidemiology,** which concerns activities related to identifying possible causes for the occurrence of diseases.

Both types of epidemiology are fundamental to the prevention and control of diseases and to the advancement of medical knowledge. Descriptive patterns of disease occurrence often lead to hypotheses about disease causation that are tested in analytic investigations. Analytic studies may yield findings that help to explain descriptive patterns and to improve surveillance efforts.

Measures of disease occurrence—the tools for descriptive epidemiology—were introduced in Chapter 2. In this chapter, these tools are used to characterize the

population distribution of tuberculosis. Toward that end, three basic questions can be asked:

1. Who develops tuberculosis?
2. **Where** does tuberculosis occur?
3. **When** does tuberculosis occur?

Collectively, these three questions serve as the basis for a descriptive investigation of tuberculosis. Answers to these questions characterize the distribution of tuberculosis by **person, place,** and **time.** As shown schematically in Figure 3–1, these features are the standard dimensions used to track the occurrence of a disease.

Person

A basic tenet of epidemiology is that diseases do not occur at random. In other words, not all persons within a population are equally likely to develop a particular condition. Variation of occurrence in relation to personal characteristics may reflect differences in level of

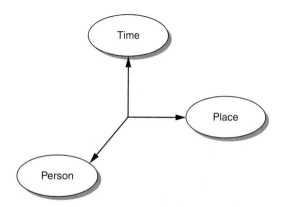

Figure 3–1. Schematic representation of the standard dimensions used to characterize disease occurrence.

exposure to causal factors, susceptibility to the effects of causal factors, or both exposure and susceptibility.

Typically, the minimal set of personal characteristics examined with respect to disease occurrence includes age, race, and gender. Because such information is routinely collected on the affected persons (cases), as well as the unaffected population from which the cases develop, epidemiologists rely on these characteristics to a great extent. The use of other attributes of interest, such as level of education and income, marital status, and occupation, is contingent on the availability of data.

The number of reported cases of tuberculosis by age in the United States during 2002 is shown in Figure 3–2. It should be emphasized that these data are derived from information reported by physicians, laboratories, and other health care providers. Tuberculosis is one of over 60 infectious diseases that currently are designated as notifiable at the national level within the United States. The Centers for Disease Control and Prevention (CDC) define a notifiable disease as follows:

A disease for which regular, frequent, and timely information on individual cases is considered necessary for the prevention and control of the disease.

The compulsory collection of information on selected infectious diseases was authorized at the national level in the United States and a number of other countries in the late 1800s. The list of nationally notifiable diseases is revised periodically in response to the emergence of pathogens that pose a threat to the health of the public. For example, the list of notifiable diseases in the United States was expanded to include West Nile encephalitis in 2002 and severe acute respiratory syndrome (SARS) in 2003.

Reporting of notifiable diseases in the United States typically begins with a clinician forwarding basic information on a newly diagnosed patient to the designated local or state health department. On a weekly basis, state and territorial officials transmit information about individual or aggregated cases of nationally notifiable diseases to the CDC. These reports follow a standard format, including information on the age, sex, and race of the patient, and date of occurrence of reported cases.

Although reporting of notifiable diseases is mandatory, and sanctions can be enforced for noncompliance, these sanctions are rarely applied. As a consequence, reporting is often incomplete, with wide-ranging estimates of completeness for various notifiable diseases. A number of factors probably affect the likelihood that a notifiable disease will be reported:

1. The clinical severity of the condition
2. Whether the affected individual consults a physician
3. The type of physician consulted (eg, private vs public provider, generalist vs specialist)
4. Any social stigma associated with the condition
5. Level of interest in the condition among clinicians
6. The physician's knowledge of reporting requirements
7. Existence of an adequate definition of the condition for surveillance purposes
8. Availability and utilization of appropriate diagnostic laboratories
9. Availability of effective disease control measures
10. Interests and priorities of local and state health officials

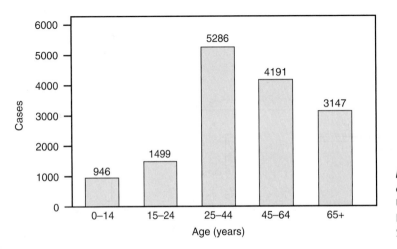

Figure 3–2. Number of reported cases of tuberculosis by age in the United States, 2002. (Data from CDC: Reported tuberculosis in the United States, 2002. September 2003.)

For a disease such as tuberculosis, in which clinical manifestations can be serious, clear diagnostic criteria and effective treatments are available, and the risk of interpersonal transmission is high, complete reporting of diagnosed cases obviously is crucial. On the other hand, interpretation of reported numbers of cases must include the possibility of incomplete notification.

Returning to the data presented in Figure 3–2, and recognizing the possibility of incomplete reporting, it appears that the age group with the highest risk of tuberculosis is 25–44 years. This conclusion is incorrect, however, because it fails to take into account the varying sizes of the source populations across the different age groups. There were over 85 million persons in the 25- to 44-year-old age group, as compared with under 67 million persons in the 45- to 64-year-old category, and under 36 million persons in the group aged 65 years or older. By calculating incidence rates, it is possible to compensate for disparities in sizes of the source populations. As illustrated in Figure 3–3, the incidence of tuberculosis rises with age, reaching a level of 8.8 cases per 100,000 persons among those 65 years of age or older. The incidence among persons in the oldest age group is over 40% higher than that for the 25- to 44-year-old age group.

A number of factors contribute to the nonrandom relationship between incidence of tuberculosis and age.

1. The long latent period between infection and development of clinical symptoms means that the ages at detection of illness are expected to be skewed toward later life.
2. Because elderly individuals lived through time periods when the disease was more common, they are more likely to have been infected than younger persons (**birth cohort effect**).
3. Older persons are more likely to have other illnesses (eg, cancer, diabetes mellitus) that may make them more susceptible to tuberculosis.
4. The decline in immune function associated with the normal aging process may increase susceptibility.
5. Elderly persons are more likely to live in closed communal settings that are conducive to the spread of tuberculosis.

An equally striking nonrandom pattern of occurrence is seen when incidence is examined as a function of race or ethnicity (Figure 3–4). The highest incidence rate of tuberculosis in the United States is found among Asians and Pacific Islanders; it is more than 18 times greater than the incidence rate for white non-Hispanics. Foreign-born persons account for about 95% of tuberculosis cases among Asians and Pacific Islanders in the United States. As exemplified by the subject of the Patient Profile, many of these individuals acquire the infection in the high-risk country of origin, but do not develop symptomatic disease until they arrive in the United States. About three out of four tuberculosis cases among Hispanics in the United States also occur in foreign-born persons. Overall, foreign-born persons account for slightly more than half of all tuberculosis cases in the United States.

The high incidence rates of tuberculosis within certain minority groups in the United States reflect the influences of other risk factors. Tuberculosis is a disease that is associated with socioeconomic disadvantage. The combination of crowded housing, poor nutrition, inadequate access to preventive and therapeutic medical services, alcoholism, and injecting drug use, as well as

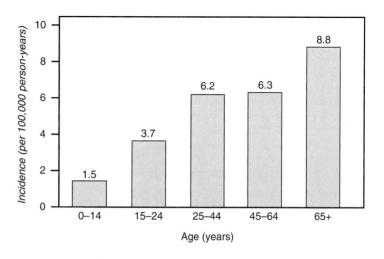

Figure 3–3. Incidence rates for reported tuberculosis, grouped by age, in the United States, 2002. (Data from CDC: Reported tuberculosis in the United States, 2002. September 2003.)

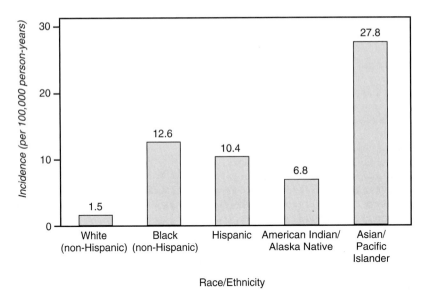

Figure 3–4. Incidence rates for reported tuberculosis, grouped by race and ethnicity, in the United States, 2002. (Data from CDC: Reported tuberculosis in the United States, 2002. September 2003.)

any predisposing medical conditions, contributes to the high risk of tuberculosis among the poor. Since black and Native American/Alaskan Native populations in the United States have comparatively large percentages of disadvantaged persons, the incidence of tuberculosis in these communities is elevated.

The distribution of tuberculosis by gender is shown in Figure 3–5. The incidence of tuberculosis is almost 60% higher among males than among females. The higher occurrence of tuberculosis among males probably is related to differences in certain high-risk behaviors (eg, heavy alcohol consumption) as well as predisposing diseases (eg, AIDS, silicosis) between males and females.

Place

Variation in the place of occurrence of a disease can be evaluated at the national level (eg, across countries), at the regional level (eg, across states), or at the local level (eg, across communities). Certain countries, particularly those in the nonindustrialized parts of the world, have comparatively high rates of tuberculosis. The estimated incidence rates of this disease across various parts of the world during 2001 are shown in Figure 3–6.

Worldwide, it is estimated that over 8 million people develop tuberculosis each year. This number is an estimate because the actual reporting of numbers of new cases of tuberculosis as well as the sizes of the source populations are incomplete in many nonindus-

trialized countries. Accordingly, this information must be interpreted with caution. Nevertheless, 95% of all new tuberculosis infections are thought to occur in the developing world.

The region of the world where the incidence rate of tuberculosis is rising most rapidly is sub-Saharan Africa,

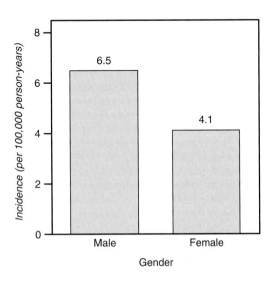

Figure 3–5. Incidence rates for reported tuberculosis, grouped by gender, in the United States, 2002. (Data from CDC: Reported tuberculosis in the United States, 2002. September 2003.)

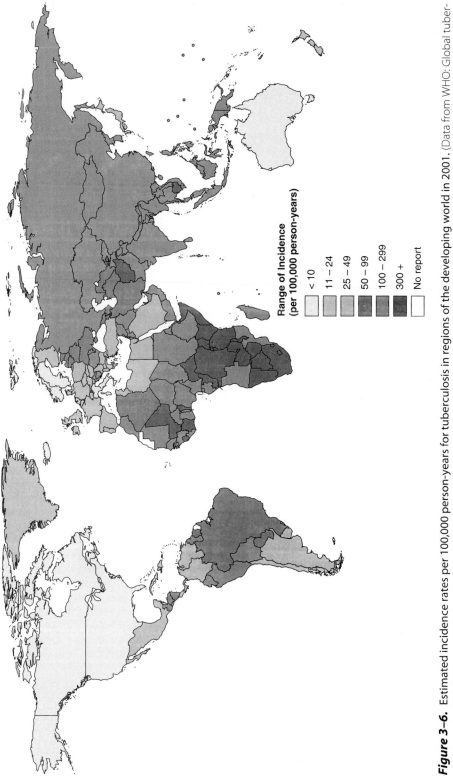

Figure 3–6. Estimated incidence rates per 100,000 person-years for tuberculosis in regions of the developing world in 2001. (Data from WHO: Global tuberculosis control. WHO Report, 2003.)

Range of Incidence
(per 100,000 person-years)

< 10
11 – 24
25 – 49
50 – 99
100 – 299
300 +
No report

which surpassed the previous leader, Southeast Asia, in 1995. The high rates of tuberculosis in nonindustrialized nations are attributable to poverty, malnutrition, crowded living conditions, inadequate preventive and therapeutic programs, and, particularly in sub-Saharan Africa, the high prevalence of infection with HIV. A growing proportion of tuberculosis occurrence worldwide is associated with HIV.

Even within an industrialized country such as the United States, variation in the incidence of tuberculosis is observed (Figure 3–7). The highest rates occur in urban areas, for example, San Francisco and New York (13 cases per 100,000 person-years). Comparatively low rates are found in rural states of the Midwestern and Western regions of the United States, such as North Dakota and Wyoming (each with less than 1 case per 100,000 person-years). These geographic patterns reflect differences in the underlying demographic characteristics of the various populations, including factors such as racial/ethnic composition and representa-

tion of immigrants from developing countries. In addition, the geographic distribution of other risk factors—poverty, malnutrition, crowded living conditions, substance abuse, and infection with HIV—probably influences the pattern of tuberculosis occurrence.

Time

The overall annual incidence of tuberculosis between 1980 and 2002 in the United States is depicted in Figure 3–8. During the first part of the 1980s, a consistent downward trend was observed, continuing a pattern that began many decades earlier. Between 1984 and 1989, the incidence of this disease remained fairly constant, with a rising incidence between 1989 and 1992. After 1992, the incidence rate began to fall again with a decline similar to that observed in the early 1980s. Another way to visualize this pattern is to compare the percentage change in incidence between the first and last years of successive 3-year time intervals (Figure 3–9).

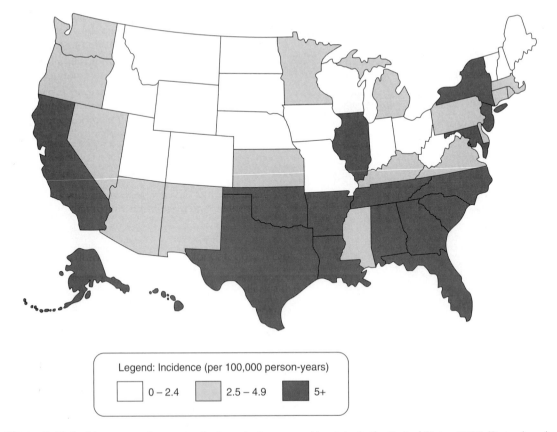

Legend: Incidence (per 100,000 person-years)

| | 0 – 2.4 | | 2.5 – 4.9 | | 5+ |

Figure 3–7. Incidence rates for reported tuberculosis, grouped by state, in the United States, 2002. (Reproduced from CDC: Reported tuberculosis in the United States, 2002. September 2003.)

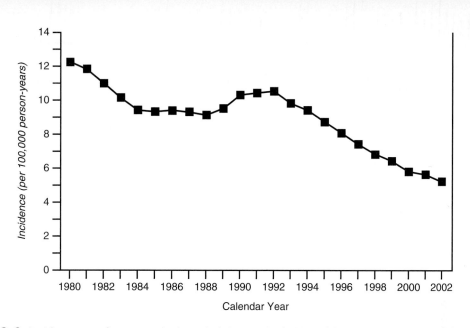

Figure 3–8. Incidence rates for reported tuberculosis by year in the United States, 1980–2002. (Data from CDC: Reported tuberculosis in the United States, 2002. September 2003.)

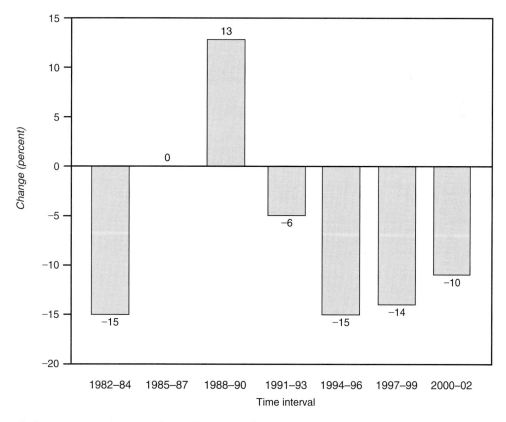

Figure 3–9. Percentage change in the incidence rates for reported tuberculosis, grouped by 3-year time intervals, in the United States, 1982–2002. (Data from CDC: Reported tuberculosis in the United States, 2002. September 2003.)

Between 1982 and 1984, the incidence of tuberculosis fell by 15%, with no change between 1985 and 1987. Between 1988 and 1990, the incidence increased by 13%, with a reversal to a 6% decrease between 1991 and 1993. Even greater decreases of 15% and 14% were observed in the next two time periods, respectively. A further reduction, albeit at a lower level (10%), occurred between 2000 and 2002.

The rise of tuberculosis occurrence in the United States during the late 1980s, followed by the subsequent fall in occurrence is a remarkable public health story. A number of factors probably contributed to the rise of this disease, including among others:

1. The emergence of a highly susceptible population of persons infected with HIV
2. Lapses in infection control practices in institutional settings
3. Increases in the number of immigrants arriving from countries with high rates of tuberculosis occurrence
4. The emergence of strains of tuberculosis resistant to multiple antibiotics
5. Failure of tuberculosis control programs to ensure that persons with active disease complete an adequate course of antibiotic therapy.

In response to the rise in the occurrence of tuberculosis in the United States, a massive public health effort was mounted to reverse this trend. The federal government appropriated substantial increases in funds to fight this disease. With the additional resources, public health agencies were able to expand programs for tuberculosis control. The essential components of these control efforts include:

1. Prompt identification of persons with active disease
2. Initiation of appropriate treatment for persons with active disease
3. Assurance that therapy is completed for persons with active disease
4. Tracing of the contacts of persons with active disease
5. Testing for infection among contacts
6. Completion of preventive therapy in eligible contacts.

The effectiveness of public health interventions was suggested by the progressive decline in incidence rates for tuberculosis after the interventions were begun. The argument that measures to control tuberculosis were responsible for the observed decline in incidence rates is strengthened by additional evidence. The rates of reduction were most substantial in areas that had the most successful control programs (as indicated by percentages of patients with elimination of organisms from sputum, completion of therapy for active cases, and tracing of contacts of active cases). Also, the proportion of organisms resistant to multiple antibiotics declined, with the greatest drop in areas with the highest rates of therapy completion. The decline in incidence rates of tuberculosis between 1992 and 2002 occurred across all age groups (Figure 3–10).

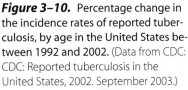 The usual rate of occurrence for a disease in a population is referred to as the **endemic rate.** A rapid and dramatic increase over the endemic rate is described as an **epidemic rate.** The development of an epidemic as a function of time is illustrated schematically in Figure 3–11. For an acute condition such as a viral illness, the epidemic may develop

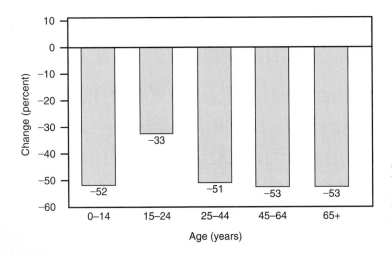

Figure 3–10. Percentage change in the incidence rates of reported tuberculosis, by age in the United States between 1992 and 2002. (Data from CDC: CDC: Reported tuberculosis in the United States, 2002. September 2003.)

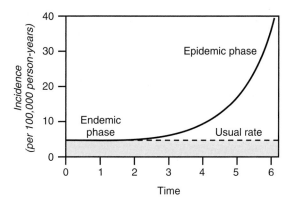

Figure 3–11. Schematic representation of the development of an epidemic of disease over time.

over a matter of days or weeks. In contrast, for a chronic illness such as lung cancer, the epidemic may emerge over a period of years to decades.

The time lag or **latent period** between exposure to a risk factor and diagnosis of a disease can be as short as a few hours (eg, staphylococcal food poisoning) or as long as decades (eg, infection to clinically active tuber-

culosis). Obviously, the greater the time between the occurrence of an initiating event and the recognition of disease, the more difficult it may be to establish the linkage between risk factor and disease occurrence. This task is made even more challenging if the risk factor is a weak determinant of the disease or if multiple different risk factors are involved.

As noted earlier, the incidence rate of tuberculosis in the United States ended a long-term continuous decline in 1984 (Figure 3–12). The solid line in Figure 3–12 depicts the number of tuberculosis cases that would have been expected if the pre-1984 rate of decline had continued. The squares in Figure 3–12 depict the actual numbers of patients with tuberculosis observed each year through 2002. It can be seen that the disparity between the actual and predicted numbers of cases is greatest in the early 1990s. After 1994, the slope of decline in the annual number of patients with tuberculosis appears similar to that prior to 1984. The rise in incidence of tuberculosis between 1984 and 1992 does not represent an epidemic in the conventional sense of a rapid rise in incidence. However, it does indicate a departure from the prior downward trend, and therefore represented a threat to the health of the public.

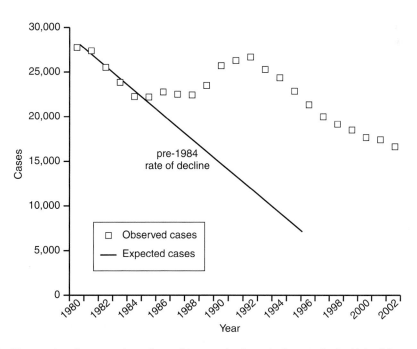

Figure 3–12. Observed and expected numbers of reported tuberculosis cases in the United States, 1980–2002. (Data from CDC: Reported tuberculosis in the United States, 2002. September 2003.)

CORRELATIONS WITH DISEASE OCCURRENCE

To develop hypotheses about possible causes of disease occurrence, the presence of a suspected risk factor can be measured in different populations and compared with the incidence of a particular disease. This type of comparison is referred to as an **ecologic study** because the analysis is at the level of an entire population rather than at the level of individual persons. Another name for this type of investigation is **correlation study,** because it seeks to determine the extent to which two characteristics (risk factor and disease occurrence) are related.

An example of ecologic data is shown in Figure 3–13. In this graph, the incidence rates of acquired immune deficiency syndrome (AIDS) in 15 states of the United States during 1997 are compared with corresponding incidence rates of tuberculosis for that same year. The states included in this analysis (Arkansas, California, Georgia, Idaho, Michigan, Mississippi, Nebraska, New Hampshire, North Carolina, Ohio, Oregon, Vermont, West Virginia, Wisconsin, and Wyoming) were selected because they represent diverse geographic areas with varying demographic characteristics.

In general, the states that had a high incidence of AIDS also had a high incidence of tuberculosis (eg, California and Georgia). At the other extreme, states

with a low incidence of AIDS also tended to have a low incidence of tuberculosis (eg, Idaho, New Hampshire, and Wyoming). As a general rule, the incidence of AIDS was about two times greater than the corresponding incidence of tuberculosis. A few exceptions occurred, such as Arkansas, in which the incidence of AIDS (9.6 cases per 100,000 person-years) was only about 35% greater than the incidence of tuberculosis (7.1 cases per 100,000 person-years). An exception in the opposite direction was Wyoming, in which the incidence of AIDS (3.3 cases per 100,000 person-years) was eight times greater than the incidence of tuberculosis (0.4 cases per 100,000 person-years).

To assess the strength of the relationship between AIDS and tuberculosis incidence, a correlation analysis was performed (see Dawson and Trapp, 2004, *Basic and Clinical Biostatistics*). The correlation coefficient was 0.91, which indicates that the incidence rate (*IR*) of AIDS and incidence rate of tuberculosis in the study are strongly and positively related. (If AIDS and tuberculosis incidence rates were perfectly correlated, the correlation coefficient would be 1. If there was no correlation between these two incidence rates, the correlation coefficient would be zero.) The **coefficient of determination,** the square of the correlation coefficient, was 0.83. This means that over four fifths of the variability in the incidence of tuberculosis could be accounted for by knowing the incidence of AIDS in these 15 states.

A linear regression analysis of these data (see Dawson and Trapp, 2004) yielded the following equation:

$$\text{Tuberculosis } IR = -0.8 + 0.57 \times (\text{AIDS } IR)$$

The graph of this regression line is depicted in Figure 3–14. In this analysis, the effect of AIDS incidence in determining the incidence of tuberculosis is highly statistically significant. In other words, it is very unlikely that the observed relationship between the incidence rates of AIDS and tuberculosis occurred by chance alone. From the regression equation it can also be seen that in the absence of AIDS (AIDS incidence = 0 cases per 100,000 person-years), the expected incidence rate of tuberculosis is –0.8 cases per 100,000 person-years. Because it is impossible to have an incidence rate less than zero, we conclude that in these states, the tuberculosis incidence rate is negligible in the absence of AIDS. For every increase of one case per 100,000 person-years in the incidence of AIDS, the incidence of tuberculosis is expected to increase by 0.57 cases per 100,000 person-years.

The relationship depicted in Figure 3–14 is very striking and suggests that the occurrence of AIDS may influence the development of tuberculosis. This type of correlation analysis, however, is best viewed as a **hy-**

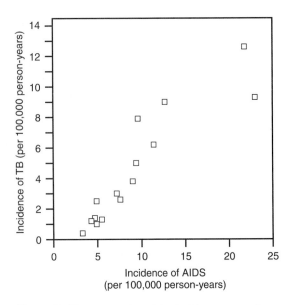

Figure 3–13. Scatterplot of the incidence rates of reported AIDS and tuberculosis (TB) in 15 states of the United States, 1997. (Data for AIDS: CDC: HIV/AIDS surveillance report. MMWR 1997;9[2]:7. Data for TB: CDC: Reported tuberculosis in the United States, 1997. July 1998.)

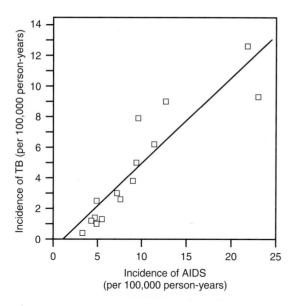

Figure 3–14. Regression line for regression of reported tuberculosis (TB) incidence on reported AIDS incidence in 15 states of the United States, 1997. (Data for AIDS: CDC: HIV/AIDS surveillance report. MMWR 1997;9[2]: 7. Data for TB: CDC: Reported tuberculosis in the United States, 1997. July 1998.)

pothesis-generating study, which means that it can be used to help formulate a hypothesis about the link between these two diseases, but it cannot establish a causal relationship between them. A correlation between incidence of AIDS and tuberculosis could occur for reasons other than a cause-and-effect relationship. For example, risk factors for both diseases (eg, injecting drug use) might be the true reason for the apparent association between AIDS and tuberculosis.

Studies that are designed to test the likelihood of a cause-and-effect relationship between a risk factor and a disease are termed **hypothesis-testing investigations.** The two approaches most commonly employed to test associations between risk factors and diseases are cohort and case–control studies. These research designs are described in Chapters 8 and 9, respectively. The effects of related variables, such as injecting drug use, can be considered in the design and analysis of these studies.

An important limitation on the epidemiologist's ability to infer a causal explanation from a correlation study is the **ecologic fallacy.** This problem may occur when a suspected risk factor and disease occurrence are associated at the population level but not at the individual subject level. In other words, populations may have high incidence rates of AIDS (risk factor) and of tuberculosis (disease occurrence) without the same persons being affected by both conditions. This type of ecologic fallacy

can be avoided only by making observations of risk factor and disease status on individual subjects. Methods of analytic epidemiology, such as cohort and case–control studies, involve observations on individuals, and thus are not subject to the hazards of ecologic reasoning. The link between the occurrence of AIDS and tuberculosis is now well established through hypothesis-testing studies, so it can be concluded that the correlation seen in Figure 3–14 is not attributable to an ecologic fallacy.

MIGRATION & DISEASE OCCURRENCE

Another useful technique in descriptive epidemiology is the examination of the effects of migration on the rate of disease occurrence. Studies of this type can help to clarify whether a disease of unknown cause is determined principally by genetic inheritance or by environmental exposure. As depicted in Figure 3–15, migration from a high-risk population to a low-risk population should not affect the occurrence of a genetically determined disease among the migrants. In contrast, migration from a high-risk population to a low-risk population is expected to be associated with a reduction in occurrence of an environmentally determined disease. Expressed in another way, migration diminishes the likelihood of exposure to environmental risk factors, and accordingly, the occurrence of disease should decrease. Of course, for diseases with long latent periods, it may take many years for the reduced rate of occurrence to become manifest.

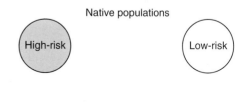
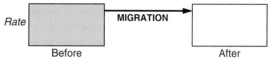
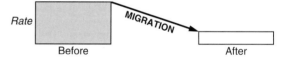

Figure 3–15. Schematic representation of the effects of migration on the rates of occurrence of genetically and environmentally determined diseases.

If environmental exposures early in life are critical, then the rate of occurrence may not be reduced among the migrants themselves (who were exposed prior to their departure), but should be diminished among their offspring born in the new location. A dramatic change in disease incidence within a single generation could not be explained on the basis of genetic changes. Approaches to the study of diseases that are thought to have genetic predispositions are presented in Chapter 11.

A number of studies have indicated that a progressive decline over time in the incidence of tuberculosis occurs among persons who migrate from high-risk areas (eg, Asia) to low-risk areas (eg, the United States and Western Europe). The basic pattern of change in incidence is shown in Figure 3–16. The incidence of tuberculosis is highest at the time of migration and falls rapidly in the next few years. The decline continues for many years, with smaller increments of change over time. The incidence among migrants does not fall to the level of the general population, however, presumably because of latent infections acquired prior to migration. Other factors that may contribute to the persistence of an elevated incidence of tuberculosis among migrants include the following:

1. Residence in migrant communities, thus maintaining a comparatively high rate of disease transmission
2. Crowded housing conditions
3. Poor nutritional status
4. Inadequate access to preventive or therapeutic medical services
5. Noncompliance with therapy

6. Presence of tuberculosis that is resistant to conventional antibiotics
7. Reinfection on return visits to the country of origin.

The overall decline in incidence of tuberculosis among migrants from high- to low-risk countries, however, provides strong circumstantial evidence about the importance of environmental determinants of this disease.

SUMMARY

In this chapter, the basic approaches to descriptive epidemiology are presented, with a focus on the patterns of occurrence of tuberculosis. Description in epidemiology begins with the assumption that diseases do not occur at random. Typically, three standard questions are posed to characterize the nonrandom distribution of a disease:

1. **Who** gets the disease?
2. **Where** does the disease occur?
3. **When** does the disease occur?

These questions concern the elements of **person, place,** and **time,** respectively.

At a minimum, the personal attributes examined in relation to disease occurrence are the distributions by age, race, and sex. The incidence of tuberculosis in the United States increases with advancing age. The racial and ethnic groups with the highest occurrence of this disease are Asians and Pacific Islanders, blacks, Hispanics, Native Americans, and Alaskan Natives. In addition, males have higher incidence rates for tuberculosis than females.

The place of occurrence of a disease may be studied at the international, regional, or local level. Tuberculosis occurs with great excess in nonindustrialized countries. Even within an industrialized country such as the United States, substantial regional and local variation in incidence is reported.

Temporal patterns can be examined across years, months, or days, depending on the time course of the disease in question. For tuberculosis, a progressive decline in incidence over time was observed in the United States until 1984, with a leveling off through 1989, followed by a rise in incidence through 1992, and then a return to falling incidence rates. The resurgence of tuberculosis in the late 1980s in the United States was attributed to a variety of factors. The contributing factors included lapses in control efforts, increased immigration of persons from countries with high incidence rates of disease, the emergence of strains resistant to multiple antibiotics, and the rising occurrence of a predisposing condition—AIDS.

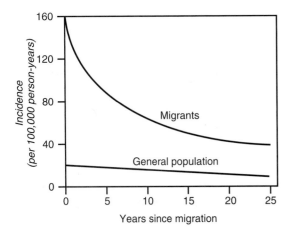

Figure 3–16. Comparison of the incidence of tuberculosis among migrants who moved from high- to low-risk countries with the incidence in the general population of the adopted country.

The concept of an epidemic as a rapid and dramatic increase in the incidence of a disease was introduced, using as an example the greater-than-expected occurrence of tuberculosis in the late 1980s. The use of ecologic (or correlation) studies was illustrated by a comparison of incidence rates of AIDS and tuberculosis in selected states. In an ecologic study, the overall amount of a risk factor (eg, AIDS) is related to the occurrence of a disease (eg, tuberculosis) across different populations. This type of correlation can be useful for generating hypotheses, but not for testing causal relationships. The influence of a background variable that is related to both the presumed risk factor and the outcome of interest can limit the utility of a correlation analysis. Furthermore, the ecologic fallacy can suggest a misleading conclusion when the risk factor and disease are related at the population level but not within particular individuals.

Finally, to distinguish genetic from environmental causes of disease, we discussed the use of studies of disease occurrence in relation to migration patterns. As applied to tuberculosis, persons who migrate from high-risk areas (eg, Asia) to low-risk areas (eg, the United States and Western Europe) experience a progressive decline in incidence over time. This pattern strongly indicates that the primary influences on the occurrence of tuberculosis are environmental.

STUDY QUESTIONS

In 2001 within the United States, the incidence of primary and secondary syphilis reversed a 10-year pattern of decline. National surveillance data were analyzed to characterize the epidemiology of syphilis (Data from CDC: Primary and secondary syphilis—United States, 2002. MMWR 2003;52: 1117.)

Questions 1–2: The incidence rates are shown by race and gender in Table 3–3. For each numbered question below, select the most appropriate group from the lettered options. Each option can be used once, more than once, or not at all.

   A. *White males*

   B. *Black males*

   C. *White females*

   D. *Black females*

   E. *All males*

   F. *All females*

   G. *All blacks*

   H. *All whites*

Table 3–3. Incidence rates (per 100,000 person-years) of primary and secondary syphilis by race and gender, United States, 2002.[a]

Gender	Race		
	White	Black	All
Male	2.2	13.5	3.8
Female	0.2	6.5	1.1
All	1.2	9.8	2.4

[a]Data from CDC: Primary and secondary syphilis—United States, 2002. MMWR 2003;**52**:1117.

   1. *The group with the greatest rapidity of new occurrences.*

   2. *The group with the lowest rapidity of new occurrences.*

Questions 3–6: Based on the information in Table 3–3, for each numbered question below, select the single best answer from the lettered options.

   3. *The black-to-white ratio of incidence rates among women is:*

     A. *6.5/0.2*

     B. *6.5/1.1*

     C. *6.5 – 0.2*

     D. *(6.5 × 2.2)/(13.5 × 0.2)*

     E. *(6.5 – 0.2)/6.5*

   4. *The male-to-female ratio of incidence rates among whites is:*

     A. *2.2/1.2*

     B. *2.2 – 0.2*

     C. *(2.2 × 6.5)/(13.5 × 0.2)*

     D. *(2.2 – 0.2)/ 2.2*

     E. *2.2/0.2*

   5. *The black-to-white excess rate of occurrence (in cases per 100,000 person-years) among males is*

     A. *3.7*

     B. *7.0*

     C. *9.7*

     D. *11.3*

     E. *13.3*

   6. *The overall male-to-female excess rate of occurrence (in cases per 100,000 person-years)*

     A. *2.0*

     B. *7.0*

     C. *2.7*

     D. *1.4*

     E. *8.6*

Questions 7–10: Based on the information in Table 3–4, for each numbered question below, select the most appropriate option from the lettered options. Each option can be used once, more than once, or not at all.

A. Phoenix, Arizona

B. Houston, Texas

C. New York, New York

D. Louisville, Kentucky

E. San Francisco, California

7. Which city has the lowest overall incidence rate?

8. Which city has the highest overall incidence rate?

9. Which city has the least gender disparity in incidence rates?

10. Which city has the greatest gender disparity in incidence rates?

Questions 11-12: For each numbered question below, select the single best answer from the lettered options.

11. For males migrating from New York to Phoenix, the incidence rate should

A. Decrease

B. Increase

C. Stay the same

D. Change, but direction cannot be determined

E. Increase, then fall below original levels

12. For females migrating from New York to Phoenix, the incidence rate should

A. Decrease

B. Increase

C. Stay the same

D. Change, but direction cannot be determined

E. Increase, then fall below original

Table 3–4. Incidence rates (per 100,000 person-years) of primary and secondary syphilis by city and gender, United States, 2002.[a]

City	Gender	
	Male	Female
Phoenix, Arizona	6.2	3.8
Houston, Texas	5.7	0.9
New York, New York	11.0	0.4
Louisville, Kentucky	11.5	10.8
San Francisco, California	78.8	1.0

[a]Data from CDC: Primary and secondary syphilis—United States, 2002. MMWR 2003;**52:**1117.

FURTHER READING

Frieden TR et al: Tuberculosis. Lancet 2003;**362:**887.

REFERENCES

Davies PDO: The world-wide increase in tuberculosis: how demographic changes, HIV infection and increasing numbers in poverty are increasing tuberculosis. Ann Med 2003;**35:** 235.

Tiruviluamala P, Reichman LB: Tuberculosis. Ann Rev Public Health 2002;**23:**403.

Clinical Background

CDC: Treatment of tuberculosis. MMWR 2003;**52**(No. RR-11):1.

Chan ED, Iseman MD: Current medical treatment for tuberculosis. BMJ 2002;**325:**1282.

Raviglione MC: The TB epidemic from 1992 to 2002. Tuberculosis 2003;**83:**4.

Descriptive Epidemiology

CDC: Reported tuberculosis in the United States, 2002. September 2003.

CDC: Trends in tuberculosis morbidity, 1992–2002. MMWR 2003;**52:**217.

Frieden TR, Driver CR: Tuberculosis control: past 10 years and future progress. Tuberculosis 2003;**83:**82.

Schneider E, Castro KG: Tuberculosis trends in the United States, 1992–2001. Tuberculosis 2003;**83:**21.

Correlations with Disease Occurrence

CDC: HIV/AIDS surveillance report. MMWR 1997;**9**(2):7.

CDC: Reported tuberculosis in the United States, 1997. July 1998.

Dawson B, Trapp RG: *Basic and Clinical Biostatistics*, 4th ed. Appleton & Lange, 2004.

Migration and Disease Occurrence

Medical Research Council Tuberculosis and Chest Diseases Unit: National survey of notifications of tuberculosis in England and Wales in 1983. BMJ 1985;**291:**658.

e-PIDEMIOLOGY

Clinical Background

http://www.hopkins-id.edu/diseases/tb/index_tb.html
http://www.pitt.edu/~super1/lecture/lec0711/index.htm

Descriptive Epidemiology

http://www.pitt.edu/~super1/lecture/lec0711/index.htm
http://www.cdc.gov/nchstp/tb/surv/surv2001/default.htm

Migration

http://www.pitt.edu/~super1/lecture/lec1341/index.htm

Medical Surveillance

KEY CONCEPTS

1. Medical surveillance is undertaken to identify changes in the distributions of diseases in order to prevent or control these conditions within a population.

2. A comparison of incidence rates across populations can help to determine characteristics of populations at higher (and lower) risk.

3. Surveillance of deaths is convenient because the information is virtually complete, standardized and inexpensive to obtain. Nevertheless, data collected from death certificates may be limited by omitted or inaccurate information.

4. Age adjustment is used to remove the influence of any age differences when comparing the disease frequencies of two populations.

5. Premature death measures the years of potential life lost to a particular disease, and therefore weighs most heavily deaths that occur at young ages.

PATIENT PROFILE

A 68-year-old female retired office manager presented with a dry, hacking cough of several months' duration. She reported a history of smoking one pack of cigarettes per day for the past 30 years. To evaluate the patient's cough, her family physician ordered a chest x-ray, which was unremarkable except for an increased density in the hilum (midcentral portion) of the lung fields. A sputum specimen was collected, and abnormally-appearing cells were noted on microscopic evaluation. Because these cells suggested a malignancy, a bronchoscopic examination was performed to allow direct visualization of the large airways. A partially obstructing mass was visible at the distal end of the right main stem bronchus. Brushings from this mass revealed cells consistent with a di-

agnosis of squamous cell carcinoma. Other diagnostic studies indicated that the cancer had spread to involve the brain and bones. Radiation therapy was administered to all sites of cancer involvement. Nevertheless, the patient's condition rapidly deteriorated, and she died less than 6 months after diagnosis.

INTRODUCTION

In this chapter, attention is focused on one of the most basic functions of epidemiology: *detection of the occurrence of health-related events or exposures in a target population.*

The goal of this detection, or **surveillance,** is to identify changes in the distributions of diseases in order to prevent or control these diseases within a population. The term surveillance literally means "to watch over," and traditionally medical surveillance activities were developed to monitor the spread of infectious diseases through a population. Today, however, surveillance programs have been applied to a wide variety of other conditions, such as congenital malformations, injuries, occupational health problems, and cancer, as well as other behaviors that affect health. Regardless of the type of outcome under consideration, medical surveillance activities involve the following key features:

1. Continuous data collection and evaluation
2. An identified target population (such as a community, a work force, or a group of patients)
3. A standard definition of the outcome of interest
4. Emphasis on timeliness of collection and dissemination of information
5. Use of data for purposes of investigation or disease control.

The goals of medical surveillance depend on the state of knowledge about the causes of the condition of interest and the extent to which effective preventive measures are known (Table 4–1). Surveillance activities can provide data about the distribution of a disease by person, place, and time. These patterns of occurrence can help shed light on possible causes of the disease. For example, if the time and place of disease occurrence are similar for two or more individuals, a shared source of illness, such as an infectious agent, may be involved. Other demographic information about affected individuals, such as age, race, and gender, typically are collected during surveillance and may provide further insight into the modes of disease acquisition. More detailed information on the personal characteristics of affected individuals can be collected through personal interviews.

In the following sections, various aspects of medical surveillance are described. By relating each of these activities to the diagnosis of lung cancer in the Patient Profile, the relationships among different types of surveillance are demonstrated.

Table 4–1. Possible goals of medical surveillance activities.

Identification of patterns of disease occurrence
Detection of disease outbreaks
Development of clues about possible risk factors
Finding of cases for further investigation
Anticipation of health service needs

SURVEILLANCE OF NEW DIAGNOSES

In the United States, the incidence of cancer is monitored by the National Cancer Institute through population-based registries that collectively comprise the Surveillance, Epidemiology, and End Results (SEER) program. **Population based** means that the target group is the general population, usually identified as residents of a particular geographic area. The term is used to contrast with other types of registries, such as those based on patients who are treated at specific hospitals or those who belong to a particular health insurance plan.

The most recently reported SEER data on the incidence of cancer are derived from 12 areas, including five entire states (Utah, Iowa, Connecticut, New Mexico, and Hawaii), six metropolitan regions (Atlanta, Detroit, Los Angeles, San Jose/Monterey, Seattle, and San Francisco), and the native population of Alaska (Figure 4–1). Although about 14% of the population of the United States resides within these 12 areas combined, this is clearly not a random sample of the nation. The areas were selected largely on the basis of the ability to maintain ongoing population-based cancer reporting systems and epidemiologic interest in the population subgroups that reside there. Collectively these registries provide reasonably representative samples of different regions of the country, rural and urban populations, and most major racial and ethnic groups.

The SEER registries use a variety of methods to locate new diagnoses of cancer. The majority of diagnoses are identified from hospital admissions through the review of pathology reports and lists of discharge diagnoses. Additional identification sources include pathology laboratories outside of hospitals, office records of physicians, outpatient treatment facilities, and death certificates. The size of the population at risk of cancer is derived for each geographic area by extrapolation from census estimates.

The 2000 annual age-adjusted incidence rates for the five most common types of cancer among men and women of all races in the United States are shown in Figure 4–2. Note that the data on breast cancer are confined to women and the data on prostate cancer are confined to men. By convention, the incidence rates for cancer are expressed per 100,000 person-years. The incidence rate for lung cancer indicates that 62 individuals within a representative sample of 100,000 persons in the United States are expected to develop lung cancer in one year.

The incidence of lung cancer is 60% higher among males (80 per 100,000 person-years) than females (50 per 100,000 person-years) in the United States. Moreover, as illustrated in Figure 4–3, the incidence of lung cancer is not constant across age groups. This disease is

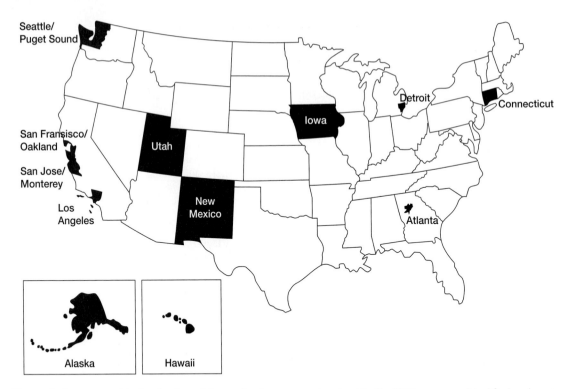

Figure 4–1. Geographic distribution of data collection centers involved in the SEER program. (Modified and reproduced from Ries LAG et al: *SEER Cancer Statistics Review, 1975–2000.* National Cancer Institute, 2003.)

extremely rare in persons under 40 years of age. After age 40, the incidence of lung cancer rises sharply, reaching a peak among persons in their 70s.

The striking relationship between age and incidence of lung cancer (and most other types of cancer) creates

a potential complication when comparing the incidence rates of population groups with different age distributions. In other words, simply because of their age, a younger group of individuals will tend to have fewer occurrences of lung cancer than an older group of peo-

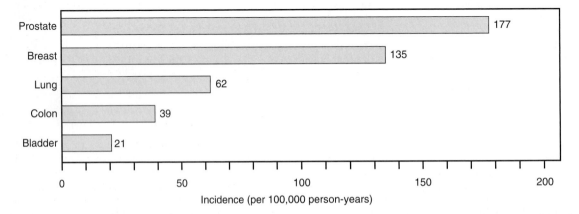

Figure 4–2. Age-adjusted incidence rates for the five leading forms of cancer among men and women of all races in the United States, 1996–2000. The rates for breast cancer are confined to women and the rates for prostate cancer are confined to men. (Data from Ries LAG et al: *SEER Cancer Statistics Review, 1975–2000.* National Cancer Institute, 2003.)

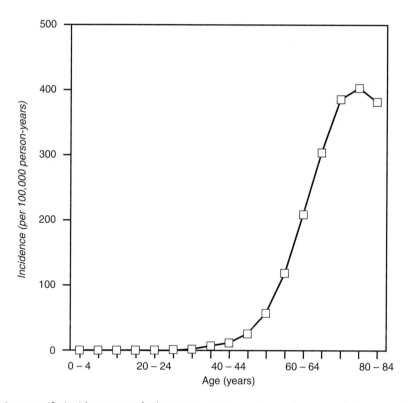

Figure 4–3. Age-specific incidence rates for lung cancer among men and women of all races in the United States, **1996–2000.** (Data from Ries LAG et al: *SEER Cancer Statistics Review, 1975–2000.* National Cancer Institute, 2003.)

ple. Failure to account for this age discrepancy would result in a distorted comparison of incidence rates for lung cancer between the two groups. To allow a comparison of incidence rates that is not influenced by age differences in the underlying populations, an age-adjustment procedure must be performed. The usual approach is referred to as **direct age adjustment** (or direct age standardization), in which *a single standard age structure is applied to the age-specific incidence rates for the groups being compared, resulting in summary rates for the groups that are not distorted by differences in age.* For direct age adjustment of cancer incidence rates in the United States, the standard age distribution currently in use by the SEER program is that of the entire population of the country in 2000.

As shown later in this chapter, blacks in the United States have an age distribution that is younger than the corresponding age distribution for whites. Because lung cancer tends to occur primarily in older adults, a comparison of overall lung cancer incidence rates for blacks and whites would be misleading, unless an adjustment is made for the underlying difference in age distribution between the races. Summary lung cancer incidence

rates for whites and blacks can be compared fairly by determining the lung cancer incidence rate that would have occurred in each racial group if it had the same age distribution as the 2000 U.S. population. The choice of the standard age distribution is arbitrary—any distribution can be used as long as it is applied equally to the groups being compared. We will focus on the topic of age adjustment in greater depth later in this chapter; a discussion of the calculation of adjusted rates can also be found in Dawson and Trapp (2004, *Basic and Clinical Biostatistics*).

RATE COMPARISONS

The age-adjusted incidence rates for leading forms of cancer in the United States are shown by race in Table 4–2. From these data, it can be seen that if the effect of age is held constant, blacks tend to have higher rates of occurrence of lung, colon, and prostate cancers than do whites. In contrast, breast and bladder cancers tend to occur with greater incidence among whites than blacks.

By dividing the incidence rate among blacks by the incidence rate among whites, a summary measure of

Table 4–2. The annual age-adjusted incidence rates per 100,000 person-years in whites and blacks for leading forms of cancer in the United States in 2000.[a]

	Incidence Rate[b]		
Type of Cancer	Blacks	Whites	Black-to-White Ratio
Prostate[c]	278	171	1.63
Breast[d]	116	141	0.82
Lung	79	63	1.25
Colon	50	38	1.32
Bladder	13	23	0.57

[a]Data from Ries LAG et al: *SEER Cancer Statistics Review, 1975–2000.* National Cancer Institute, 2003.
[b]Directly age adjusted to the 2000 population of the United States.
[c]Male only.
[d]Female only.

disparity in rates of occurrence is obtained. An index of the racial disparity in cancer incidence is the ratio of black-to-white incidence rates, or **rate ratio** (*RR*). If blacks and whites have the same rate of disease occurrence, the rate ratio would have a value of unity (*RR* = 1). When blacks have an elevated incidence rate compared with whites, the black-to-white rate ratio is greater than one (*RR* > 1). In contrast, when blacks have a lower incidence rate than whites, the rate ratio is less than one (*RR* < 1). The further the rate ratio is from unity, the greater the disparity in incidence rate between the races.

The black-to-white rate ratio of 1.25 for lung cancer indicates that the incidence of this cancer in black persons is about 25% greater than it is in white persons (Figure 4–4). In contrast, the rate ratio of 0.57 for bladder cancer indicates that the incidence rate of this cancer in blacks is more than 40% lower than it is in whites. These patterns suggest that the factors that in-

fluence the development of lung cancer and the factors that influence the development of bladder cancer are distributed differently between the races. These predisposing conditions, termed **risk factors,** could include genetic susceptibility to the cancers in question as well as exposure to environmental agents. The most common epidemiologic approaches to evaluating risk factors are discussed in Chapters 8 (Cohort Studies) and 9 (Case-Control Studies). Approaches to the study of genetic susceptibility are presented in Chapter 11.

Variations in incidence rates across demographic groups can provide important information about the causation of specific types of cancers. For example, cigarette smoking has been linked to the development of lung and bladder cancers, and among males a larger proportion of blacks than whites smoke. Therefore at least among males, the racial difference in prevalence of cigarette smoking may account for the increased occurrence of lung cancer among blacks. However, the higher incidence rate of bladder cancer among whites (particularly among males) suggests that factors other than cigarette smoking must be involved in the development of this disease.

SURVEILLANCE OF DEATHS

Another index used to measure the population distribution of a disease is the mortality rate, which characterizes the rapidity with which deaths from the disease occur over time. The **mortality rate** is determined by the combined forces of the rate of new diagnoses (**incidence rate**) and the likelihood of death following diagnosis (**case fatality**). For diseases such as lung cancer, which have a high case fatality (ie, a low rate of cure or recovery), mortality rates give a reasonable approximation of incidence rates. As shown in Figure 4–5, the overall age-adjusted mortality rate for lung cancer is about 90% as large as the corresponding incidence rate. For a cancer with a more favorable prognosis, such as thyroid cancer, there will be a greater disparity between mortality and incidence rates (Figure 4–6). The age-

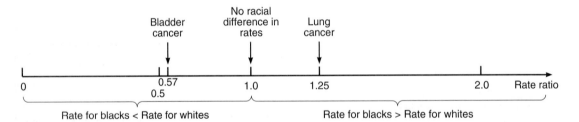

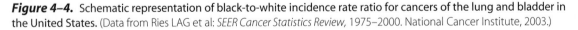

Figure 4–4. Schematic representation of black-to-white incidence rate ratio for cancers of the lung and bladder in the United States. (Data from Ries LAG et al: *SEER Cancer Statistics Review, 1975–2000.* National Cancer Institute, 2003.)

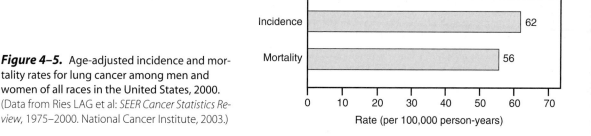

Figure 4–5. Age-adjusted incidence and mortality rates for lung cancer among men and women of all races in the United States, 2000. (Data from Ries LAG et al: *SEER Cancer Statistics Review*, 1975–2000. National Cancer Institute, 2003.)

adjusted mortality rate for thyroid cancer is only about 7% as large as the corresponding incidence rate, because most persons who develop this disease do not die from it.

Despite the potential disparity between incidence and mortality rates, the distribution of deaths from a disease by person, place, and time still can be useful for surveillance purposes. Pragmatic advantages to the use of information on mortality for surveillance purposes are listed below:

1. Widely collected, virtually complete data: registration of deaths is compulsory in most industrialized countries, and few deaths are not reported

2. Standardized nomenclature: the International Classification of Diseases is used to promote uniformity in reporting of causes of death

3. Modest cost: recording of deaths is relatively inexpensive.

Statistics on mortality thus serve as a convenient tool for epidemiologic surveillance, particularly when incidence data are not available. For example, as already noted, the SEER program covers only about 14% of the population of the United States, but death registration is compulsory throughout the nation. Accordingly, statistics on mortality can provide a more complete picture of the geographic distribution of cancer than can be determined from incidence data alone. A map of age-adjusted mortality rates for lung cancer for males and females of all races in the United States illustrates this point (Figure 4–7).

The process of collecting information on deaths in the United States begins with completion of a death certificate. Background demographic data (eg, age, birthdate, birthplace, race, sex, marital status, place of residence, occupation, and education) usually are recorded by the funeral director. A physician is required to certify the conditions responsible, in whole or in part, for the patient's death. For registration purposes, a distinction is made among

1. Immediate cause of death
2. Conditions that led to the immediate cause of death
3. Underlying cause of death.

Only the underlying cause of death is tabulated in official statistics. The underlying cause of death is defined as (1) the disease or injury that initiated the train of morbid events leading directly to death, or (2) the circumstances of the accident or violence that resulted in the fatal injury. For each of the causes of death listed on the certificate, the physician records the length of time between onset and death. Other required information includes whether an autopsy was performed, the place of death, and the manner of death (ie, natural, unintentional injury, homicide, suicide, or unknown).

Overall, only about 10% of death certificates indicate that an autopsy was performed on the deceased individual (the decedent). For people who die from cancer, stroke, chronic obstructive pulmonary disease, or diabetes mellitus, an autopsy is performed for fewer than 1 person in 20. The causes of death with the high-

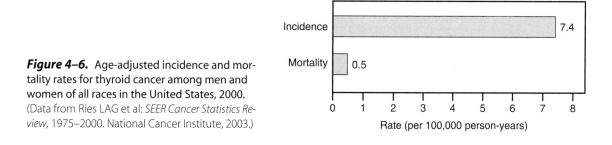

Figure 4–6. Age-adjusted incidence and mortality rates for thyroid cancer among men and women of all races in the United States, 2000. (Data from Ries LAG et al: *SEER Cancer Statistics Review*, 1975–2000. National Cancer Institute, 2003.)

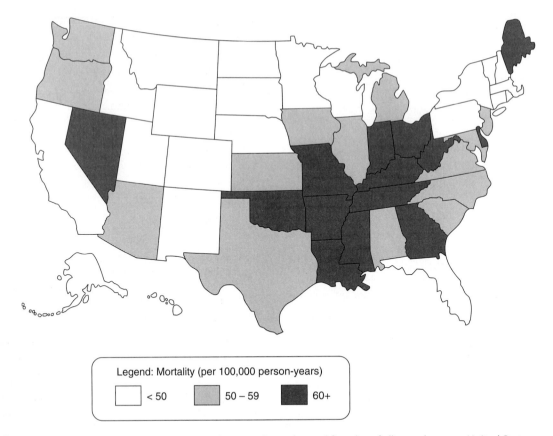

Figure 4–7. Age-adjusted lung cancer mortality rates for males and females of all races by state, United States, 1996–2000. (Data from Ries LAG et al: *SEER Cancer Statistics Review*, 1975–2000. National Cancer Institute, 2003.)

est percentages of subsequent autopsies are homicides (97%), suicides (56%), and unintentional injuries (49%). Medical examiners and coroners are responsible for investigating sudden or unanticipated deaths—such as those resulting from homicide, suicide, or unintentional injuries—as well as deaths arising unexpectedly from natural causes. The investigation includes collecting information on the circumstances surrounding the death, and where appropriate, measuring the decedent's alcohol and drug levels. The information reported by medical examiners and coroners usually is not available at the time of initial certification of death, and therefore is added later as an amendment.

Death certificates are filed with a local registrar, who checks for completeness of the information provided and then forwards the certificates to the state vital records office. The aggregated certificates are coded, numbered, and stored at the state level, and certificates for nonresidents are forwarded to their state of residence. The composite death information from each state is transferred to the National Center for Health Statistics for compilation into a national data base. The process of collecting information on deaths in the United States is summarized in Figure 4–8.

As noted, there are a number of advantages to the use of death registrations for purposes of medical surveillance. At the same time, it must be recognized that there are limitations to the information obtained in this manner:

1. Most physicians receive little formal instruction about how to fill out death certificates. As a result, the medical information reported is often incomplete or inaccurate.

2. In many situations, the certifying physician may have little particular knowledge of the decedent, leading to further errors in reporting or omissions of important conditions.

3. The use of only one underlying cause of death in official tabulations can lead to a very incomplete

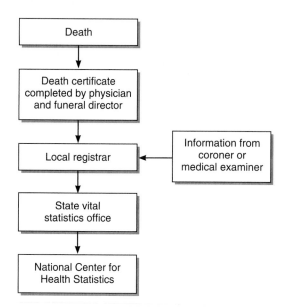

Figure 4–8. Flow diagram for processing of information about deaths in the United States.

picture of the contributions of various conditions to mortality. For example, in instances in which hypertension is reported on a death certificate, it is listed as the underlying cause of death only 10% of the time.

4. Concern for the confidentiality of the decedent may cause some physicians to omit sensitive diagnoses. There is evidence, for instance, that acquired immune deficiency syndrome (AIDS) has been underreported as an underlying cause of death.

5. When standard classifications of disease are periodically updated, the rules about assigning underlying causes of death can change, resulting in abrupt, artificial changes in the mortality trends for certain diseases.

6. With the many steps involved in collecting, editing, coding, and processing of death certificates, summary mortality data for a given year are not reported, even in preliminary form, until about 2 years later.

For any particular application, the appropriateness of using death registrations for purposes of medical surveillance is determined by balancing the advantages of universal coverage, convenience, and accessibility against the limitations of inaccurate and incomplete information, as well as delays in availability. Circum-

stances in which this type of information is likely to prove most useful include:

1. Monitoring historical trends in the burden of a disease and forecasting future expectations

2. Identifying population subgroups with disproportionate burdens of disease

3. Generating hypotheses about risk factors for a disease

4. Prioritizing the allocation of health care resources

5. Monitoring progress toward meeting health status objectives for a population.

AGE ADJUSTMENT

Mortality rates for all causes of death in the United States are shown by age and race in Figure 4–9. For both whites and blacks, mortality rates are high during the first year of life, are low during childhood, adolescence, and young adulthood, and then rise rapidly with increasing age. At every age depicted, however, the death rates for blacks exceed those of whites.

Therefore it might be surprising that the **crude death rate** (total deaths per total person-years) for blacks (774 deaths/100,000 person-years) is lower than the corresponding rate for whites (895 deaths/100,000 person-years). As indicated in Figure 4–10, the black-to-white ratio of crude mortality rates is 0.86, suggesting that blacks have a lower risk of death than do whites. This apparent paradox is explained by differences in the underlying age distributions of blacks and whites. On average, black persons in the United States tend to be younger than white persons (Figure 4–11). For example, only 7.8% of blacks in the United States are 65 years or older, compared with 13.4% of whites. Thus a smaller proportion of the black population experiences the high mortality associated with advanced age. To obtain an undistorted summary comparison of mortality for blacks and whites, the age differential between the races must be eliminated.

As noted previously, the usual approach to removing the influence of age from a comparison of summary rates is direct age adjustment. This technique involves the following steps:

1. Select a standard age structure. By convention, the standard distribution used for age adjustment of mortality rates in the United States is the age distribution of the total population of the country in 2000.

2. Multiply the age-specific mortality rates for each group being compared by the corresponding age-specific numbers of persons in the standard popu-

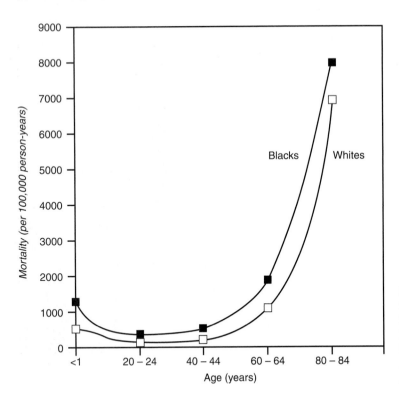

Figure 4–9. Mortality rates for all causes of death in the United States, by age and race, 2001. (Data from National Center for Health Statistics: National Vital Statistics Report. Monthly Vital Statistics Report. Vol 52, 2003.)

lation. The result is the expected number of deaths for that age category.

3. Sum the expected numbers of deaths across all age categories to yield a total number of expected deaths for each group being compared.

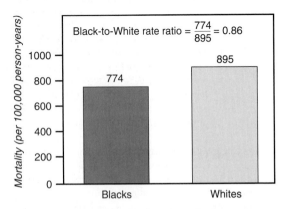

Figure 4–10. Crude mortality rates for blacks and whites in the United States, 2001. (Data from National Center for Health Statistics: National Vital Statistics Report. Vol 52, 2003.)

4. Divide the total number of expected deaths in each group by the total size of the standard population to yield the summary age-adjusted mortality rate.

When this direct age-adjustment procedure is performed on the age-specific death rates for blacks and whites in the United States for 2001, the summary mortality rates shown in Figure 4–12 are obtained. Note that the age-adjusted rates are higher than the crude rates for blacks (Figure 4–10), since the standard population has an older age distribution than does the black population. For whites, the reverse phenomenon is observed; the age-adjusted rate is lower than the crude rate because the white population has an older distribution of ages than the standard population.

The numerical values of the age-adjusted rates are not particularly meaningful by themselves, because the values will vary according to the standard age distribution used. The utility of the age-adjusted rates is that they allow comparisons across groups, such as the black-to-white rate ratio, by removing any age disparity between the groups being compared. It can be seen from Figure 4–12 that the age-adjusted mortality rate for blacks is almost 30% greater than it is for whites (rate ratio = 1.32). Thus the age-adjusted mortality rate ratio provides a summary measure that is consistent

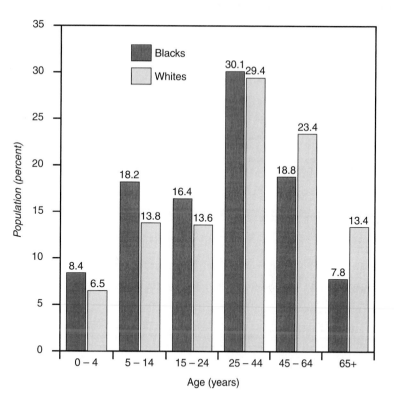

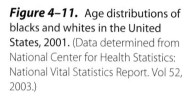

Figure 4–11. Age distributions of blacks and whites in the United States, 2001. (Data determined from National Center for Health Statistics: National Vital Statistics Report. Vol 52, 2003.)

with the increase in black mortality shown in Figure 4–9. Through the use of an adjustment technique, the distorting effect of differing underlying age distributions has been removed from the contrast of summary mortality rates.

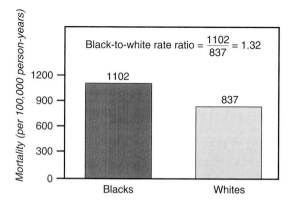

Figure 4–12. Age-adjusted (2000 U.S. population standard) total mortality rates for blacks and whites in the United States, 2001. (Data from National Center for Health Statistics: National Vital Statistics Report. Vol 52, 2003.)

MORTALITY PATTERNS

In addition to variation by age and race, mortality in the United Sates also varies by other characteristics. Age-adjusted mortality rates for whites and blacks for calendar years 1980 through 2001 are shown in Figure 4–13. Within each race, the age-adjusted mortality rates tended to decline, and the percentage decline was similar for whites (17%) and blacks (16%) over this time period. The fall in mortality rates was fairly continuous and progressive among whites. For blacks, however, there was a substantial decline between 1980 and 1982, with relatively level rates between 1982 and 1995, followed by a progressive decline thereafter.

As shown in Figure 4–14, black males have the highest age-adjusted mortality rate, followed in succession by white males and black females, with the lowest death rates observed among white females. Within both racial groups, males have higher mortality rates than females. For both genders, blacks have higher mortality rates than whites.

Table 4–3 lists the annual age-adjusted mortality rates for all persons in the United States according to the 10 leading causes of death. Four of the five most common causes of death in this country result from long-term, chronic processes: heart diseases, malignant

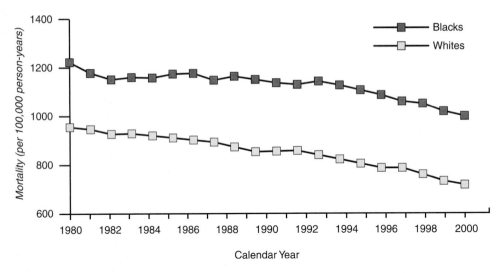

Figure 4–13. Age-adjusted total mortality rates by calendar year and race in the United States, 1980–2001. (Data from National Center for Health Statistics: National Vital Statistics Report. Vol 52, 2003.)

neoplasms (cancer), cerebrovascular disease (stroke), and chronic respiratory diseases.

Age-adjusted mortality rates for the individual causes of death vary by race and sex. Blacks have higher death rates than whites for 7 of the 10 leading causes of death (Figure 4–15). The relative increase in mortality among blacks is greatest for nephritis/nephrosis (black-to-white RR = 2.4), followed by septicemia (RR = 2.3), diabetes mellitus (RR = 2.1), stroke (RR = 1.4), heart disease and cancer (RR = 1.3), and influenza and pneumonia (RR = 1.1). Unintentional injuries occur with similar age-adjusted death rates among blacks and whites (RR = 1.0). Only chronic respiratory diseases and Alzheimer's disease (RR = 0.7) are responsible for lower age-adjusted rates of death among blacks than whites.

As depicted in Figure 4–16, males have higher age-adjusted mortality rates for 8 of the 10 leading causes of death in the United States. The relative increase in mortality among males is greatest for unintentional injuries (male-to-female RR = 2.2); followed by homicide, diseases of the heart, malignant neoplasms, and nephritis/nephrosis (RR = 1.5); chronic respiratory diseases, influenza, and pneumonia (RR = 1.4); and diabetes melli-

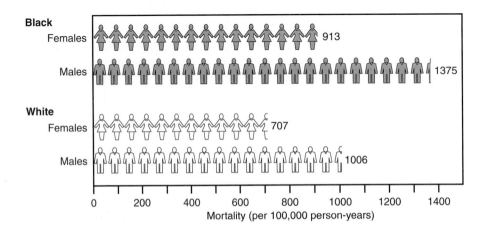

Figure 4–14. Age-adjusted mortality rates for all causes of death by race and sex in the United States, 2001. (Data from National Center for Health Statistics: National Vital Statistics Report. Vol 52, 2003.)

Table 4–3. Age-adjusted mortality rates per 100,000 person-years for the 10 leading causes of death in the United States in 2001.[a]

Rank	Cause of Death	Mortality Rate[b]
1	Diseases of heart	248
2	Malignant neoplasms	196
3	Cerebrovascular diseases	58
4	Chronic respiratory disease	44
5	Unintentional injuries	36
6	Diabetes mellitus	25
7	Influenza and pneumonia	22
8	Alzheimer's disease	19
9	Nephiritis/nephrosis	14
10	Septicemia	11

[a]Data from National Center for Health Statistics: National Vital Statistics Report, 2001. Vol **52[3],** 2003.
[b]Directly adjusted to the 2000 population of the United States.

tus and septicemia ($RR = 1.2$). No gender difference in age-adjusted death rates was observed for stroke ($RR = 1.0$). Only for Alzheimer's disease did males have a lower age-adjusted mortality rate than females ($RR = 0.8$).

Trends over time in the overall age-adjusted mortality rates for the 10 leading causes of death between 1999 and 2001 are displayed schematically in Figure 4–17. Over this relatively brief period, declines in death rates occurred for diseases of the heart (–7%); stroke, influenza, and pneumonia (–6%); chronic respiratory diseases (–4%); and malignant neoplasms (–2%). Concurrent percentage increases in age-adjusted; mortality rates occurred for Alzheimer's disease (+16%); nephritis/nephrosis (+8%); and unintentional injuries, diabetes mellitus, and septicemia (+1%).

Returning to lung cancer, the focus of the Patient Profile, the age-adjusted mortality rate from this disease is the highest for any form of cancer in the United States (Figure 4–18). Lung cancer accounts for more than one fourth of all deaths from malignant neoplasms in the United States. Between 1975 and 1990 the age-adjusted mortality rate from lung cancer increased steadily in the United States (Figure 4–19). Between 1990 and 1993, lung cancer mortality remained level, with a decline thereafter. Even with the recent declines in mortality, over the period 1975 through 1995 the rate of deaths from this disease increased by almost 40%. Although males account for almost 60% of all deaths from lung cancer, the percentage increase in age-adjusted mortality between 1973 and 1995 was much greater for females (129%) than for males (10%). Among males, the age-adjusted death rates for lung cancer rose from 1975 to 1984, reached a plateau from

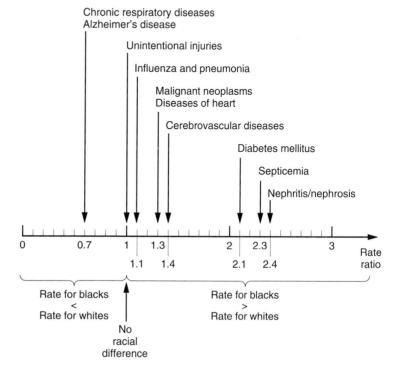

Figure 4–15. Black-to-white ratios of age-adjusted mortality rates for the 10 leading causes of death in the United States, 2001. (Data from National Center for Health Statistics: National Vital Statistics Report. Vol 52, 2003.)

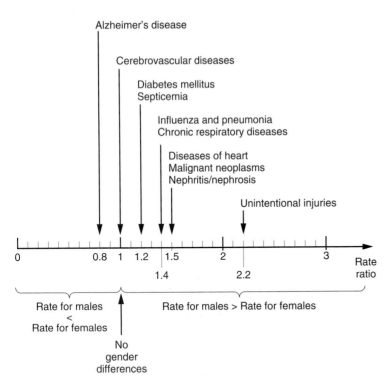

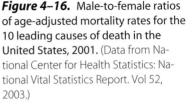

Figure 4–16. Male-to-female ratios of age-adjusted mortality rates for the 10 leading causes of death in the United States, 2001. (Data from National Center for Health Statistics: National Vital Statistics Report. Vol 52, 2003.)

1984 to 1991, and declined after 1991. For females, the age-adjusted death rates climbed persistently from 1975 through 1995 and were relatively level thereafter.

As shown in Figure 4–20, the age-adjusted mortality from lung cancer varies considerably by race and sex in the United States. Among both whites and blacks, there is a considerably greater mortality rate from this disease among males. Black males have a more than 30% higher death rate from lung cancer than white males. In contrast, black females have about a 5% lower age-adjusted mortality rate from lung cancer than do white females.

PREMATURE LOSS OF LIFE

Mortality rate is a convenient and easily understood measure of the burden of a disease on a population. However, by weighing the impact of all deaths equally, mortality rate does not convey the extent to which persons are dying prematurely. In this context, **premature death** means a death that occurs earlier than would have been expected in the absence of the disease. Clearly, causes of death that tend to occur among young people result in a much greater loss of life expectancy than do causes of death that tend to occur among the elderly. For example, in 2001 the life ex-

pectancy at birth was 77 years, compared with only 12 years for persons aged 75 years or older. It may seem paradoxical that persons born in 2001 were expected to live only to age 77, whereas persons born in 1926 were expected to live to age 89 (77 + 12 years). Remember, however, that the older persons had already survived to age 75 years by 2001, and thus had escaped all of the risks of death between birth and 75 years that the newborns still faced.

A death at birth and a death at age 75 contribute equally to mortality rate. It is clear, however, that the death of a newborn results in a loss of 77 years of life expectancy, compared with a loss of only 12 years of life expectancy for the death of a 75 year old. In a sense then, the death of a newborn contributes more than six times the amount of premature loss of life than the death of a 75 year old. This is not to say that the life of a newborn is "more important" than that of a 75 year old. Rather, it simply means that preventing a death has very different consequences for longevity, depending on the age of the person. To the extent that the benefits of health interventions are assessed by their impact on longevity, those that reduce deaths among young persons will appear relatively more important.

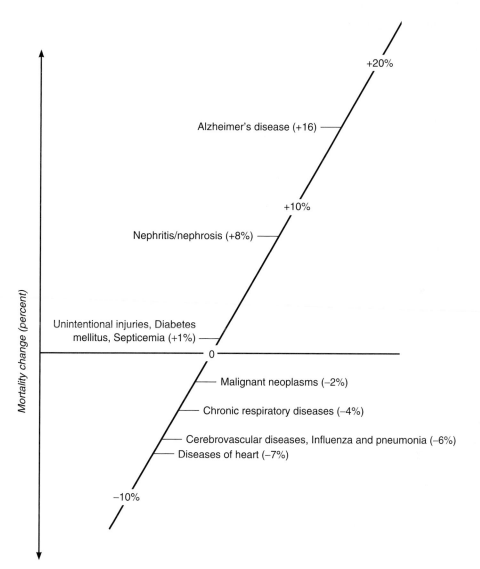

Figure 4–17. Percentage changes in age-adjusted mortality rates for leading causes of death in the United States, 1999–2001. (Data from National Center for Health Statistics: National Vital Statistics Report. Vol 52, 2003.)

One approach to estimating the impact of a cause of death on premature loss of life is the **person-years of life lost,** which is calculated in the following manner:

1. Identify the age at death for each decedent
2. Given the decedent's age, estimate the years of life expectancy that were lost because of the death

3. Sum the years of life expectancy lost over all decedents.

Selected leading contributors to person-years of life lost in the United States are summarized in Figure 4–21. In 2000, there were 2.4 million deaths, which resulted in a total of about 35 million person-years of life lost. Heart disease, which tends to occur among the elderly, accounted for 30% of all deaths, but only

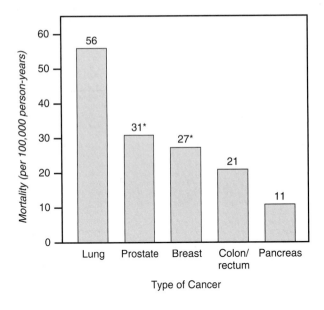

Figure 4–18. Age-adjusted mortality rates for the five leading forms of cancer in the United States, 2000. The rate for breast cancer is confined to women and the rate for prostate cancer is confined to men. (Data from Ries LAG et al: *SEER Cancer Statistics Review, 1975–2000.* National Cancer Institute, 2003.)

22% of the person-years of life lost. In contrast, injuries, which tend to occur among the young, accounted for only 4% of all deaths, but almost 9% of person-years of life lost.

The person-years of life lost from selected leading causes of death from cancer are shown in Figure 4–22. The leading contributor is lung cancer, which accounts for almost one third of all of the person-years of life lost to cancer. Breast cancer and large bowel malignancies

each account for more than 10% of the person-years of life lost to cancer.

Another measure of premature loss of life is the **years of potential life lost before age 75 years** (YPLL < 75), which is calculated in the following manner:

1. The difference between age 75 years and the age of death is calculated for each decedent.
2. These differences are summed over all decedents.

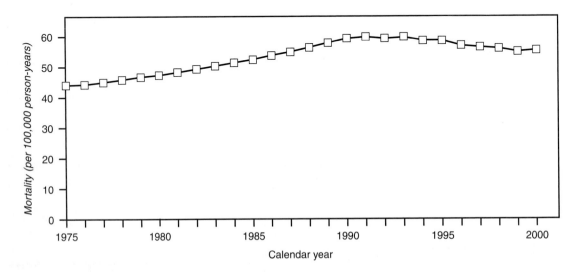

Figure 4–19. Age-adjusted mortality rates for lung cancer by calendar year in the United States, 1975–2000. (Data from Ries LAG et al: *SEER Cancer Statistics Review, 1975–2000.* National Cancer Institute, 2003.)

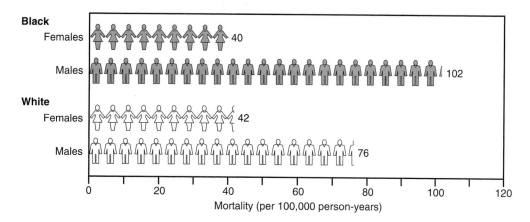

Figure 4–20. Age-adjusted mortality rates for lung cancer by race and sex in the United States, 2000. (Data from Ries LAG et al: *SEER Cancer Statistics Review, 1975–2000.* National Cancer Institute, 2003.)

3. This summation is divided by the number of persons under age 75 years in the source population of persons.

4. The resulting estimate is multiplied by 1000 or 100,000, depending on the units desired.

The overall YPLL < 75 in the United States during 2001 was 7564 per 100,000 person-years. The YPLL < 75 for selected underlying causes of death are shown in

Figure 4–23. The leading contributor to YPLL < 75 was cancer, which accounted for 22% of the total and a similar percentage of all deaths (23%). The proportionate contribution of unintentional injuries was much greater to YPLL < 75 (14%) than to deaths (4%). Similarly, suicide and homicide also accounted for larger proportionate shares of total YPLL < 75 (5% and 4%, respectively) than of all deaths (about 1% each). The larger contributions of unintentional injuries, suicide,

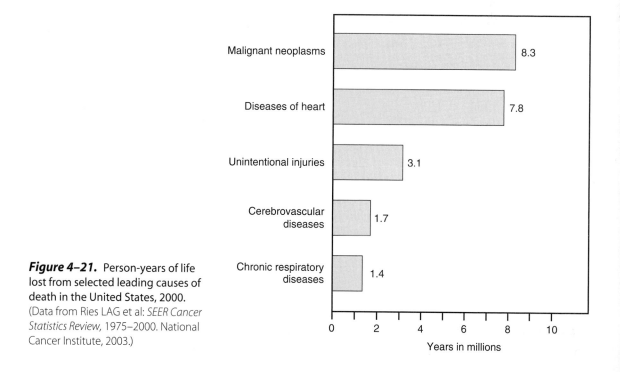

Figure 4–21. Person-years of life lost from selected leading causes of death in the United States, 2000. (Data from Ries LAG et al: *SEER Cancer Statistics Review, 1975–2000.* National Cancer Institute, 2003.)

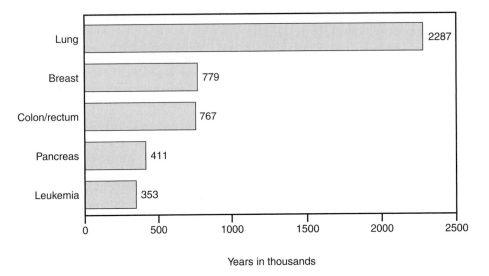

Figure 4–22. Person-years of life lost from selected leading causes of death from cancer in the United States, 2000. (Data from Ries LAG et al: *SEER Cancer Statistics Review,* 1975–2000. National Cancer Institute, 2003.)

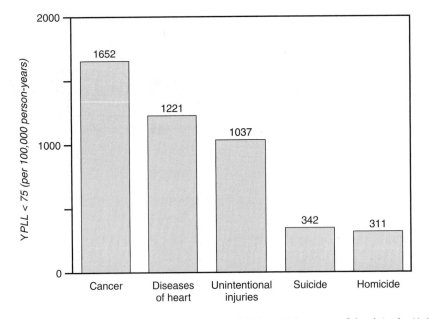

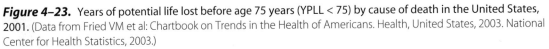

Figure 4–23. Years of potential life lost before age 75 years (YPLL < 75) by cause of death in the United States, 2001. (Data from Fried VM et al: Chartbook on Trends in the Health of Americans. Health, United States, 2003. National Center for Health Statistics, 2003.)

and homicide to YPLL < 75 resulted from the comparatively young ages at which these fatalities tend to occur.

SURVEILLANCE OF RISK FACTORS

In the preceding section, attention was focused on surveillance of medical events, such as new diagnoses or deaths from specific diseases. Surveillance techniques also can be used to characterize patterns of risk factor distribution by person, place, and time. The Behavioral Risk Factor Surveillance System (BRFSS), which is supported by the Centers for Disease Control and Prevention, collects this type of information. The BRFSS was initiated in 1984 to provide statewide data on life-style characteristics that could affect health status. Data are collected by the health departments of most states using a standard protocol. Adult respondents are sampled randomly and are briefly interviewed over the telephone.

The most important risk factor for the development of lung cancer is cigarette smoking. Data collected by the BRFSS can be used to describe smoking patterns within the general population. The overall prevalence of cigarette smoking in the United States in 2002, as determined by the BRFSS, was 23%. As shown in Figure 4–24, the estimated prevalence of cigarette use varied by state of residence, with the highest reported level in Kentucky (33%). Utah had the lowest reported level of any state (13%). The low frequency of cigarette smoking in Utah is attributable to the high proportion of residents who are practicing Mormons, and whose religious beliefs include abstinence from tobacco and alcohol. Given the marked differential in cigarette smoking in Utah and Kentucky, it is not surprising that between 1996 and 2000, the age-adjusted lung cancer mortality rate in Utah (26 cases per 100,000 person-years) was only about one third as high as that in Kentucky (79 cases per 100,000 person-years).

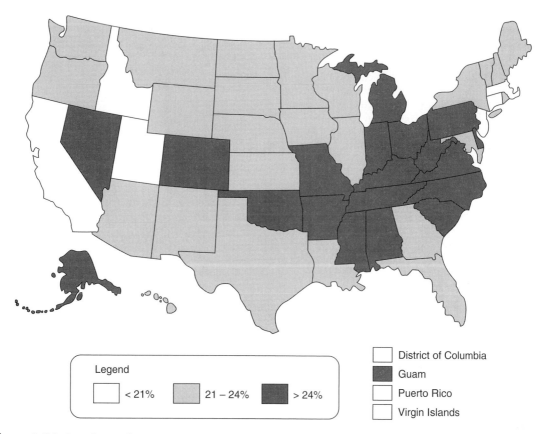

Figure 4–24. Prevalence of cigarette smoking, by state, United States, 2002. (Data from CDC: Behavioral Risk Factor Surveillance System, 2003.)

Another system used to collect information on risk factors and health status in the United States is the National Health Interview Survey (NHIS). The NHIS is a continuous nationwide household survey that uses data collected through personal interviews. In 2001, data were collected on 100,000 persons. The overall prevalence of current cigarette smoking among adults (≥ 25 years of age) in the United States during that year as determined by the NHIS was 22%.

The NHIS prevalence estimates for cigarette smoking are shown by race and sex in Figure 4–25. These data indicate that cigarette use is most common among black males, followed by white males, black females, and finally white females. In general, this pattern is consistent with the race and sex distribution of lung cancer mortality rates depicted in Figure 4–20. Although the prevalence of cigarette smoking has been declining overall, smoking remains the single most preventable cause of death in the United States. Progress toward meeting the national objective of reducing the prevalence of this behavior can be monitored through risk factor surveillance systems such as the BRFSS and the NHIS.

SUMMARY

In this chapter, lung cancer was used as a focus for consideration of the role of **surveillance** in epidemiology. Surveillance was defined as the detection of the occurrence of health-related events or exposures in a target population. Successful surveillance activities require continuity over time, standardized methodology, and timeliness of data collection and dissemination.

Surveillance data can be used in different ways, depending on the type of information collected. Persons newly diagnosed with a disease can yield information on incidence rates, deaths from a disease can be used to describe mortality rates, indices of premature death can be used to assess the impact of a disease on longevity, and prevalence of risk factors can be used to predict future disease occurrence or to assess the status of prevention initiatives.

Surveillance activities in the United States related to lung cancer include collection of data on newly diagnosed persons (through population-based cancer registries), deaths (through death certificates), and prevalence of cigarette smoking (through population-based personal interview surveys).

The utility of **age adjustment** was demonstrated for the control of differences in underlying age structure, when comparing summary rates of lung cancer incidence or mortality across population subgroups.

Key findings from surveillance related to lung cancer in the United States are as follows:

1. Lung cancer has the third highest incidence rate among all forms of cancer, trailing only breast cancer among women and prostate cancer among men. Malignancies of the lung are the leading cause of death from cancer.

2. The incidence of lung cancer increases sharply between 40 and 70 years of age.

3. The overall age-adjusted incidence rate of lung cancer is about 25% higher in blacks than in whites. Contrast of age-adjusted mortality rates reveals a 32% higher rate among blacks.

4. The age-adjusted mortality rate for lung cancer is about 90% of the corresponding incidence rate, indicating a high case fatality. The lung cancer age-adjusted mortality increased by over 40% between 1973 and 1995.

5. Age-adjusted mortality rates for lung cancer vary widely across states, as do the corresponding prevalences of cigarette smoking.

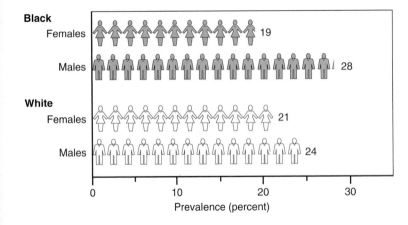

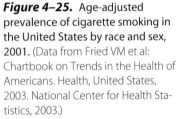

Figure 4–25. Age-adjusted prevalence of cigarette smoking in the United States by race and sex, 2001. (Data from Fried VM et al: Chartbook on Trends in the Health of Americans. Health, United States, 2003. National Center for Health Statistics, 2003.)

6. Lung cancer accounts for about one third of the premature mortality from cancer and about 7% of total premature loss of life.

7. The comparatively high age-adjusted mortality rate for lung cancer among black males is paralleled by a comparatively high prevalence of cigarette smoking.

Several features of the Patient Profile illustrate these descriptive patterns of lung cancer distribution: (1) the patient was 68 years of age at presentation, a comparatively high-risk age for lung cancer occurrence, (2) she was a long-term cigarette smoker, thereby substantially increasing her risk for developing this disease, and (3) the rapidity of her death following diagnosis is consistent with the high case fatality of this disease. With the generally poor treatment results for lung cancer, the greatest promise for controlling the impact of this disease is by preventing people from starting to smoke cigarettes and encouraging current smokers to quit.

1. The lowest overall rapidity of new occurrences.
2. The highest overall incidence rate.
3. The greatest male-to-female ratio of incidence rates among blacks.
4. The smallest male-to-female ratio of incidence rates among whites.
5. The lowest black-to-white ratio of incidence rates among females.
6. The least level of racial disparity in incidence rates.
7. Mortality rate is closest to incidence rate.
8. Mortality rate is furthest from incidence rate.
9. Median survival occurs between 1 and 5 years.
10. Greatest percentage of overall fatalities occur between 1 and 5 years.
11. Highest case fatality.
12. Lowest case fatality.

STUDY QUESTIONS

Questions 1–12: Recent data on the incidence and survival of selected cancers in the United States are presented in Table 4–4. For each numbered question below, select the most appropriate cancer from the following lettered options. Each option can be used once, more than once, or not at all.

    A. Oral cavity
    B. Esophagus
    C. Pancreas
    D. Bladder
    E. Brain

FURTHER READING

Alberg AJ, Samet JM: Epidemiology of lung cancer. Chest 2003;**123**:21S–49S.

REFERENCES

Introduction

Berkelman RL, Buehler JW: Surveillance. In: *Oxford Textbook of Public Health*, 2nd ed., Vol 2. Holland WW, Detels R, Knox G (editors). Oxford University Press, 1991.

Teutsch SM, Churchill RE: *Principles and Practice of Public Health Surveillance*. Oxford University Press, 1994.

Table 4–4. Incidence rates (per 100,000 person-years) by race and sex and overall survival rates at one and five years for selected cancers, United States.[a]

Type of Cancer	Incidence[b]				Survival[c]	
	White Males	White Females	Black Males	Black Females	1 year	5 years
Oral cavity	15	6	21	5	83	59
Esophagus	8	2	11	4	42	12
Pancreas	12	9	18	13	19	4
Bladder	41	10	20	8	91	83
Brain	9	6	5	3	53	34

[a]Data from Ries LAG et al: *SEER Cancer Statistics, 1975–2000*. National Cancer Institute, 2003.
[b]For 2000, age-adjusted to the 2000 population of the United States.
[c]For persons diagnosed in 1995.

Thacker SB, Stroup DF: Future directions for comprehensive public health surveillance and health information systems in the United States. Am J Epidemiol 1994;**140:**383.

Surveillance of New Diagnoses

Ries LAG et al: *SEER Cancer Statistics Review,* 1975–2000. National Cancer Institute, 2003.

Surveillance of Deaths

Messite J, Stellman SD: Accuracy of death certificate completion. JAMA 1996;**275:**794.

Stroup NE et al: Sources of routinely collected data for surveillance. In: *Principles and Practice of Public Health Surveillance.* Teutsch SM, Churchill RE (editors). Oxford University Press, 1994.

Age Adjustment

Dawson B, Trapp RG: *Basic and Clinical Biostatistics,* 4th ed. Appleton & Lange, 2004.

Mortality Patterns

National Center for Health Statistics: National Vital Statistics Report, 1996. Vol 52, 2003.

Premature Loss of Life

National Center for Health Statistics: Health, United States, 1998 with Socioeconomic Status and Health Chartbook, 1998.

Ries LAG et al: *SEER Cancer Statistics Review,* 1975–2000. National Cancer Institute. 2003.

Surveillance of Risk Factors

CDC: Behavioral Risk Factor Surveillance System, 2003.

Fried VM et al: Chartbook on Trends in the Health of Americans. Health, United States, 2003. National Center for Health Statistics, 2003.

e-PIDEMIOLOGY

Patient Profile

http://www.lungcanceronline.org/info/index.html

Introduction

http://www.cdc.gov/epo/dphsi/phs/overview.htm

Surveillance of New Diagnoses

http://www.pitt.edu/~super1/lecture/cdc0271/index.htm
http://seer.cancer.gov/csr/1975_2000/
http://www.pitt.edu/~super1/lecture/lec3011/index.htm

Surveillance of Deaths

http://www.pitt.edu/~super1/lecture/lec3731/index.htm

Age Adjustment

http://www.pitt.edu/~super1/lecture/lec0491/index.htm

Mortality Patterns

http://www.cdc.gov/nchs/data/nvsr/nvsr52/nvsr52_03.pdf
http://www.cdc.gov/nchswww/products/pubs/pubd/hus/hus.htm

Premature Loss of Life

http://www.cdc.gov/nchswww/products/pubs/pubd/hus/hus.htm

Surveillance of Risk Factors

http://www.cdc.gov/brfss
http://www.cdc.gov/nchs/nhis.htm

Disease Outbreaks

5

KEY CONCEPTS

1. A disease outbreak is an epidemic that occurs suddenly and within a relatively confined geographic area.

2. The occurrence of a disease outbreak requires a pathogen in sufficient quantities, a mode of transmission, and a pool of susceptible persons.

3. The two primary modes of transmission of pathogens in disease outbreaks are person-to-person spread and common source of exposure.

4. Criteria for determining whether a disease outbreak should be investigated include, among others: the number and severity of persons affected, uncertainty about cause, and level of public concern.

5. The attack rate is a measure of the number of persons affected by the disease outbreak among persons at risk.

6. Food-borne pathogens can give rise to disease outbreaks through a common source exposure.

7. Emerging infectious disease refers to an infection that has newly appeared in a population, or has existed but is rapidly increasing in incidence or geographic spread.

8. Certain emerging pathogens, such as severe acute respiratory syndrome (SARS)–related coronavirus, West Nile virus, and Ebola virus are responsible for highly publicized recent outbreaks of disease with high case-fatalities.

9. In 2001, the threat of bioterrorism was realized when Bacillus anthracis was mailed to at least five locations, resulting in 22 cases of anthrax and five deaths.

PATIENT PROFILE

A 23-year-old male student presented at 10:30 PM on January 17 at the college infirmary complaining of a sudden onset of abdominal cramping, nausea, and diarrhea. Although the patient was not in severe distress and had no fever or vomiting, he was weak. A number of other students, all with the same symptoms, visited the college infirmary over the next 20 hours. All patients were treated with bed rest and fluid replacement therapy. They recovered fully within 24 hours of the onset of illness.

INTRODUCTION

The concept of an epidemic as a dramatic rise in the occurrence of a disease was introduced in Chapter 3. When an epidemic occurs suddenly and in a relatively limited geographic area, it is described as a **disease outbreak.** The emergence of a disease outbreak requires immediate action to determine the origin of the problem, and ultimately to prevent other persons from becoming affected.

In many outbreak situations, distinctive clinical features of the affected individuals may suggest the underlying cause (sometimes termed pathogen). A working hypothesis can lead to prompt identification of the causal agent and implementation of control measures. Ideally, the choice of control strategy is predicated on knowledge of the source of the causal agent and how it is spread.

In other circumstances, however, the clinical features of affected individuals do not suggest a particular pathogen. An urgent response is required, although the investigator does not yet have a specific working hypothesis about the cause. Consequently, the first phase of investigation involves the collection of basic descriptive information to better characterize the illness and its pattern of occurrence. With this background descriptive data in hand, investigators can generate hypotheses and design specific analytical studies to identify the causal factor of the illness.

The development and maintenance of a disease outbreak typically require each of the following three characteristics:

1. The presence of a pathogen in sufficient quantities to affect multiple persons
2. An appropriate mode of transmitting the pathogen to susceptible persons
3. An adequate pool of susceptible persons who are exposed to the pathogen.

These three features are presented schematically in Figure 5–1.

Some outbreaks are self-limited and terminate without any intervention. In other situations, however, the outbreak will continue unless action is taken to prevent

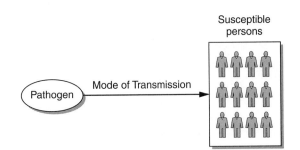

Figure 5–1. Schematic representation of factors required for the development and maintenance of a disease outbreak.

further spread. An effective control strategy should address one or more of the three conditions necessary for an epidemic. Specifically, the following interventions could terminate an outbreak:

1. Removal or elimination of the source of the pathogen
2. Blockage of the transmission process
3. Elimination of susceptibility (eg, through vaccination or medication).

Epidemiologists often distinguish between two primary modes of transmission in acute outbreaks of disease: (1) person-to-person spread and (2) common-source exposure.

As the name implies, person-to-person spread occurs when the causal agent is transmitted from one individual to another. As described in Chapter 3, tuberculosis is propagated in this manner, with the pathogen conveyed from an infectious person to a susceptible individual via airborne particles. The investigation of an outbreak of tuberculosis is likely to reveal an initial (or index) case, and a number of subsequent cases that develop among the close contacts of the infectious person. An effective control strategy would involve isolation of the index case and treatment of the index case with antibiotics until the individual involved is no longer infectious, and antibiotic therapy for infected close contacts.

A common-source exposure occurs when the causal agent is transmitted to affected individuals by some shared feature of the environment. For example, contaminated food can be the source of pathogenic bacteria for persons who ingest the food. Appropriate control measures for this type of outbreak would involve removal of the contaminated food and review of food preparation practices to prevent future outbreaks. Common-source outbreaks are not limited to infectious pathogens. For example, chemical contamination of shared food, air, or water can result in an outbreak of disease.

Outbreaks of disease are fairly common, and not all episodes can be investigated. In deciding whether an investigation is warranted, it is useful to consider the following factors:

1. Apparent number of persons affected
2. Presence of unusual or severe clinical symptoms
3. Lack of an obvious explanation for disease occurrence
4. Perceived need to implement control measures
5. Level of public concern
6. Potential for contributing to medical knowledge.

The situation depicted in the Patient Profile did not involve a life-threatening condition, and the symptoms were rather typical of an acute gastrointestinal illness. On the basis of these criteria alone, an investigation of this outbreak would not be justified. On the other hand, a relatively large number of individuals were affected, the cause was uncertain, and members of this college community were concerned about further spread of the epidemic. For these reasons, an investigation of the outbreak was undertaken.

THE EPIDEMIC

This epidemic of apparent gastroenteritis occurred on the campus of a liberal arts college in the northeastern United States. The temporal association of cases led to the working hypothesis that the cause of this epidemic was a microbial pathogen from a common source. It was suspected that there was one vehicle for transmission of the disease agent, and as the epidemic quickly reached a temporal peak, that the vehicle was quickly exhausted or removed. The epidemic was investigated by public health authorities.

THE INVESTIGATION

Existing information was gathered quickly, first at the infirmary and then at the college administration office. The index case presented to the infirmary at 10:30 PM on January 17, and by 8 PM on January 18, 47 affected students were examined. A quantitative measure of the extent of an outbreak is the **attack rate** (*AR*). The *AR* is calculated using the following equation:

$$\text{Attack rate } (\textbf{\textit{AR}}) = \frac{\text{Number of new cases}}{\text{Persons at risk}} \times 100$$

Note that the *AR* is a measure of risk, as defined in Chapter 2. Accordingly, a period of time must be specified in the estimation of an *AR*.

Knowledge that the college enrollment was 1164 allows the *AR* for the outbreak of the gastrointestinal disease to be calculated. The *AR* for the period from 10:30 PM January 17 to 8:00 PM January 18 was

$$\text{Attack rate}_{\text{(all students)}} = \frac{47}{1164} \times 100 = 4.0\%$$

It was readily apparent, however, that the population at risk could be defined more narrowly because all students who reported to the infirmary lived in dormitories on campus, but only about two thirds of all enrolled students lived in those dormitories. In other words, the one third of students who lived outside of dormitories did not appear to be at risk of disease. Because these students were not entered into the numera-

tor of the equation, their inclusion in the denominator makes the calculation potentially misleading. A more precise estimate of the *AR,* based on the 756 students at risk in the dormitories, was

$$\text{Attack rate}_{\text{(dorm residents)}} = \frac{47}{756} \times 100 = 6.2\%$$

By defining the population at risk more precisely, the estimated *AR* increased by more than 50%.

Because the patients' dormitories were recorded on infirmary records, the *AR*s could be calculated by dormitory and by gender (dormitories were separated by gender). These data are presented in Table 5–1. The striking difference in the *AR*s clearly suggested that the residents of two dormitories (1 and 12) were at greater risk than residents of the other 12 dormitories. A combined *AR* for the two dormitories at greater risk can be contrasted with the other 12 as follows:

$$\text{Attack rate}_{\text{(dorms 1, 12)}} = \frac{(19+13)}{(80+62)} \times 100 = 22.5\%$$

The *AR* for the remaining 12 dormitories was

$$\text{Attack rate}_{\text{(remaining dorms)}} = \frac{(47-32)}{(756-142)} \times 100$$
$$= \frac{15}{614} \times 100 = 2.4\%$$

Table 5–1. The dormitory of residence of the 47 known cases and the attack rate, as well as the population and sex of the occupants of each dormitory.

Dormitory	Sex	Population at Risk	Number of Cases	Attack Rate (*AR* %)
1	F	80	19	23.8
2	F	62	2	3.2
3	F	89	0	0
4	F	61	1	1.6
5	F	53	5	9.4
6	M	35	0	0
7	M	63	0	0
8	F	103	4	3.9
9	M	35	1	2.9
10	M	37	0	0
11	F	34	1	2.9
12	M	62	13	21.0
13	M	32	1	3.1
14	M	10	0	0
Total	—	756	47	6.2

A ratio of these attack rates may be calculated as follows:

$$\text{Risk ratio} = \frac{AR_{(\text{dorms 1, 12})}}{AR_{(\text{remaining dorms})}} = \frac{22.5\%}{2.4\%} = 9.4$$

This risk ratio means that the AR in dormitories 1 and 12 was 9.4 times greater than in the remaining 12 dormitories.

A different ratio could be constructed using only the number of cases. Such a ratio would be 32 cases (dormitories 1 and 12) divided by the 15 cases in the remaining 12 dormitories. This ratio is 32/15, or 2.1. It should be clear, however, that this latter ratio is not an appropriate comparison since it does not take into account the differing sizes of the populations at risk in the dormitories. There were only one fourth as many students at risk in dormitories 1 and 12, and so the same number of cases would not be expected to occur in these two dormitories as occurred in the other 12. If the residents of dormitories 1 and 12 experienced the same risk as other dormitory residents, then the expected number of cases in dormitories 1 and 12 would be

$$\text{Expected cases}_{(\text{dorms 1, 12})}$$
$$= \text{Students at risk}_{(\text{dorms 1, 12})} \times AR_{(\text{remaining dorms})}$$
$$= 142 \times \frac{15}{614} = 3.5$$

The frequency data in Table 5–1 can also be used to calculate rates by gender. For males, the AR was

$$AR_{(\text{males})} = \frac{(1+13+1)}{(35+63+35+37+62+32+10)} \times 100$$
$$= \frac{15}{274} \times 100$$
$$= 5.5\%$$

A similar calculation for females yielded an AR of 6.6%. The ratio of attack rates for females to males was 1.2, indicating that there was not much difference in risk of acquiring this disease by gender.

Visits to some of the campus dormitories by the investigators soon revealed that not all students who became ill had visited the infirmary. Thus it became important to obtain additional data regarding the nature and extent of the outbreak, which it was hoped would be less biased by differences in care-seeking behavior. Questionnaires were prepared and distributed by hand to all students living in seven dormitories chosen to provide a representative sample of the student population. The results from this survey are presented in Table 5–2. A different picture of this epidemic emerged from these results. The overall AR could now be calculated as

$$\text{Attack rate} = \frac{110}{304} \times 100 = 36.2\%$$

Note that the denominator for this AR is 304, which was the number of returned questionnaires, and not 411, which was the total number of eligible students. Because nonrespondents could not be classified according to disease status (in the numerator of the AR calculation), their inclusion in the denominator makes the AR calculation invalid. In the initial infirmary data, the

Table 5–2. Responses to the questionnaire survey by dormitory.[a]

Dormitory	Population	Questionnaires Returned		Number of Ill Students
		Number	Percent	
5	53	49	92.5	13
6	35	26	74.3	13
7	63	28	44.4	15
8	103	65	63.1	21
9	35	19	54.3	5
12	62	44	71.0	22
Nurses' residence[b]	60	60	100	17
Unidentified[c]	—	13	—	4
Total	411	304	74.0	110

[a]Dormitories 1–4, 10, 11, 13, and 14 were not surveyed.
[b]Nurses' dormitory was located off campus.
[c]Dormitory of residence was not entered on 13 questionnaires.

*AR*s for dormitories 6 and 12 were 0% and 21%, respectively. From the survey responses, however, these dormitories did not appear to have different *AR*s:

$$AR_{(dorm\ 6)} = \frac{13}{26} \times 100 = 50\%$$

$$AR_{(dorm\ 12)} = \frac{22}{44} \times 100 = 50\%$$

In other words, the infirmary records and the questionnaire data gave two very different perspectives on the distribution of the outbreak by place of residence. The explanation for this discrepancy was not immediately apparent, but could have reflected differences in approaches to data collection. The infirmary data were useful in the initial phase of the investigation because they were readily available. On the other hand, these data could have been influenced by various factors, such as variation in the severity of illness and care-seeking behavior. The student survey tended to avoid these problems.

The true *AR* of gastroenteritis on campus was not known. The best estimate was 36.2%, as determined from the student survey, but this *AR* could have been incorrect as only 74% of the survey questionnaires were returned (see Table 5–2). If the illness experience of the nonrespondents differed appreciably from the three fourths of students who responded, then the estimated *AR* could have been incorrect. It is possible, for example, that students who were not affected by the illness were less motivated to respond to the survey. Under these circumstances, the calculated *AR* of 36.2% would be higher than the true *AR* for all students. The extent to which the estimated and true *AR*s differ reflects **bias,** or lack of validity. Another potential source of bias could have arisen in the selection of the dormitories to be surveyed. To the extent that these dormitories were systematically different from the remaining nonsurveyed dormitories, bias could have been introduced into the estimation of the true *AR*. Furthermore, if students misreported their illness experience, either intentionally or unintentionally, a distorted apparent pattern of the outbreak could have emerged.

The concept of bias will be discussed at length in Chapter 10. Suffice it to say that minimizing the amount of bias in any study is desirable. To reduce the potential for bias in the present context, the amount of missing information must be minimized. Because the investigators could not force students to respond, it would be unrealistic to expect complete participation. Nevertheless, various strategies could be used to increase the response level (eg, the use of reminders and peer support). The pattern of response rates shown in Table 5–2 was clearly nonrandom, with particularly low response levels in dormitories 7, 8, and 9. Focused efforts to increase participation among residents of those dormitories might have helped to increase confidence in the validity of the findings.

Several factors could explain why the *AR*s estimated from infirmary records were low. Some students may have experienced mild illness that did not require medical attention, and others may have sought care elsewhere. Also, it was discovered that dormitories 1 and 12, which initially appeared to have the highest *AR*s, were located adjacent to the infirmary, and therefore access to this facility was more convenient for these residents.

The survey data indicated a much higher *AR* and more widespread nature of the disease than originally suspected; in fact, more than one third of all students appeared to be involved. In addition, the abrupt onset of disease and the clustering of cases in time suggested a common-source exposure. Data collected during the survey indicated that no large gatherings of students, such as parties or sports events, had recently occurred. Attention then was directed at meals, as most students ate at the college cafeteria. Included in the survey were questions concerning the source of meals eaten on January 16 and 17. Information from the survey is summarized in Table 5–3. Data are presented in a format that is typical for food histories. *AR*s are presented for those who ate and those who did not eat each meal. For example, 152 students ate breakfast on January 16, and of these 52 reported that they became ill. Thus the *AR* was $(52/152) \times 100 = 34.2\%$. *AR*s were calculated in a similar manner for all meals on these days.

The relationship between eating a particular meal and developing illness was assessed by contrasting *AR*s in those who ate the meal and those who did not. Not surprisingly, most *AR*s were approximately 36%, with little difference between those who did or did not eat a particular meal. The exception was found for the January 17 lunch meal. A ratio of *AR*s (risk ratio) for eaters and noneaters of this meal was calculated as follows:

$$RR_{(1/17\ lunch)} = \frac{AR_{(1/17\ lunch\ eaters)}}{AR_{(1/17\ lunch\ noneaters)}} = \frac{42.2\%}{5.8\%} = 7.3$$

This risk ratio indicates that those who ate this meal were more than seven times as likely to have become ill as those who did not eat this meal. Similar risk ratios were calculated for the other meals and were close to 1.0. For example, the risk ratio for dinner on January 17 was 37.5/32.6 = 1.2.

Having identified the meal at which the students most probably were exposed to the causal pathogen and knowing each student's time of onset of symptoms, it was possible to calculate the **incubation period,** in this

Table 5–3. Analysis of meal-specific exposure histories of the respondents to the questionnaire.

	Students Who Ate Specific Meal				Students Who Did Not Eat Specific Meal			
	Ill	Well	Total	AR (%)	Ill	Well	Total	AR (%)
January 16								
Breakfast	52	100	152	34.2	51	94	145	35.2
Lunch	89	150	239	37.2	20	44	64	31.3
Dinner	87	150	237	36.7	23	44	67	34.3
January 17								
Breakfast	56	105	161	34.8	42	89	131	32.1
Lunch	106	145	251	42.2	3	49	52	5.8
Dinner	78	130	208	37.5	31	64	95	32.6

case the time between eating the meal and the onset of symptoms, for 101 ill students. The distribution of these incubation periods is shown in Table 5–4 and is presented graphically in Figures 5–2 and 5–3. In Figure 5–2, the number of cases that occurred is shown by time in hours between exposure and onset of illness. In Figure 5–3, the cumulative percentage distribution of cases is presented by incubation period. *The median incubation period is the time by which 50% of the cases have occurred.* The median incubation period in Figure 5–3 is 10 hours. A follow-up survey was directed at obtaining information about the noon meal of January 17. Data from the follow-up study are presented in Table 5–5.

To identify the food(s) responsible for the outbreak, dietary histories were analyzed. The questionnaires provided information about particular foods that 251 students ate at the noon meal on Friday, January 17. If students were uncertain about whether they ate the food in question, they were not included in the analysis of that particular food. As a consequence, the total of those who ate and those who did not eat each specific item did not equal 251 for all items.

The ratios of ARs yielded values greater than 1.0 for certain items, indicating that the risk of illness was greater among students who ate that item than among those who did not eat the item. For other items the val-ues were less than 1.0, indicating that risk of illness was lower among those who ate the item in question. For example, the risk ratio was 0.7 for fish chowder, 1.0 for fruit salad, and 8.0 for lamb stew pie. It was clear from these data that the risk ratio for illness was considerably higher for those who ate lamb stew pie than for those who did not. This information suggested that lamb stew pie was the most likely source of exposure to the pathogen. Further investigation of the preparation of the lamb stew pie indicated that it was prepared the previous day (January 16), refrigerated, and warmed on the morning it was served.

Although no specific laboratory studies were performed, the etiologic agent that caused this outbreak could be inferred from available information. The illness was marked by gastrointestinal symptoms of limited duration, usually without fever or vomiting; the median incubation period was 10 hours; and a meat dish was presumed to be the most likely source of the pathogen. Based on these observations, the etiologic agent probably was *Clostridium perfringens.* When ingested from inadequately cooked foods, particularly stews, meats, or gravies, type A strains of this bacterium produce a toxin that causes gastrointestinal symptoms. The incubation period, which may range from 8 to 22 hours, is typically 10–12 hours. The absence of fever differentiated this particular gastrointestinal illness from shigellosis or salmonellosis, and the absence of vomiting distinguished this illness from food poisoning by staphylococcal bacteria or chemical agents.

Because food poisoning from *C perfringens* does not involve person-to-person transmission, it is not necessary to isolate affected patients. Supportive treatment should include oral administration of fluids and electrolytes, or intravenous therapy in severe cases. Antibiotic treatment is not required. Taking measures to reduce bacterial proliferation in food sources can prevent outbreaks of food poisoning from *C perfringens.* Thorough cooking of meats and stews at an adequate temperature is essential. Dividing stews into small cooking

Table 5–4. Distribution of incubation periods.

Incubation Period (Hours)	Number of Students	Cumulative Number of Students
8	22	22
9	11	33
10	18	51
11	8	59
12	42	101

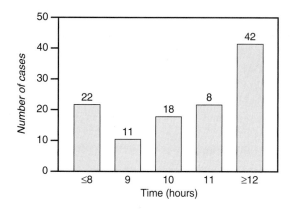

Figure 5–2. Distribution of number of cases by time from eating suspect meal to development of symptoms.

portions helps ensure uniform heating and decreases the need to store and reheat leftovers.

FOOD-BORNE DISEASE

As indicated in the preceding example, large outbreaks of disease can result from a common-source exposure to contaminated food. More than 200 different known diseases of humans are transmitted through food. When such outbreaks are investigated in the United States, the data typically are collected by state or local health agencies and reported to a national surveillance system coordinated by the Centers for Disease Control and Prevention (CDC).

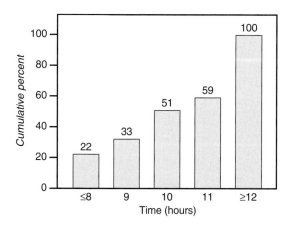

Figure 5–3. Cumulative percentage distribution of cases by time from eating suspect meal to development of symptoms.

As shown in Figure 5–4, the number of persons reported with food-borne disease is a small percentage of the total number of persons exposed to contaminated food within the population. The area of the largest square represents the total number of persons who are exposed to contaminated food. Among those persons, some, but not all, experience illness. Of those with symptoms, only a portion will seek medical attention, and an even smaller fraction will have diagnostic specimens obtained. Some of those specimens will have diagnostic tests performed, of which a proportion will confirm a pathogen, a fraction of which will be reported officially.

Given this chain of selective factors, it is clear that national surveillance data yield an incomplete picture of the true occurrence of food-borne disease. It is estimated that there are about 76 million persons who contract food-borne illnesses in the United States each year. Of these individuals, about 325,000 are hospitalized and 5000 die.

Recognizing the limitations of surveillance data, this information still represents our best window into the population experience. In 2001, 1238 food-borne disease outbreaks were reported to the CDC, involving 25,035 affected persons. Of the total reported outbreaks, only 445 (36%) had a confirmed agent, involving 14,090 affected persons.

As shown in Figure 5–5, bacterial agents accounted for over half of the reported food-borne outbreaks with known causes, followed by viruses, chemicals, parasites, and multiple agents. The mean number of affected persons varied by type of agent (Figure 5–6), with the largest average reported outbreak size for viral and bacterial agents, and the least for chemical agents.

More detailed information on the reported food-borne outbreaks involving bacterial pathogens in the United States during 2001 is shown in Table 5–6. *Salmonella enteritidis* was responsible for the largest numbers of reported outbreaks and affected persons. *Clostridium perfringens,* the pathogen responsible for the outbreak described in the Patient Profile, accounts for the next largest number of reported outbreaks and affected persons, followed by *Staphylococcus aureus, Escherichia coli* serotype O157:H7, *Campylobacter jejuni, Salmonella typhimurium,* and *Shigella sonnei.*

Brief descriptions of key features of the common bacterial food-borne diseases are presented in Table 5–7. Some of these attributes are very characteristic of specific pathogens. For example, *S enteritidis* infection typically results from the consumption of raw or undercooked eggs, *E coli* O157:H7 infection usually arises from the eating of undercooked ground beef, and *C jejuni* infection is most commonly associated with dining on undercooked chicken. The incubation periods from exposure to symptom development range from a few

Table 5–5. Food-specific histories of students who ate lunch at the college cafeteria on January 17.

Food or Beverage	Students Who Ate Specific Food or Beverage				Students Who Did Not Eat Specific Food or Beverage			
	Ill	Well	Total	AR (%)	Ill	Well	Total	AR (%)
Fish chowder	16	36	52	30.8	87	103	190	45.8
Lamb stew pie	95	56	151	62.9	7	82	89	7.9
Tuna noodle casserole	12	57	69	17.4	92	80	172	53.5
Pineapple Jell-O salad	58	54	112	51.8	39	69	108	36.1
Fruit salad	32	39	71	45.1	63	82	145	43.4
Cabbage salad	4	5	9	44.4	95	126	221	43.0
Plain Jell-O with vanilla sauce	19	29	48	39.6	80	102	182	44.0
Plain Jell-O without vanilla sauce	62	77	139	44.6	39	56	95	41.1
Milk	91	127	218	41.7	12	13	25	48.0
Coffee	10	31	41	24.4	89	103	192	46.4
Tea	23	19	42	54.8	78	114	192	40.6

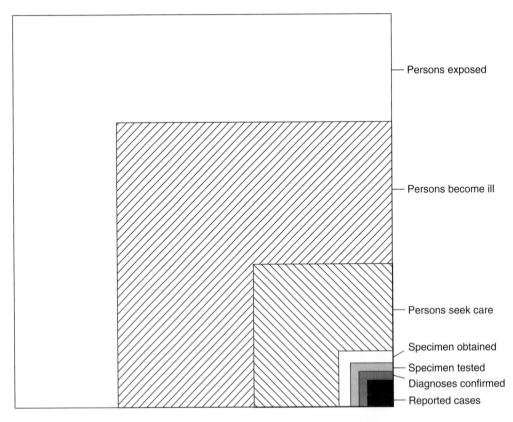

Figure 5–4. Schematic diagram of the amount of food-borne disease officially reported in relation to the larger populations of persons at successive levels of the identification process.

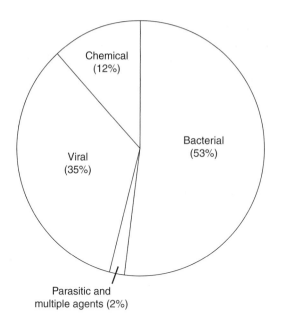

Figure 5–5. Distribution of reported food-borne outbreaks with known causes by type of agent, United States, 2001. (Data from Foodborne Outbreak Response and Surveillance Unit: 2001 Summary Statistics, CDC, 2003.)

hours for *S aureus* food poisoning to several days (eg, *E coli* O157:H7 and *C jejuni* infections). Bloody diarrhea is associated with *E coli* O157:H7 and *Shigella* infections, whereas the diarrhea related to the other illnesses is not bloody. Some of these outbreaks also have a characteristic seasonality to their occurrence. For example, as shown in Figure 5–7, the reported outbreaks of *S enteritidis* were heavily concentrated in the months of April through July.

The national information on food-borne diseases just described was collected through **passive surveillance.** That is to say that those responsible for collecting the information did not go out into the community to obtain it. Rather, they *relied upon existing information that was reported to them voluntarily by laboratories and health care providers.* The advantages of passively collected information are that it is timely and inexpensive to collect. The principal limitations of this type of information are that it may be incomplete and inaccurate.

In contrast, **active surveillance** refers to *a system in which those responsible for collecting the information go into the community (usually defined geographically) to obtain it.* Information can be collected from interviews, examinations, and special testing, as well as routine data sources. Compared with passive surveillance, the advantages of active data gathering are that it tends to be more complete and accurate. On the other hand, information obtained through active surveillance typically takes more time and expense to amass.

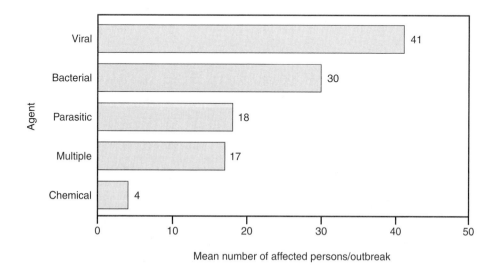

Figure 5–6. Mean numbers of affected persons per reported food-borne outbreak by type of agent, United States, 2001. (Data from Foodborne Outbreak Response and Surveillance Unit: 2001 Summary Statistics, CDC, 2003.)

Table 5–6. Most commonly reported bacterial food-borne pathogens, United States, 2001.[a]

Bacterium	Number of Outbreaks	Total Affected Persons	Mean Affected Persons/Outbreak
Salmonella enteritidis	40	1594	40
Clostridium perfringens	30	1193	40
Staphylococcus aureus	23	646	28
Escherichia coli O157:H7	16	275	17
Campylobacter jejuni	13	247	19
Salmonella typhimurium	12	501	42
Shigella sonnei	9	91	10

[a]Data from Foodborne Outbreak Response and Surveillance Unit: 2001 Summary Statistics, CDC, 2003.

An active surveillance system for food-borne disease was established in the United States in 1996 and is referred to as the Food-borne Diseases Active Surveillance Network (FoodNet). By 2002, this system was expanded to nine states with an aggregate population of over 37 million persons (13% of the national population). Ten specific pathogens (eight bacteria and two parasites) were included in the most recent surveillance data. Over the period 1996 though 2002, declines in incidence were seen for *Campylobacter* (24%), *S typhimurium* (31%), *Listeria* (38%), and *Yersinia* (43%). *Shigella, S enteritidis,* and *E coli* O157:H7 did not have consistent trends over this period of time. As shown in Figure 5–8, infections with *Campylobacter* and *Salmonella* had much greater incidence in early childhood than at older ages.

Overall, about one in six persons with a positive culture were hospitalized, although this varied widely by pathogen. *Listeria,* for example, accounted for less than 1% of all diagnoses, but it had the most serious conse-quences, with 90% of cases hospitalized and a case fatality of 20%.

The epidemiology of food-borne disease has changed over time for a variety of reasons. First, there have been changes in dietary habits within the population. Over the past two decades in the United States, the consumption of whole milk and red meat has declined, whereas the intake of poultry, fresh vegetables, and fruits has increased. The availability of domestic fresh fruits and vegetables has been supplemented by importing these commodities from tropical countries. Food-borne outbreaks of disease caused by a variety of *Salmonella* species have been traced to imported fruits and vegetables, and many other outbreaks probably go undetected because the imports are widely distributed.

Another trend that has affected the epidemiology of food-borne disease is the rising consumption of food in commercial establishments. Pathogens such as Norwalk virus can be spread from an infected food handler to a consumer through contaminated food. Training in hy-

Table 5–7. Key features of the commonly reported bacterial food-borne diseases.

Agent	Typical Vehicle	Incubation Period	Mechanism	Symptoms
Salmonella enteritidis	Undercooked eggs	12–72 hours	Tissue invasion, inflammation	Fever, diarrhea, cramping
Clostridium perfringens	Undercooked meats, gravy	8–22 hours	Enterotoxin	Abdominal pain, cramping, diarrhea
Staphylococcus aureus	Undercooked meats, gravy, eggs	2–6 hours	Preformed toxin	Nausea, vomiting, cramping, diarrhea
Escherichia coli O157:H7	Undercooked ground beef	72–216 hours	Enterotoxin	Bloody diarrhea, cramping, occasional renal failure
Campylobacter jejuni	Undercooked chicken	48–120 hours	Tissue invasion, inflammation	Diarrhea, abdominal pain, fever
Salmonella typhimurium	Undercooked meats, poultry, eggs	12–48 hours	Tissue invasion, inflammation	Diarrhea, fever, abdominal pain
Shigella sonnei	Salads, diary products, poultry	12–48 hours	Tissue invasion, enterotoxin	Fever, diarrhea (often bloody), cramping

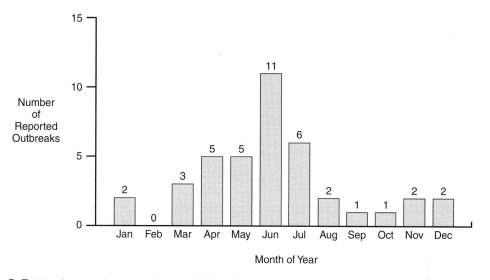

Figure 5–7. Distribution of reported *S enteritidis* food-borne outbreaks by month of the year, United States, 2001. (Data from Foodborne Outbreak Response and Surveillance Unit: 2001 Summary Statistics, CDC, 2003.)

giene and sanitation often is minimal in this industry because the food handlers are low paid, poorly educated, and have a rapid turnover in employment. For many of these individuals, sick leave may not be available, so they may work while ill with infectious diseases.

Yet another factor that has influenced the epidemiology of food-borne disease is the growing presence of large-volume food production facilities. With a trend toward mass-produced foods that are distributed to consumers in remote locations, food-borne diseases may affect large numbers of persons in a variety of locations. Consequently, the classic hallmarks of food-borne disease outbreaks—high attack rates, short incubation periods, and clustering of affected persons in

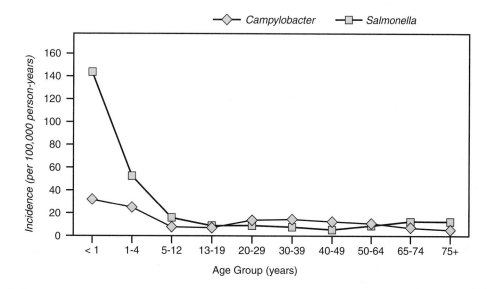

Figure 5–8. Incidence rates of *Campylobacter* and *Salmonella* infections by age group, United States, 2001. (Data from CDC: FoodNet Annual Report, 2001.)

time and space—may not occur, making the outbreak difficult to detect. Once an outbreak is suspected, however, the search for the underlying cause typically follows the basic approach outlined in the preceding section.

EMERGING INFECTIOUS DISEASES

Outbreaks of disease sometimes arise within a population when it is exposed to a new pathogen. The term **emerging infectious disease** is applied to *an infection that has newly appeared in a population or has existed but is rapidly increasing in incidence or geographic range.* Two of the more dramatic examples are the infectious diseases related to human immunodeficiency virus (HIV) and severe acute respiratory syndrome (SARS) coronavirus. There are, however, many other examples, including Lyme disease, hantavirus pulmonary syndrome, hemolytic uremic syndrome, Ebola hemorrhagic fever, and West Nile encephalitis.

Although evolutionary processes can give rise to new infectious agents, most emerging infections probably result from previously existing but obscure pathogens. A number of factors can promote the emergence of these preexisting pathogens:

1. Ecologic changes
2. Shifts in human populations
3. International travel and commerce
4. Changes in technological or industrial practices
5. Microbial adaptation
6. Lapses in the public health system.

Ecologic changes can contribute to emerging infections by placing people into close contact with pathogens not previously encountered by some or all human populations. In addition, ecologic changes can result in conditions that increase the size of a microbial population. The role of ecologic changes in the emergence of an infectious disease is well illustrated by Lyme disease, a systemic illness with characteristic skin rash, joint pain, and in advanced stages, neurologic and cardiac manifestations. This condition is caused by the spirochete *Borrelia burgdorferi,* which was first isolated and identified in 1982. This spirochete is borne by a particular deer tick. The first outbreak of Lyme disease was detected in the Connecticut town after which the disease is named. The emergence of Lyme disease in New England probably occurred as a consequence of reforestation of land that had been previously cleared for agricultural purposes. As the forests returned, the deer population grew, in turn allowing the expansion of the tick population and transmission of the spirochete to humans through tick bites.

Not all ecologic changes that contribute to emerging infections are caused by human activity. Natural changes in ecology can also give rise to emerging infections, as illustrated by the hantavirus pulmonary syndrome (HPS). Hantavirus is named for a river in South Korea in which the virus was originally discovered. It is suspected that outbreaks of disease caused by the Hantaan virus occurred in Asia for many centuries, and that the virus was responsible for the condition known as Korean hemorrhagic fever, which affected thousands of soldiers involved in the Korean War during the 1950s. Until 1993, however, hantavirus was not known to cause disease in the United States or to cause an adult respiratory distress syndrome. Beginning with an influenza-like illness, HPS progresses rapidly to respiratory failure, with a high case fatality.

The first outbreak of HPS was detected in the Four Corners region of the southwestern United States during 1993. A new strain of hantavirus was identified, and the reservoir for this pathogen was shown to be the deer mouse, *Peromyscus maniculatus.* The population of this deer mouse in the Four Corners region rose 10-fold between 1992 and 1993, a result of the end of a 6-year drought. The mouse's predators had decreased during the drought, and with an ample food supply after the drought, the mouse population exploded, expanding the reservoir for the hantavirus and increasing the likelihood of contact with humans.

Emerging infections can be traced to human societal changes, such as migration from high- to low-risk areas. As described in Chapter 3, the resurgence of tuberculosis in the United States during the late 1980s was attributable in part to migrants arriving from high-prevalence countries, such as those in Asia and Latin America.

For centuries, international travel has been a means by which pathogens are introduced into previously unexposed populations. There are many examples, including the importation of yellow fever from Africa to the Americas during the sixteenth and seventeenth centuries. Another historical illustration is the spread of cholera during the nineteenth century from India to the Middle East and then to Europe. However, the opportunities for global spread of infections have multiplied in recent years. First, the volume of international travel has expanded, increasing the number of person-to-person contacts. Second, the speed of international travel by airplane makes it more likely that infected individuals will be contagious on arrival at their destinations. When modes of transit were considerably slower than today, there was greater opportunity for an infection to run its course before an infected traveler reached a destination. Third, as noted in the previous section, the growing globalization of food and other markets increases the number of opportunities to convey pathogens from one country to another.

There is no more impressive example of the role of international travel in the spread of an emerging infectious disease than that of SARS. This disease caused by a newly emerged coronavirus and characterized by fever and atypical pneumonia, arose in November 2002 in Guangdong Province in southern China. A physician in Guangdong became infected while caring for patients and subsequently traveled to Hong Kong. He stayed overnight at a hotel, and the next day he was admitted to a hospital where he subsequently died. While staying at the hotel, however, his infection was spread to 12 other persons.

The chain of transmission of SARS at the hotel in Hong Kong is illustrated in Figure 5–9. The affected physician (person A) spread the disease to ten other persons who stayed on the same floor of the hotel and to two others who were on other floors. After being infected, these contacts then traveled around the world to Viet Nam, Singapore, Canada, the United States, and Ireland, where they then spread the disease to others. Collectively, over 400 cases of SARS in eight countries could be traced directly or indirectly to the affected physician. When the global chain of transmission was broken in July 2003, a total of over 8000 persons were

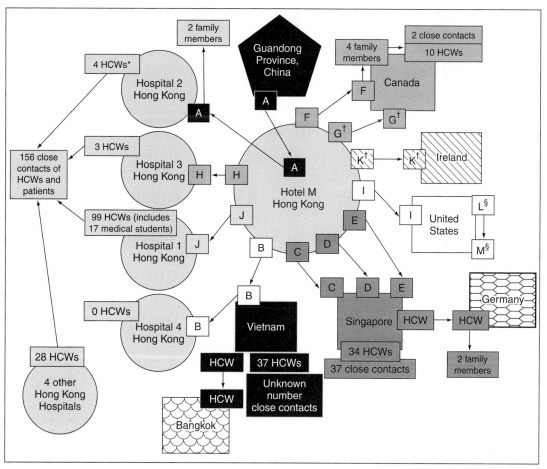

* Health-care workers.
†All guests except G and K stayed on the 9th floor of the hotel. Guest G stayed on the 14th floor, and Guest K stayed on the 11th floor.
§Guest L and M (spouses) were not at Hotel M during the same time as index Guest A but were at the hotel during the same times as Guests G, H, and I, who were ill during this period.

Figure 5–9. Chain of transmission of the severe acute respiratory syndrome (SARS) from an index case (A) to contacts in the same hotel, Hong Kong, 2003. (Adapted from CDC: Update: outbreak of Severe Acute Respiratory Syndrome—worldwide, 2003. MMWR 2003;**52**:241.)

infected and 774 deaths had occurred in 29 countries. With such a rapidly fatal illness, it would have been difficult to spread SARS around the world so quickly in the absence of airplane travel.

The spread of infectious disease across wide geographic areas can occur without person-to-person transmission. For instance, technologic changes now allow food and other products to be produced in mass quantities and to be distributed widely, thereby enhancing the spread of emerging infections. A recent multistate outbreak of *Escherichia coli* O157:H7 infections illustrates this phenomenon. In 1993, a physician in the State of Washington first noted and reported the hemolytic uremic syndrome in a cluster of children who had presented to local emergency rooms with bloody diarrhea. Investigation by state health officials and officials from three other western states identified more than 500 affected persons. Their illnesses were linked to the consumption of hamburgers at a particular chain of fast-food restaurants. Cultures of stool from affected persons revealed *E coli* O157:H7, an organism that lives in the intestines of healthy cattle, can contaminate meat during slaughter, and is a pathogen to humans. This organism was isolated from 11 lots of hamburger, collectively accounting for over a million ground beef patties. The affected hamburger was traced back to five slaughterhouses in the United States and one in Canada, which were the likely sources of the contaminated meat.

Evolutionary changes in microbes also can give rise to emerging infections. Antibiotic resistance is one such mechanism of adaptation. The problem of multidrug-resistant tuberculosis was described in Chapter 3. Other current examples of pathogens for which antibiotic resistance may impede disease control efforts include penicillin-resistant *Streptococcus pneumoniae* and nosocomial enterococci resistant to vancomycin. In addition to antibiotic resistance, evolutionary changes to established pathogens can limit their control in other ways. Many viruses mutate rapidly, yielding new strains of pathogens with surface antigens that differ from those of existing strains; this phenomenon is known as **antigenic drift.** Reinfection with the new viral strain can arise because its antigens are not recognized by the immune system of the host. In rare instances, a new variant of a pathogen may even result in an entirely new clinical syndrome. The manifestations of streptococcal toxic shock syndrome and necrotizing fasciitis linked with group A streptococcal infection may represent this type of phenomenon.

The failure of public health measures also can give rise to emerging infections. For instance, a nonfunctioning water filtration plant in Milwaukee, Wisconsin resulted in contamination of the municipal water supply with *Cryptosporidium* in 1993. This pathogen is a protozoan that infects epithelial cells of the gastrointestinal, biliary, and respiratory tracts of humans and other animals. In humans, the primary manifestations of illness are diarrhea and cramping abdominal pain. Among immunodeficient persons, including those with acquired immune deficiency syndrome (AIDS), infection can follow a fulminant course, even leading to death. The outbreak in Milwaukee produced illness in more than 400,000 individuals, 4400 of whom required hospitalization.

Certain emerging infectious diseases have garnered considerable public attention because of the severity of the respective illnesses. A few examples are presented in Table 5–8, with summaries of recent outbreaks. Ebola virus is a member of the *Filoviridae* family of viruses. It is native to Africa and probably resides within an animal reservoir, with spread to humans by contact with infected animals. Ebola virus then is transmitted between people by contact with contaminated secretions or blood. The resulting infection has an incubation period of 2 to 21 days, with symptoms of fever, headache, muscle and joint pains, diarrhea, rash, and bleeding. The reported case fatalities range from 50% to 90% of affected persons.

West Nile virus is a member of the *Flaviviridae* family of viruses. It was first recognized in the West Nile

Table 5–8. Summary of outbreaks of selected viral emerging diseases.

Agent	Location	Year(s)	Number of Cases	Number of Deaths	Case Fatality (%)
Ebola virus	Uganda	2000–01	425	224	53
	Gabon	2001–02	60	50	83
	Republic of Congo	2003	143	128	90
West Nile virus	United States	2001	66	9	14
		2002	4156	284	7
		2003	8912	211	2
SARS-associated coronavirus	Global	2002–03	8098	774	10

district of Uganda (after which it was named) in 1937. Disease from this agent was not observed in the Western Hemisphere until 1999. The primary amplifying hosts for the virus are birds, with mosquitoes of the species *Culex pipiens* serving as vectors for transmission. Humans and horses are infected incidentally through bites from infected mosquitoes.

In humans, West Nile disease has an incubation period of 2 to 14 days, with symptoms of fever, malaise, headache, rash, and muscle weakness. About 1% of affected persons develop severe neurological disease, which may include inflammation of the brain or spinal cord and a paralysis that is similar to poliomyelitis. The case fatality rate generally is 10% or less. As shown in Figure 5–10, West Nile virus spread across the United

States in successive annual outbreaks between 1999 and 2003. Initially, it began in the northeast, with subsequent expansion to the south and midwest, and eventually to the far west.

SARS is caused by SARS-associated coronavirus, and as indicated earlier, it first appeared in southern China in November 2002. It is thought to have arisen as a genetic mutation of a virus that affects nonhuman animals. It is easily spread by person-to-person transmission via inhalation of the virus. The incubation period is 2 to 7 days, and the symptoms are characterized by fever, dry cough, and respiratory distress that can progress to respiratory failure. The distribution of SARS cases by week of onset in 2002–2003 is shown in Figure 5–11. It can be seen that the initial peak of cases

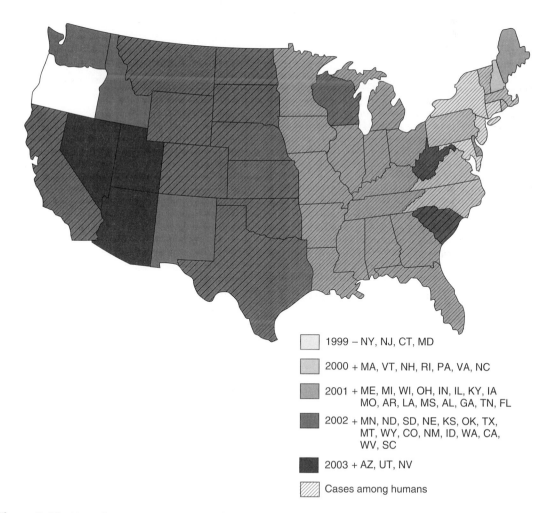

Figure 5–10. Map of states reporting West Nile virus infection in birds, mosquitoes, animals, or humans by year of first detection, United States, 1999–2003. (Data from CDC: West Nile Virus: Statistics, Surveillance and Control, 2003.)

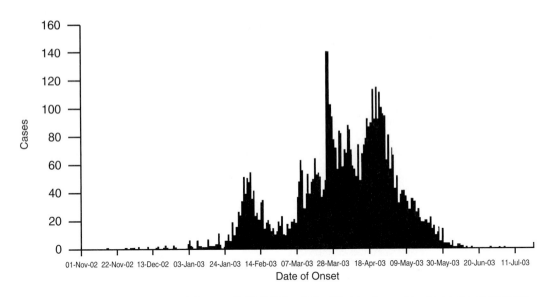

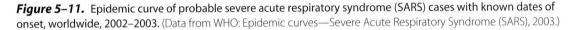

*This graph does not include 2,527 probable cases of SARS (2,521 from Beijing, China), for whom no dates of onset are currently available.

Figure 5–11. Epidemic curve of probable severe acute respiratory syndrome (SARS) cases with known dates of onset, worldwide, 2002–2003. (Data from WHO: Epidemic curves—Severe Acute Respiratory Syndrome (SARS), 2003.)

occurred in early February 2003, followed by successive peaks in March and April related to secondary spread of the infection.

At present, vaccines do not exist for these three cited emerging viral diseases. Therefore prevention of spread represents the first line of defense against these infections. In order for preventive measures to be effective, new cases must be recognized quickly and reported to public health authorities. In the cases of Ebola and SARS, in which transmission occurs by person-to-person contact, appropriate infection control practices are critical. Immediate isolation of infected individuals, along with standard hygienic precautions (eg, hand cleansing), and appropriate barrier protection are indicated. For West Nile virus, protection against mosquito bites is critical. Appropriate measures include draining standing water where mosquitoes breed, covering skin surfaces with clothing and insect repellant, and avoiding outdoor activities from dusk to dawn when mosquitoes tend to feed. Education of the public and health care professionals about these disease control strategies is critical to containing the spread of these emerging diseases.

BIOTERRORISM

All of the outbreaks described in the preceding sections were related to the natural occurrence of disease. Intentional exposure of humans to infectious agents also can

result in disease, although such episodes historically have been uncommon events.

The threat of intentional exposure changed dramatically in 2001 when a series of letters containing *Bacillus anthracis* were mailed to the offices of various news media organizations and elected officials in the United States. **Bioterrorism** *is the use of biological agents by individuals or groups in order to create fear or cause illness or death.* These acts can be motivated by political, religious, social, or other ideological objectives.

The intentional outbreak of anthrax in the United States during 2001 provides some important lessons about bioterrorism. In brief, at least five letters containing spores of *B anthracis* were mailed from Trenton, New Jersey to offices in Florida, New York City, and Washington, DC. Four of the envelopes were recovered, two of which were postmarked on September 18 and the other two were postmarked on October 9. The letters made reference to the terrorist attack on the World Trade Center on September 11, 2001. All of the letters contained spores of *B anthracis* of the Ames strain, although the specific source of the material involved was not determined. The spores were contained within a powder, and it is estimated that the material may have included hundreds of billions of spores.

As shown in Figure 5–12, a total of 22 cases of bioterrorism-related anthrax were identified. Two distinct clusters of cases were observed around the time of

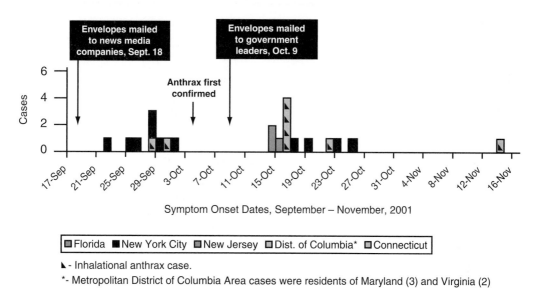

Figure 5–12. Epidemic curve for 22 confirmed and suspected cases of bioterrorism-related anthrax, United States, 2001. (Data from Jernigan DB et al: Investigation of bioterrorism-related anthrax, United States, 2001: epidemiologic findings. Emerg Infect Dis 2003;**8**:1019.)

delivery of the two separate mailings. The first cluster occurred between September 22 and October 1 and predominantly involved cutaneous disease. The second cluster was between October 14 and 25 and primarily involved inhalational anthrax.

Together, the two clusters included 11 cases of confirmed inhalational anthrax and 11 cases of cutaneous anthrax (7 confirmed and 4 suspected). Five of the inhalational anthrax patients died (case fatality = 45%), but none of the cutaneous anthrax patients died (case fatality = 0%). The affected individuals resided in seven different states (New York, 7 cases; New Jersey, 6; Maryland, 3; Florida and Virginia, 2 each; and Connecticut and Pennsylvania, 1 each). Twelve of the affected persons were mail handlers, among whom inhalational anthrax was the predominant form of disease (67%). For the mail handlers with known times of exposure, the incubation period for inhalational anthrax was 4.5 days. The second largest occupational category of exposure was work at a media company (6 cases), where cutaneous anthrax predominated (83%).

This anthrax episode illustrates several of the reasons that biological agents may be attractive to terrorists:

1. **Stability:** The agent was sent through the mail, surviving transport over distance, handling, and time.
2. **Infectivity:** The agent was "weaponized" by using material with a high concentration of spores, uniform particle size, low electrostatic charge, and re-

duction of clumping. Also, the recipients were highly susceptible to contracting the disease.
3. **Low visibility:** The use of the postal service allowed the terrorist to be virtually invisible at the time of release.
4. **Ease of delivery:** The agent was mailed at low cost from a remote location, with a delay in the time of exposure making it difficult, if not impossible, to trace the perpetrator.

The anthrax attacks also demonstrate the impact that a bioterrorist event can have on the public health system. The ability to deliver antibiotics to large numbers of potentially exposed individuals was critical to preventing further infection. A total of 33,000 persons were placed on antibiotics by public health authorities, with 10,000 requested to complete a 60-day course. The number of people who took antibiotics of their own volition is unknown. The United States Army Medical Research Institute of Infectious Diseases performed 19,000 assays for anthrax during the outbreak, and state and local health departments performed countless analyses on suspicious white powders.

Other consequences of the anthrax attacks included disruption of mail delivery to the US Capitol for weeks. The decontamination of the Hart Senate Office building took over 3 months to complete at a cost of over $23 million. The total cost to the nation of the anthrax attacks is beyond reckoning.

The fact that only 22 persons became ill, and of those only 5 died, is a tribute to the rapid and effective responses of the clinicians and public health workers involved. Good communication was essential between the physicians caring for the patients and the officials investigating and attempting to control the outbreak. For example, the morbidity and mortality could have been far worse if the index case was not diagnosed so quickly by an astute clinician and quickly linked by investigators to a potential exposure from a suspicious letter received at work.

Even before the anthrax episode of 2001, the threat of biological terrorism was recognized. In 1999, the United States Congress initiated an effort to enhance capabilities to respond to bioterrorism. The CDC was designated to coordinate planning, and in that context, conducted a public health assessment of potential biological terrorism agents. The following criteria were used in that assessment:

1. **Public health impact**—based upon illness and death
2. **Delivery potential to large populations**—based upon stability of the agent, the ability to mass produce and distribute, and the potential for human-to-human transmission
3. **Public perception**—based upon fear and public disruption
4. **Special preparedness needs**—based on requirements for surveillance, testing, and vaccine or antibiotic stockpiles.

Using these criteria, a set of three priority categories was established for public health preparedness, as summarized below:

A. Agents with the greatest potential for mass casualties and that require broad-based preparedness

B. Agents with some potential for mass casualties, but lower morbidity and mortality and less public perception

C. Agents that do not present a high risk at present but could emerge as future threats.

While all of these agents warrant consideration from the perspective of public health preparedness, only those highest-risk agents (Category A) are presented here. The criteria used in the evaluation and the corresponding weights assigned to each of these agents are summarized in Table 5–9. The agents with the highest potential for causing death are *B anthracis, Y pestis, C botulinum,* and viral hemorrhagic fevers. The ability to disseminate the agent to large populations was deemed greatest for *B anthracis.* The ability to generate public fear was highest for smallpox, anthrax, and viral hemorrhagic fevers. Special preparations are required for all of these agents, with slightly lower ranking for viral hemorrhagic fevers because effective vaccines and antibiotics are not available for these agents.

Clinical features of the Category A agents are presented in Table 5–10. In general, very low levels of exposure are required to produce infection. The incubation periods and durations of illness are particularly short for anthrax, plague, and botulism. The initial symptoms of all of these diseases are nonspecific, and parallel those associated with influenza. The risk of death is relatively high for all of these agents, although somewhat lower for tularemia and variable for the viral hemorrhagic fevers.

Most of the agents on the Category A list are infrequent natural causes of disease in the United States. For those that are part of the regular notifiable disease reporting process, the numbers of cases observed over the 8-year period from 1992 through 1999 are presented in Figure 5–13. The most common naturally occurring

Table 5–9. Criteria and weighting[a] for Category A biological threat agents.[b]

Condition	Agent	Public Health Impact		Dissemination to Large Population	Public Fear	Special Preparation
		Disease	Death			
Smallpox	Variola major	+	++	+	+++	+++
Anthrax	Bacillus anthracis	++	+++	+++	+++	+++
Plague[b]	Yersinia pestis	++	+++	++	++	+++
Botulism	Clostridium botulinum	++	+++	++	++	+++
Tularemia	Francisella tularensis	++	++	++	+	+++
Viral hemorrhagic fevers[c]	Multiple	++	+++	+	+++	++

[a]Agents were ranked from highest threat (+++) to lowest (+).
[b]Modified from Rotz LD et al: Public health assessment of potential biological terrorism agents. Emerg Infect Dis 2002;**8**:225.
[c]Pneumonic plague.
[d]*Filoviruses* (Ebola, Marburg) or *Arenaviruses* (eg, Lassa, Machupo).

Table 5-10. Characteristics of infections caused by Category A biological threat agents.

Disease	Infective Dose	Incubation Period (days)	Initial Symptoms	Duration of Illness (days)	Case-Fatality
Smallpox	1–10 virions	7–17	Fever, malaise, rash	28+	High
Anthrax	8000–15,000 spores	1–6	Fever, malaise, fatigue	3–5	High
Plague	100 organisms	2–4	Fever, chills, cough	2–6	High
Botulism	100 ng toxin	1–3	Fever, weakness, cramping, nausea	2–3	High
Tularemia	10–50 organisms	1–14	Fever, cough	14+	Moderate
Viral hemorrhagic fevers	1–10 particles	2–21	Fever, malaise, muscle, joint pains	7–16	Moderate to High

disease was tularemia, with a mean annual number of new cases exceeding 100. Botulism accounted for the next largest number of reports, with fewer than 50 cases per year on average, followed by plague with about 10 cases per year. During the entire 8-year period, only one case of anthrax was observed and there were no cases of smallpox.

The relative rarity of these conditions under natural circumstances can help raise suspicion of a terrorist-related incident when an outbreak occurs, as was illustrated in the anthrax episode of 2001. Other features of the natural occurrence of these diseases may differ from those of an intentional exposure, thereby providing clues to the origin. For instance, in the United States, tularemia occurs naturally with greatest frequency in

midwestern states. Tularemia in a different location, such as an urban setting on the west coast, would clearly suggest an unnatural pattern of exposure. Similarly, under normal circumstances plague tends to occur almost exclusively in western states, and food-borne botulism is particularly common in Alaska among the native population. Outbreaks of these diseases in other parts of the country might suggest the possibility of bioterrorism.

Seasonality is an important feature of endemic tularemia and plague, both of which predominate during the summer months. Outbreaks of these diseases at other times of the year might signal an intentional exposure. Other demographic patterns within the affected population also might be helpful in distinguishing nat-

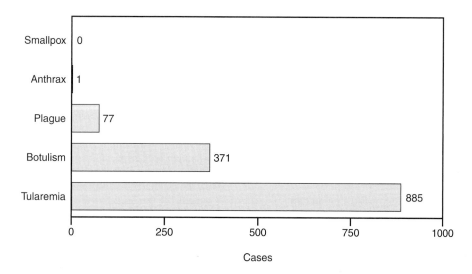

Figure 5-13. Numbers of reported endemic cases of disease caused by Category A bioterrorism agents, United States, 1992–1999. (Data from Chang M et al: Endemic, notifiable bioterrorism-related diseases, United States, 1992–1999. Emerg Infect Dis 2003;**9**:556.)

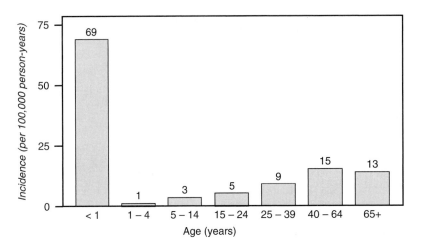

Figure 5–14. Average annual incidence rates of food-borne botulism by age, United States, 1992–1999. (Data from Chang M et al: Endemic, notifiable bioterrorism-related diseases, United States, 1992–1999. Emerg Infect Dis 2003;**9**:556.

urally occurring events from bioterrorist episodes. For example, food-borne botulism occurs with the highest incidence in infants, as illustrated in Figure 5–14. In a food-borne botulism outbreak without a predilection for affecting young children, the possibility of an intentional exposure might be considered.

In considering the future likelihood of bioterrorism, most experts suggest that the issue is not *whether* such episodes will occur, but *when, where, and how* they will happen. There is ample opportunity for access to these deadly agents, given the high levels of past production around the world and the ease with which they can be produced in the future. Moreover, the delivery of these agents can be simple, efficient, inexpensive and difficult to trace, as illustrated by the anthrax attacks of 2001. As long as there are conflicts between people, one must assume that the risk of bioterrorism persists. As with all threats to the health of the public, priority must be given to preventing disease occurrence, detecting it quickly when it occurs, treating those affected, and controlling the spread of disease to other individuals.

SUMMARY

The investigation of **disease outbreaks** (sudden and geographically limited epidemics) is an essential role of epidemiology. The primary goals of an outbreak investigation are the identification of the causal agent (the pathogen) and the prevention of further cases. The propagation of a disease outbreak requires a pathogen, a viable mode of transmission, and an adequate pool of susceptible persons. Elimination of one or more of these three components will terminate the outbreak.

Two basic modes of transmission are **person-to-person** spread and **common-source** exposure. Infectious illnesses can be transmitted by either mode, whereas non-infectious environmental pathogens usually produce disease outbreaks through a common-source transmission.

Not all disease outbreaks warrant investigation. The decision to investigate an outbreak typically is based on the severity of illness, the number of affected persons, uncertainty about the pathogen, and the perceived need to control further spread of the disease. Investigations usually are conducted by local, state, or federal public health officials.

In this chapter, the principles and methods of outbreak investigation are illustrated by the evaluation of an episode of food poisoning on a college campus. This outbreak attracted attention because almost 50 students sought medical care for acute gastrointestinal symptoms in a period of less than 24 hours.

A measure of the risk of developing an illness over a specified period of time is the **attack rate** (*AR*). Based on infirmary records, the *AR* among all students was estimated to be 4%, but among those residing in dormitories, the estimated *AR* was 6%. The *AR* did not differ by gender, but students residing at two dormitories had higher *AR*s than residents of the other 12 dormitories.

To collect more detailed, and perhaps more complete, information than could be obtained from infirmary records, investigators conducted a survey of residents based on a representative sample of dormitories. The survey results indicated a much higher *AR* for dormitory residents (36%) than had been estimated from infirmary records (6%). The possibility of **bias** (systematic error) in both estimates must be considered. Nevertheless, the results of the survey suggested that (1) the outbreak was widespread among dormitory residents and (2) the prior definition of high-risk dormitories based on infirmary records might be inaccurate.

Comparison of *ARs* for persons who ate and did not eat specific foods indicated a strong association between eating a particular food and the risk of gastrointestinal illness. The distribution of times from ingestion to the onset of symptoms (incubation period) revealed a median interval of about 10 hours. A follow-up survey revealed that lamb stew pie was the most suspect common-source exposure for this outbreak.

Although cultures of the foods and specimens from affected individuals were not obtained, the nature of the symptoms, the median incubation period, and the presumed source of exposure implicated *C perfringens* as the pathogen. Knowledge of the factors that contribute to the proliferation and transmission of this bacteria was used to control the outbreak; such knowledge could be used to prevent similar episodes in the future.

At the national level, information on food-borne outbreaks is collected through **passive surveillance,** involving the voluntary submittal of information by physicians and laboratories to the CDC. Although this information likely represents a small portion of the total outbreaks, it provides data quickly and at limited cost. This information suggests that bacterial agents are the most common sources of food-borne infection, followed by viruses. *S enteritidis* was the most commonly reported pathogen, followed by *C perfringens.* Typical sources of infection vary by agent, as do the symptoms.

An **active surveillance** system for selected food-borne diseases also exists in the United States and has been useful for tracking the incidence of these infections. The traditional epidemiology of food-borne outbreaks—high attack rates, short incubation periods, and clustering of affected individuals in time and place—is changing for a number of reasons. The composition of the typical diet has shifted, with decreased consumption of red meat and increased consumption of poultry, fresh fruits, and vegetables. Consequently, exposure to pathogens associated with the latter products is rising. The increased consumption of food from commercial establishments also has resulted in greater opportunities for transmission of infections from food handlers to consumers. Increasing numbers of facilities that produce food in massive quantities, combined with the use of distribution systems that deliver foods to geographically remote markets, tend to diminish any clustering in time and space of persons who are infected with pathogens borne by these foods.

Emerging infections can be defined as infections that are appearing in a population for the first time or that have existed in a population but are rapidly increasing in incidence or geographic range. A number of factors contribute to the emergence of certain infections:

1. Man-made or natural changes in the environment (eg, accounting for Lyme disease and HPS)
2. Demographic shifts in populations (eg, accounting for the spread of HIV)
3. Increased international travel and commerce (eg, the rapid global spread of severe acute respiratory syndrome [SARS])
4. Technologic and industrial changes (eg, accounting for the rise of hemolytic uremic syndrome in the Northwest in 1993)
5. Adaptation of microbes (eg, accounting for antibiotic-resistant organisms)
6. Lapses in the public health system (eg, accounting for infections due to water-borne *Cryptosporidium*).

Recent outbreaks involving several emerging infectious diseases were highlighted. Infection with Ebola virus, which has occurred in multiple African countries, causes a highly fatal hemorrhagic fever. West Nile virus has spread from its origins in Africa to the United States, where it has migrated across the country over the past few years. This seasonal disease is transmitted by infected mosquitoes and occasionally results in serious neurologic consequences. SARS is caused by a coronavirus that originated in China in late 2002 and creates a highly contagious atypical pneumonia that can lead to respiratory failure.

Bioterrorism is the intentional use of biologic agents for causing fear, as well as human illness and death. Although occasional episodes have occurred in the past, the anthrax attacks of 2001 underscored the threat of bioterrorism. This episode involved the mailing of at least five envelopes containing weapons-grade material containing *B anthracis.* A total of 22 persons were infected, resulting in five deaths.

The CDC has identified a series of agents that pose the greatest threats to public health from bioterrorism. These so-called Category A pathogens include those responsible for smallpox, anthrax, plague, botulism, tularemia, and viral hemorrhagic fevers. Patterns of occurrence that differ from those of the naturally occurring infections may give rise to the suspicion of an intentional exposure.

Effective responses to an attack by bioterrorists include the prompt recognition, treatment, and where appropriate, isolation of cases. If possible, the source of the infection should be identified in order to limit any further exposure. Other persons who were potentially exposed should be identified, monitored and treated with appropriate preventive or therapeutic measures.

STUDY QUESTIONS

An outbreak of Ebola hemorrhagic fever occurred in Uganda between August 2000 and January 2001. Contact tracing from three laboratory-confirmed patients identified the chains of transmission for 27 cases (Francesconi P et al: Ebola hemorrhagic fever transmission and risk factors of contacts, Uganda. Emerg Infect Dis 2003;**9**:1430).

Questions 1–3: For each numbered question below, select the single best answer from the lettered options.

1. The distribution of dates of onset was from September 18 through October 28, with the following numbers of cases in successive weeks of the outbreak: 3, 3, 4, 4, 9, 3, 1. The sentinel cases for this outbreak most likely occurred in which week?

    A. 1

    B. 3

    C. 5

    D. 7

    E. Cannot be determined

2. The incidence rate probably was highest in which week?

    A. 1

    B. 3

    C. 5

    D. 7

    E. Cannot be determined

3. A total of 22 patients died. The case-fatality (in %) was:

    A. 2

    B. 22

    C. 66

    D. 81

    E. Cannot be determined

A study was conducted among a total of 83 contacts of patients, 20 of whom became ill and 63 remained well. Information was collected on the types of interactions between patients and their contacts, as shown in Table 5–11.

Questions 4–10: From the information provided in Table 5–11, answer the following questions, selecting the single best answer from the lettered options.

4. The most frequent type of contact was

    A. Sharing meals

    B. Washing clothes

    C. Exposure to body fluids

    D. Sleeping in same hut

    E. Touching body

5. Which type of contact had the lowest attack rate?

    A. Sharing meals

    B. Washing clothes

    C. Exposure to body fluids

    D. Sleeping in same hut

    E. Touching body

6. Which type of contact had the highest attack rate?

    A. Sharing meals

    B. Washing clothes

    C. Exposure to body fluids

    D. Sleeping in same hut

    E. Touching body

7. Which type of contact had the lowest risk ratio?

    A. Sharing meals

    B. Washing clothes

    C. Exposure to body fluids

Table 5–11. Interaction histories for contacts of patients with Ebola hemorrhagic fever.[a]

Interaction with patient	Contact			No Contact		
	Ill	Well	Total	Ill	Well	Total
Sharing meals	6	9	15	14	54	68
Washing clothes	11	24	35	9	39	48
Exposure to body fluids	15	15	30	5	48	53
Sleeping in same hut	11	17	28	9	46	55
Touching body	19	51	70	1	12	13

[a]Data from Francesconi P et al: Ebola hemorrhagic fever transmission and risk factors of contacts, Uganda. Emerg Infect Dis 2003;**9**:1430.

D. *Sleeping in same hut*

E. *Touching body*

8. *Which type of contact had the highest risk ratio?*

A. *Sharing meals*

B. *Washing clothes*

C. *Exposure to body fluids*

D. *Sleeping in same hut*

E. *Touching body*

9. *Which type of contact appears to confer the highest risk of transmission?*

A. *Sharing meals*

B. *Washing clothes*

C. *Exposure to body fluids*

D. *Sleeping in same hut*

E. *Touching body*

10. *Given these study results, which of the following infection control practices would be most effective?*

A. *Handwashing and use of gloves*

B. *Sterilize plates and utensils*

C. *Wear surgical masks*

D. *Daily washing of clothing*

E. *Boiling all drinking water*

FURTHER READING

Oldfield EC: Emerging foodborne pathogens: keeping your patients and your families safe. Rev Gastroenterol Disord 2001;**1:**177.

REFERENCES

Introduction

Reingold AL: Outbreak investigations—A perspective. Emerg Infect Dis 1998;**4:**21.

Food-Borne Disease

CDC: Preliminary FoodNet data on the incidence of foodborne illnesses—selected site, United States, 2002. MMWR 2003;**52:**340.

Mead PS et al: Food-related illness and death in the United States. Emerg Infect Dis 1999;**5:**607.

Woteki CE, Kineman BD: Challenges and approaches to reducing foodborne illness. Ann Rev Nutr 2003;**23:**315.

Emerging Infectious Diseases

CDC: Update: outbreak of Severe Acute Respiratory Syndrome—worldwide, 2003. MMWR 2003;**52:**241.

Huhn GD et al: West Nile virus in the United States: an update on an emerging infectious disease. Am Fam Physician 2003;**68:**653.

Bioterrorism

Chang M et al: Endemic, notifiable bioterrorism-related diseases, United States, 1992–1999. Emerg Infect Dis 2003;**9:**556.

Henderson DA et al: *Bioterrorism: Guidelines for Medical and Public Health Management.* American Medical Association, 2002.

Jernigan DB et al: Investigation of bioterrorism-related anthrax, United States, 2001: epidemiologic findings. Emerg Infect Dis 2002;**8:**1019.

Rotz LD et al: Public health assessment of potential biological terrorism agents. Emerg Infect Dis 2002;**8:**225.

e-PIDEMIOLOGY

Further Reading

http://vm.cfsan.fda.gov/~mow/intro.html

Introduction

http://www.bmj.com/epidem/epid.b.shtml
http://www.pitt.edu/~super1/lecture/lec8401/index.htm

The Investigation

http://www.pitt.edu/~super1/lecture/lec0161/index.htm
http://vm.cfsan.fda.gov/~mow/chap11.html
http://www.pitt.edu/~super1/lecture/lec0311/index.htm
http://www.pitt.edu/~super1/lecture/lec9601/index.htm
http://www.pitt.edu/~super1/lecture/lec6151/index.htm
http://www.pitt.edu/~super1/lecture/lec8401/index.htm
http://www.pitt.edu/~super1/lecture/lec8411/index.htm

Food-Borne Disease

http://vm.cfsan.fda.gov/~mow/app2.html
http://www.cdc.gov/foodborneoutbreaks/guide_fd.htm
http://www.phppo.cdc.gov/phtn/casestudies/graphics/ecolis.pdf
http://www.phppo.cdc.gov/phtn/casestudies/graphics/gass.pdf
http://www.pitt.edu/~super1/lecture/lec9701/index.htm

Emerging Infectious Diseases

http://www.pitt.edu/~super1/lecture/lec1511/index.htm
http://www.pitt.edu/~super1/lecture/lec4281/index.htm
http://www.pitt.edu/~super1/lecture/lec10131/index.htm
http://www.pitt.edu/~super1/lecture/lec10141/index.htm
http://www.pitt.edu/~super1/lecture/lec10361/index.htm

Bioterrorism

http://www.bt.cdc.gov/documents/PPTResponse/agentsglenfinal.pdf
http://www.cdc.gov/ncidod/EID/vol8no10/02-0353.htm
http://www.pitt.edu/~super1/lecture/lec11591/index.htm

Diagnostic Testing

KEY CONCEPTS

1. The sensitivity of a diagnostic test is the likelihood that persons with the disease of interest will have positive test results.

2. The specificity of a diagnostic test is the likelihood that persons who do not have the disease of interest will have negative test results.

3. Positive predictive value measures the likelihood of having the disease of interest among those whose diagnostic test results are positive.

4. Negative predictive value is the likelihood of not having the disease of interest among those whose diagnostic test results are negative.

5. Likelihood ratios can be used to measure the extent to which the likelihood of the disease of interest is changed by the results of a diagnostic test.

6. The area under a receiver operating characteristic (ROC) curve can be used to assess the performance of a diagnostic test.

7. Screening for a particular disease is conducted in order to detect the disease at an earlier stage than would occur through routine methods.

8. An error in the evaluation of a screening test, known as lead time bias, can occur when persons with disease detected by screening appear to live longer simply because of the earlier recognition of their illnesses.

9. An error in the evaluation of a screening test, known as length-biased sampling, can occur when persons with disease detected by screening appear to live longer simply because they have more slowly progressing illnesses.

PATIENT PROFILE

A 54-year-old high school teacher visited her family practitioner for an annual checkup. She reported no illnesses during the preceding year, felt well, and had no complaints. The hot flashes she had experienced a year ago had resolved without treatment. The physician performed a physical examination, comprising breast, pelvic (including a Papanicolaou smear), and rectal examinations; all were unremarkable. The physician recommended that the patient have a mammogram, which was scheduled for 1 week later.

The results of the mammogram were not normal, and the radiologist suggested that a breast biopsy be performed. The family practitioner notified the patient of the abnormal mammogram and referred her to a surgeon, who concurred that physical examination of the breast was normal. Based on the mammographic abnormality, however, the surgeon and the radiologist agreed that fine-needle aspiration (FNA) of the abnormal breast under radiologic guidance was indicated. Evaluation of the FNA specimen by a pathologist

revealed cancer cells, and the patient was sched-
uled for further surgery the following week.

CLINICAL REASONING

The practice of clinical medicine is the artful application of science. A seemingly straightforward chain of decisions by the physicians in the Patient Profile ultimately led to the diagnosis of breast cancer and subsequent treatment. In practice, however, the process of clinical reasoning can be extremely complex. Each decision made by the clinicians in the Patient Profile included the possibility that information was incorrect. Sir William Osler eloquently described the difficulties of clinical decision making in 1921:

> *The problems of disease are more complicated and difficult than any others with which the trained mind has to grapple. . . . Variability is the law of life. As no two faces are the same, so no two bodies are alike, and no two individuals react alike and behave alike under the abnormal conditions which we know as disease. This is the fundamental difficulty in the education of the physician, and one which he (or she) may never grasp. . . . Probability is the guide of life.*

The clinical decision-making process is based on probability. For example, in the Patient Profile the clinician knew that a 54-year-old woman with a normal breast examination had a low probability of having breast cancer (~0.3%). An abnormal screening mammogram increased the likelihood of having breast cancer to perhaps 13%. The radiologist may have predicted a slightly lower or higher probability of breast cancer being present based on the particular mammographic findings. A positive FNA test increased the probability of having breast cancer to about 64%. Again, based on the characteristics of this patient's FNA specimen, such as the appearance of the nucleus or the nuclear/cytoplasmic ratio, the estimate of the

probability of breast cancer being present may be raised or lowered slightly. Furthermore, different pathologists may reach different conclusions when interpreting the same microscopic specimen: some pathologists may state that cancer cells are definitely present, whereas others may report that the specimen is suspicious for the presence of cancer.

Figure 6–1 is a diagrammatic representation of stages in the diagnostic process that ultimately led to a diagnosis of breast cancer in the woman in the Patient Profile. The likelihood of confirming the existence of a particular disease at any point in time is given on the horizontal axis. At the far left, the probability of the presence of disease is 0, and at the far right, the probability is 100%. Based on each new meaningful piece of information, the likelihood that a particular disease is present moves toward 0 or 100%. In the Patient Profile, the probability of breast cancer for the patient increased from near 0 to almost 67% during the diagnostic work-up. *The purpose of a diagnostic test is to move the estimated probability of the presence of a disease toward either end of the probability scale,* thereby providing information that will alter subsequent diagnostic or treatment plans. When the estimated probability of a disease being present is close to 0, the disease can be ruled out; when the estimated probability is close to 100%, the presence of disease is confirmed.

Although diagnostic procedures such as x-rays or biopsies are often considered laboratory tests, almost all approaches to gathering clinical information can be regarded as tests. A patient's responses to questions during history taking or the presence or absence of physical findings influence the clinician's estimation of the probability of a particular disease being present. In the Patient Profile, if the patient's sister and mother had been previously diagnosed with breast cancer, the patient's likelihood of having breast cancer prior to any tests could have been as high as 1%. If a palpable breast lump had been present on physical examination, the likelihood that the patient had cancer could have been estimated to be 20–40% prior to the mammogram. Experienced diagnosticians

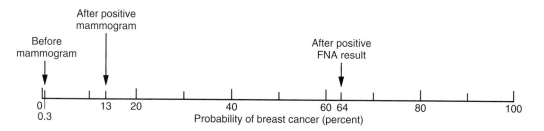

Figure 6–1. Schematic diagram of the estimated probabilities of breast cancer in a 54-year-old woman without a palpable breast mass: before a mammogram, after a positive mammogram, and following a positive FNA test result.

typically form hypotheses early in an encounter with a patient and then direct the history and physical examination in an effort to refine the estimated probabilities of a relatively small number of diseases.

Tests may be performed for many reasons. In the preceding discussion, attention was focused on determining the probability that a disease was present. Tests also may be used to assess the severity of an illness, predict disease outcome, or monitor response to therapy. Regardless of the purpose of a test, it is important to remember that the test is used to estimate the probability of an outcome.

SENSITIVITY AND SPECIFICITY

In a perfect world, medical tests would always be correct. For example, women could undergo a diagnostic test that would unequivocally determine whether breast cancer was present and the test would have no side effects. A positive test result would indicate that cancer was present and a negative test result would indicate that cancer was absent. In reality, however, every test is fallible.

Consider a test that has only positive or negative results. After the test is performed, one of four possible scenarios will occur, as demonstrated in Figure 6–2. For the purposes of this discussion, "true" disease status is determined by the most definitive diagnostic method, referred to as a "gold standard." For example, the gold standard for breast cancer diagnosis might be histopathologic confirmation of cancer in a surgical specimen. In cell *a* of Figure 6–2, the disease of interest is present and the test result is positive, a true-positive result. In cell *d,* the disease is absent and the test result is negative, a true-negative result. In both of these cells, the test result agrees with the actual status of the disease. Cell *b* represents individuals without the disease who have a positive test result. Since these test results incorrectly suggest that the disease is present, they are considered to be false-positives. Individuals in cell *c* have the disease but have negative test results. These results are designated false-negatives because they incorrectly suggest that the disease is absent.

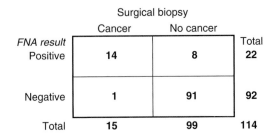

	Surgical biopsy		
	Cancer	No cancer	
FNA result			Total
Positive	14	8	22
Negative	1	91	92
Total	15	99	114

Figure 6–3. Comparison of FNA test results with findings from surgical excisional biopsies in women without palpable breast masses. (Data reproduced, with permission, from Bibbo M et al: Stereotaxic fine needle aspiration cytology of clinically occult malignant and premalignant breast lesions. Acta Cytol 1988;**32**:193.)

Any diagnostic test can be evaluated in this manner. The first step in the evaluation of a test is determining the "true" status of the disease. For the FNA test, we could compare results obtained from FNA with results obtained if every woman subsequently underwent a surgical excisional biopsy procedure (ie, removal and histopathologic examination of the tissue in question). This procedure, the gold standard, is considered to represent the true status of the disease.

Just such a comparison of FNA results with excisional biopsy was made in 114 consecutive women with normal physical examinations and abnormal mammograms; patients received an FNA followed by a surgical excisional biopsy of the same breast (Bibbo et al, 1988). The results of the comparison are given in Figure 6–3.

Sensitivity and **specificity** are terms used to describe the validity of the FNA test relative to the surgical excisional biopsy.

The sensitivity of a test is defined as the percentage of persons with the disease of interest who have positive test results. Sensitivity is calculated as follows:

$$\text{Sensitivity} = \frac{\text{True-positives}}{\text{True-positives}+\text{False-negatives}} \times 100$$

$$= \frac{a}{a+c} \times 100$$

Substituting data from Figure 6–3, the sensitivity of the FNA test is

$$\text{Sensitivity} = \frac{\text{True-positives}}{\text{True-positives}+\text{False-negatives}} \times 100$$

$$= \frac{14}{14+1} \times 100 = 93\%$$

	"Truth"	
	Disease	No disease
Test result		
Positive	*a* True-positive	*b* False-positive
Negative	*c* False-negative	*d* True-negative

Figure 6–2. Format for comparison of the results of a diagnostic test with the "true" status of a disease.

The greater the sensitivity of a test, the more likely the test will detect persons with the disease of interest. For the FNA test, 93% of all the patients with breast cancer had positive test results. Tests with great sensitivity are useful clinically to rule out the presence of a disease. That is, a negative result would virtually exclude the possibility that the patient has the disease of interest.

Specificity of a test is defined as the percentage of persons without the disease of interest who have negative test results. Specificity is calculated as follows:

$$Specificity = \frac{True\text{-}negatives}{True\text{-}negatives + False\text{-}positives} \times 100$$

$$= \frac{d}{d+b} \times 100$$

Substituting data from Figure 6–3, the specificity of the FNA test is

$$Specificity = \frac{True\text{-}negatives}{True\text{-}negatives + False\text{-}positives} \times 100$$

$$= \frac{91}{91+8} \times 100 = 92\%$$

The greater the specificity of a test, the more likely it is that persons without the disease of interest will be excluded from consideration of having the disease. Very specific tests often are used to confirm the presence of a disease. If the test is highly specific, a positive test result would strongly suggest the presence of the disease of interest.

POSITIVE & NEGATIVE PREDICTIVE VALUE

Sensitivity and specificity are descriptors of the accuracy of a test. Two measures concerning the estimation of the probability of the presence or absence of disease are the **positive predictive value** (PV^+) and the **negative predictive value** (PV^-).

The PV^+ is defined as the percentage of persons with positive test results who actually have the disease of interest. The PV^+ therefore allows us to estimate how likely it is that the disease of interest is present if the test is positive. Referring again to Figure 6–2, the PV^+ is calculated as follows:

$$PV^+ = \frac{True\text{-}positives}{True\text{-}positives + False\text{-}positives} \times 100$$

$$= \frac{a}{a+b} \times 100$$

The PV^+ is the percentage of persons with positive test results who have the disease. The calculation of the PV^+ for the FNA test described in Figure 6–3 is

$$PV^+ = \frac{True\text{-}positives}{True\text{-}positives + False\text{-}positives} \times 100$$

$$= \frac{14}{14+8} \times 100 = 64\%$$

The average probability of breast cancer among women in this sample prior to the FNA test was 15 affected women out of 114 total women, or 13%. After the FNA test, the probability of breast cancer for a woman with a positive test result increased to 64%.

The PV^- is defined as the percentage of persons with negative test results who do not have the disease of interest. The general formula for the calculation of PV^- is:

$$PV^- = \frac{True\text{-}negatives}{True\text{-}negatives + False\text{-}negatives} \times 100$$

$$= \frac{d}{d+c} \times 100$$

For the FNA test data in Figure 6–3, the PV^- is

$$PV^- = \frac{True\text{-}negatives}{True\text{-}negatives + False\text{-}negatives} \times 100$$

$$= \frac{91}{91+1} \times 100 = 99\%$$

Before the FNA was performed, the average likelihood of not having breast cancer among women in this sample was 99 unaffected women out of 114 total women, or 87%. After a negative FNA result, the probability of not having breast cancer increased to 99%.

Now that the post-FNA probability of disease has been calculated for either a positive or negative test result, the usefulness of the FNA test for a patient with a nonpalpable breast lesion can be considered. A positive test result increased the probability of breast cancer from 13% to 64%. Whether the probability of breast cancer is 13% or 64%, further work-up is indicated. Both before and after a positive FNA result, the clinician would conclude that the likelihood of breast cancer was too great to forego a test such as a surgical biopsy, which would provide the most definitive diagnosis.

A negative test result, however, would reduce the probability that breast cancer is present to 1% (100% - PV^- = 1%). The decision could be made to defer surgical biopsy and repeat mammographic and physical examinations in several months for women with abnormal mammograms but normal FNAs, accepting a 1 in 100 risk of mistakenly delaying treatment of an existing cancer. A more aggressive approach would be to perform a surgical biopsy on every woman with an abnormal mammogram. The basis of this decision would be that a probability of breast cancer of 1% is too high *not* to proceed with a surgical biopsy. The advantage of performing an FNA on patients with abnormal mammograms is that the vast majority of these women could be spared the increased morbidity and expense associated with a surgical biopsy.

In addition to recognizing that all tests are fallible, it is important to appreciate that the usefulness of a test changes as the clinical situation changes. Specifically, the pretest probability of the presence of disease in an individual, or the prevalence of disease in a population, greatly influences the predictive value. The concept of variable test performance can be illustrated by comparing the use of FNA in women with mammographically detected breast lesions but without palpable breast masses to the use of FNA in women with breast masses found on physical examination (Figure 6–4).

Note that the prevalence of breast cancer in these two groups, which is the same as the average pretest probability of the presence of disease, was higher among the women with palpable masses (38%) than among the women without palpable masses (13%). Although the FNA test had identical specificity and sensitivity in these two clinical situations, the PV^+ of the test was 64% for women without palpable masses, but 88% for women with palpable masses. The PV^+ rose with an increase in the pretest probability of disease. Therefore, it was easier to confirm the presence of breast cancer in a woman with increased baseline likelihood of disease.

The PV^- was 99% when FNA was used for women without palpable masses, but decreased to 96% when used for women with palpable masses. The PV^- decreased as the pretest probability of the presence of disease increased; it becomes easier to exclude a disease as the pretest prevalence of disease decreases. The differences in predictive value between these two populations result only from the difference in the pretest probability of the presence of disease.

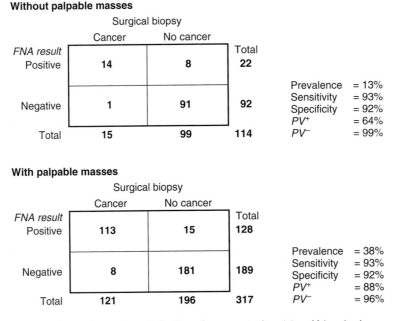

Without palpable masses

Surgical biopsy

FNA result	Cancer	No cancer	Total
Positive	14	8	22
Negative	1	91	92
Total	15	99	114

Prevalence = 13%
Sensitivity = 93%
Specificity = 92%
PV^+ = 64%
PV^- = 99%

With palpable masses

Surgical biopsy

FNA result	Cancer	No cancer	Total
Positive	113	15	128
Negative	8	181	189
Total	121	196	317

Prevalence = 38%
Sensitivity = 93%
Specificity = 92%
PV^+ = 88%
PV^- = 96%

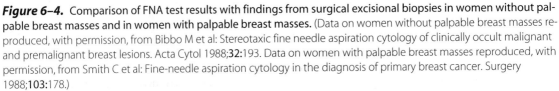

Figure 6–4. Comparison of FNA test results with findings from surgical excisional biopsies in women without palpable breast masses and in women with palpable breast masses. (Data on women without palpable breast masses reproduced, with permission, from Bibbo M et al: Stereotaxic fine needle aspiration cytology of clinically occult malignant and premalignant breast lesions. Acta Cytol 1988;**32**:193. Data on women with palpable breast masses reproduced, with permission, from Smith C et al: Fine-needle aspiration cytology in the diagnosis of primary breast cancer. Surgery 1988;**103**:178.)

Does the difference in predictive values described in Figure 6–4 have clinical implications? As discussed previously, among women with nonpalpable lesions, a negative FNA test result ($PV^- = 99\%$) could reduce the probability of the presence of disease to 1%, and therefore obviate the need for a surgical biopsy. In the group with palpable masses, after a negative FNA test result, the probability of breast cancer still would be 4%, which might warrant further testing, for example, a surgical biopsy. If neither a positive nor a negative test result would change subsequent management, the use of FNA among women with palpable lumps should be questioned.

CUTOFF POINTS

In this chapter the use of FNA was analyzed as a method for detecting breast cancer, assuming that the test's report would indicate either "cancer present" or "cancer absent." The dichotomous classification of clinical findings as positive or negative is commonplace and useful. Examples of dichotomous results are a positive or negative history of pain in a breast, the presence or absence of a palpable breast mass on physical examination, and a normal or abnormal alkaline phosphatase level (a serum marker of bone or liver disease). In reality, however, test results often occur along a continuum. Breast pain, for example, can be negative, intermittent, or continuous. The size of a breast mass is usually measured in centimeters. A serum alkaline phosphatase level may range along a continuous scale. In general, the more extreme the value of a continuous test result, the greater the likelihood that the result reflects a laboratory error or an abnormality in the patient.

The results of the FNA test often are classified as follows:

1. Insufficient material to adequately assess presence or absence of malignant cells
2. Benign (no malignant cells present)
3. Suspicious (atypical cells present but not definitely malignant)
4. Malignant cells present.

Whether each of these four possible results is considered a positive or negative test result influences the assessment of test performance. In both the clinical series of patients with breast abnormalities presented above (see Figure 6–4), the patients with inadequate specimens were considered to have negative test results. Another important decision concerning FNA is whether to classify women with suspicious or atypical results as positive or negative. The ramifications of this decision were explored in an evaluation of the test among women with palpable breast masses. That evaluation of

FNA, shown in Figure 6–5, employs two different assumptions: (1) suspicious FNA results were considered to be positive, and (2) suspicious FNA results were considered to be negative. Note that the sensitivity of FNA decreased and the specificity increased when women with suspicious FNA findings were considered to have negative test results.

This is an example of changing the **cutoff point,** which is the point at which a test result is considered to change from negative to positive. In Figure 6–5, in which suspicious FNA results were treated as positive, the cutoff point was considered to be between normal FNAs and suspicious FNAs. When suspicious FNA results were considered to be negative, a cutoff point between a suspicious FNA result and a malignant FNA result was chosen. *Moving the cutoff point changes the test's sensitivity, specificity, and positive and negative predictive values, and hence the way in which the test is used.*

As illustrated in Figure 6–5, with a cutoff point set between the categories of benign and suspicious, a negative FNA result would reduce the probability of breast cancer, but with the resulting chance of breast cancer at 4%, a biopsy may still be warranted. A positive FNA result would increase the likelihood of cancer to 88%, but still would not absolutely confirm the diagnosis. Alternatively, by setting the cutoff point between the categories of suspicious and malignant (a more stringent requirement for a test result to be considered positive), the PV^+ of the test becomes 100%. This could be useful clinically, because women with a positive FNA result would require no further diagnostic tests prior to definitive treatment (at a minimum, removal of the breast mass). Indeed, many clinicians believe that a positive FNA test result precludes the need for surgical excisional biopsy, thereby saving the patient an additional procedure and reducing the cost of treatment.

LIKELIHOOD RATIOS

Another set of measures is useful in the interpretation of diagnostic tests. These measures are referred to as **likelihood ratios** (*LR*). *An LR is the probability of a particular test result for a person with the disease of interest divided by the probability of that test result for a person without the disease of interest.* For tests such as FNA, which can be classified into dichotomous results, *LR*s are defined for either positive or negative test results. The *likelihood ratio for a positive test result* (*LR⁺*) *is the probability of a positive test result for a person with the disease of interest divided by the probability of a positive test result for a person without the disease.* Mathematically, the *LR⁺* is calculated as

$$LR^+ = \text{Sensitivity} / (1 - \text{Specificity})$$

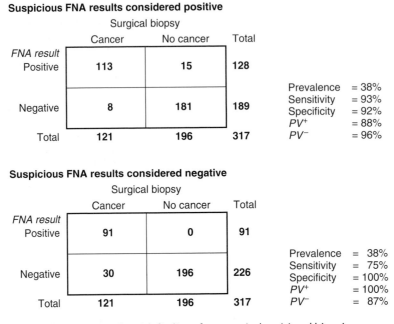

Suspicious FNA results considered positive

	Surgical biopsy		
	Cancer	No cancer	Total
FNA result			
Positive	113	15	128
Negative	8	181	189
Total	121	196	317

Prevalence = 38%
Sensitivity = 93%
Specificity = 92%
PV^+ = 88%
PV^- = 96%

Suspicious FNA results considered negative

	Surgical biopsy		
	Cancer	No cancer	Total
FNA result			
Positive	91	0	91
Negative	30	196	226
Total	121	196	317

Prevalence = 38%
Sensitivity = 75%
Specificity = 100%
PV^+ = 100%
PV^- = 87%

Figure 6–5. Comparison of FNA test results with findings from surgical excisional biopsies among women with palpable breast masses. (Data reproduced, with permission, from Smith C et al: Fine-needle aspiration cytology in the diagnosis of primary breast cancer. Surgery 1988;**103**:178.)

in which sensitivity and specificity are expressed as proportions rather than as percentages. The smallest possible value of the LR^+ occurs when the numerator is minimized (sensitivity = 0), producing an LR^+ of zero. The maximum value of the LR^+ occurs when the denominator is minimized (specificity = 1, so 1 - specificity = 0), resulting in an LR^+ of positive infinity. An LR^+ of one indicates a test with no value in sorting out persons with and without the disease of interest, since the probability of a positive test result is equally likely for affected and unaffected persons. Values of the LR^+ greater than one correspond to situations in which persons affected with the disease of interest are more likely to have a positive test result than unaffected persons. The larger the value of the LR^+, the stronger the association between having a positive test result and having the disease of interest.

The likelihood ratio for a negative test result (LR^-) *is the probability of a negative test result for a person with the disease of interest divided by the probability of a negative test result for a person without the disease.* Mathematically, the LR^- is calculated as

$$LR^- = (1 - \text{Sensitivity}) / \text{Specificity}$$

in which sensitivity and specificity again are expressed as proportions rather than as percentages. The smallest

value of the LR^- occurs when the numerator is minimized (sensitivity = 1, so 1 - sensitivity = 0), resulting in an LR^- of zero. The largest value of the LR^- occurs when the denominator is minimized (specificity = 0), resulting in an LR^- of positive infinity. Just as with the LR^+, an LR^- with a value of one indicates a test with no value in sorting out persons with and without the disease of interest, as the probability of a negative test result is equally likely among persons affected and unaffected with the disease of interest. The smaller the value of the LR^-, the stronger the association between having a negative test result and not having the disease of interest.

The calculation of LR^+ and LR^- can be illustrated by data on the FNA test as applied to women without palpable breast masses (see Figure 6–3). In this example, the LR^+ is

$$LR^+ = \text{Sensitivity} / (1 - \text{Specificity})$$
$$= 0.93 / (1 - 0.92) = 0.93 / 0.08 = 11.63$$

and the LR^- is

$$LR^- = (1 - \text{Sensitivity}) / \text{Specificity}$$
$$= (1 - 0.93) / 0.92 = 0.07 / 0.92 = 0.08$$

One of the desirable properties of the likelihood ratios is that they do not vary as a function of the prevalence of disease. This can be shown with the data presented in Figure 6–4. For women without palpable breast masses, the prevalence of disease is 13%. As just calculated, the LR^+ is 11.63 and the LR^- is 0.08. For women with palpable breast masses, the prevalence of disease is much greater—38%. The LR^+, however, is still given by

$$LR^+ = \text{Sensitivity} / (1 - \text{Specificity})$$
$$= 0.93 / (1 - 0.92) = 0.93 / 0.08 = 11.63$$

and the LR^- is still given by

$$LR^- = (1 - \text{Sensitivity}) / \text{Sepcificity}$$
$$= (1 - 0.93) / 0.92 = 0.07 / 0.92 = 0.08$$

Thus, in contrast to predictive values, the likelihood ratios do not vary according to the prevalence of disease.

As indicated above, the sizes of the two likelihood ratios indicate the strength of the linkage between a test result and the likelihood of disease. A diagnostic test with a large LR^+ value increases the suspicion of disease for patients with positive test results. The larger the size of the LR^+, the better the diagnostic value of the test. Although somewhat arbitrary, an LR^+ value of 10 or greater is often perceived as an indication of a test of high diagnostic value. The FNA test with an LR^+ of 11.63, therefore, satisfies this criterion.

Similar reasoning applies to the LR^- except in the opposite direction. A diagnostic test with a small LR^- value decreases the suspicion of disease for patients with negative test results. The smaller the size of the LR^-, the better the diagnostic value of the test. Again, on somewhat arbitrary grounds, an LR^- value of 0.1 or less is often perceived as an indication of a test with high diagnostic value. The FNA test with an LR^- of 0.08, therefore, satisfies this criterion as well.

LRs can be used to derive a direct measure of the extent to which the likelihood of the presence of disease is changed by the results of a diagnostic test. Begin by considering the likelihood that a person has the disease of interest before the test is performed. This is referred to as the **pretest probability of disease.** For a specific patient, the pretest likelihood of disease is based on the available clinical information about the patient. For example, the patient in the Patient Profile was in her mid-50s, with a normal breast examination and an abnormal mammogram. The treating physicians could estimate the pre-FNA test likelihood of breast cancer for this patient either by referring to published studies of women with similar presenting characteristics or by referring to their own clinical experience. The information presented in Figure 6–3 is based on one published series involving patients with clinical characteristics similar to the patient in the Patient Profile. Among these 114 women, 15 had breast cancer. In other words, the pretest probability of the presence of disease in this sample was $15/114 = 0.13$. Therefore, based on this information the best initial estimate of the pretest probability of the presence of disease for the patient is 0.13.

Next, we convert the pretest probability of disease into **pretest odds of disease.** The pretest odds of disease are defined as the estimate before diagnostic testing of the probability that a patient has the disease of interest divided by the probability that the patient does not have the disease of interest. In the present example, the pretest odds are given by

$$\frac{\text{Pretest}}{\text{odds}} = \frac{\text{Pretest}}{\text{probability}} \Big/ (1 - \text{Pretest probability})$$
$$= 0.13 / (1 - 0.13) = 0.13 / 0.87 = 0.15$$

Next the **posttest odds of disease** are calculated. The posttest odds of disease are defined as the estimate after diagnostic testing of the probability that a patient has the disease of interest divided by the probability that the patient does not have the disease of interest. The posttest odds of disease are calculated as the product of the pretest odds of disease and the LR^+. Therefore in the present example the posttest odds are

$$\text{Posttest odds} = \text{Pretest odds} \times LR^+$$
$$= 0.15 \times 11.63$$
$$= 1.76$$

Finally, the posttest probability of disease is calculated as

$$\frac{\text{Posttest}}{\text{probability}} = \text{Posttest odds} / (1 + \text{Posttest odds})$$
$$= 1.76 / (1 + 1.76)$$
$$= 1.76 / 2.76 = 0.64$$

In other words, as a result of obtaining a positive test result, the estimated probability of the presence of disease has risen from 0.13 to 0.64, an almost fivefold increase in the estimated likelihood of disease.

ROC CURVES

As noted in the section on cutoff points, FNA is an example of a diagnostic test for which the results are classified in discrete categories of possible outcome. These include inadequate specimen for evaluation, benign, suspicious, and malignant. The cutoff point between positive and negative test results can be set to have either a restrictive definition of positive test results (malignant cells present) or a more inclusive definition of positive test results (either suspicious or malignant cells present). The change in cutoff point was shown to affect the sensitivity, specificity, and predictive values of the FNA test, and therefore the clinical value of the information obtained.

Other types of diagnostic tests, such as serum levels of enzymes, produce results along a continuous scale of measurement. In such a situation, there are many more options about where to set the cutoff point between a positive and a negative test result. Along the continuous scale of measurement, different cutoff points will result in differing levels of sensitivity or specificity. As a general rule, as the cutoff point rises, the sensitivity will increase, with a corresponding decrease in the specificity. A convenient summary of this relationship can be shown in a graph referred to as a **receiver operating characteristic (ROC) curve.** This curve derives its name from its first application—measuring the ability of radar operators to distinguish radar signals from noise. For the purposes of diagnostic testing, a graph is constructed with sensitivity (sometimes labeled as the true-positive rate) on the vertical axis, and 1 – specificity (sometimes labeled as the false-positive rate) on the horizontal axis. At each cutoff point, sensitivity and 1 – specificity will be calculated. These results then can be graphed along the full range of cutoff points, producing the ROC curve. A hypothetical example of an ROC curve is shown in Figure 6–6. In this graph, the performance of the diagnostic test is shown by the solid line. The dashed diagonal line represents a reference of a test with no diagnostic value. At every point along this dashed line, the sensitivity is equal to 1 – specificity. Note that when the sensitivity is equal to 1 – specificity, the numerator of the LR^+ is equal to its denominator. That is to say, at every point along this dashed diagonal line the LR^+ is equal to one, and a positive test result is equally likely for persons with and without the disease of interest. A diagnostic test that is clinically useful, therefore, will have an ROC curve that is far from this dashed diagonal line.

Another way of thinking about the ROC curve for a diagnostic test is to consider the vertical axis (sensitivity) the "signal" and the horizontal axis (1 – specificity) the "noise." Toward the left-hand portion of Figure 6–6 there is a steep rise in sensitivity (signal), with a corresponding modest increase in 1 – specificity (noise). In other words, substantial gains can be made in sensitivity, with only modest reductions in specificity—a very favorable trade-off. However, toward the right-hand portion of Figure 6–6 the slope of the ROC

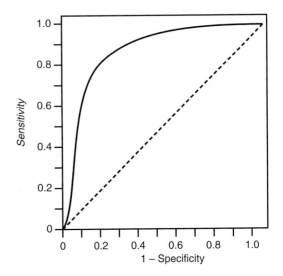

Figure 6–6. A hypothetical example of an ROC curve. The solid line represents the performance of the diagnostic test of interest; the dashed diagonal line serves as a reference of a test with no diagnostic value.

curve is very flat, indicating relatively little improvement in signal for substantial increases in noise—a very unfavorable trade-off.

A summary index of overall test performance can be calculated as the area under the ROC curve. The greater the area, the better the test performance. The highest possible value for the area under an ROC curve is 1, which is equivalent to a perfect test. In contrast, the area under the dashed diagonal line, corresponding to a test that does not distinguish between persons with and without the disease of interest, is 0.5.

Given these extremes, obviously it is desirable for the area under an ROC curve to be closer to 1 than to 0.5. This principle also can be used to compare the relative values of two different diagnostic tests for a particular disease. This point is illustrated in Figure 6–7, in which the performance of two hypothetical diagnostic tests, A and B, are contrasted. The area under the ROC curve is greater for test A than for test B, indicating superior diagnostic value.

SCREENING TESTS

In the Patient Profile, a mammogram was recommended to the patient as a **screening test** for breast cancer. The purpose of a mammogram is to detect breast cancer earlier in the course of the disease than would otherwise occur if the test

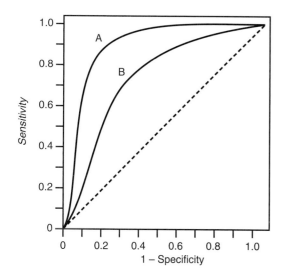

Figure 6–7. ROC curves comparing the performance of two hypothetical diagnostic tests (A and B) for a particular disease. The dashed diagonal line serves as a reference of a test with no diagnostic value. The area under the curve for test A is greater than the area under the curve for test B, indicating superior diagnostic value for test A.

were not performed. Figure 6–8, a schematic representation of the course of disease over time, illustrates the possibility of detecting the presence of disease earlier using a screening test, thereby allowing for more effective treatment and prolonged survival. Inherent in this schematic diagram are two important concepts: (1) a screening test can identify individuals with a disease before the presence of disease is detected by routine diagnosis (eg, when symptoms occur), and (2) treatment at the time of detection by screening, as opposed to the time of routine diagnosis, results in an improved chance of survival.

Breast cancer is a prototypical example of a progressive disease. As with most neoplasms, a breast cancer is

believed to begin as a single malignant cell, which grows rapidly and forms a proliferating tumor. Over time, breast cancer cells can spread through the lymphatic system to the axillary lymph nodes and eventually to other parts of the body via the lymphatic system, the vascular system, or both. Detection of breast cancer earlier in the course of the disease decreases the likelihood that the cancer will spread to lymph nodes and other sites.

It has long been known that length of survival from time of diagnosis of breast cancer is related to the size of the tumor and the extent of spread to adjacent and remote sites. When mammography was first introduced, it was obvious that cancerous lesions in the breast—even those that could not be felt by even the most skilled clinician—could be detected with a mammogram. Researchers postulated that by screening asymptomatic women with mammography, breast cancer could be detected at an earlier stage, and therefore affected women as a group would experience increased survival. This logic seems infallible, but two important biases—**lead-time bias** and **length-biased sampling**—must be considered when evaluating any screening program.

As illustrated in Figure 6–9, *lead-time bias is an increase in survival as measured from detection of disease to death, without lengthening of life.* Note in Figure 6–9 that the person detected with screening and the person detected without screening die at exactly the same time, but the time from diagnosis until death is greater for the screened patient because the cancer was recognized at an earlier point in time. The time from early diagnosis by screening to routine diagnosis is defined as the lead time.

Length-biased sampling occurs when disease detected by a screening program is less aggressive than disease detected without screening. On average, breast cancers detected by a screening program may be less aggressive than cancers that are diagnosed when symptoms appear. This occurs because less aggressive cancers typically grow at a slower pace than more aggressive malignancies, and therefore the length of time

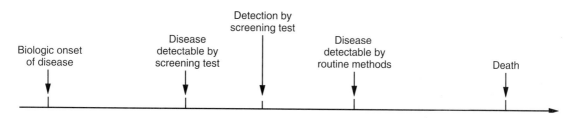

Figure 6–8. The natural history of a disease over time, including the preclinical stage in which a screening test can detect the presence of disease.

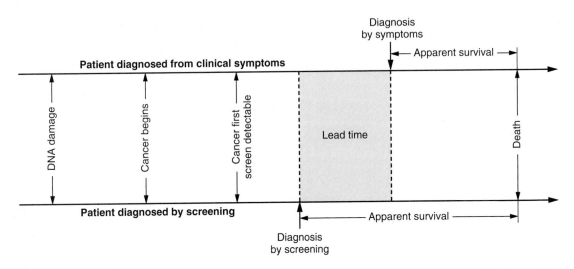

Figure 6–9. A comparison of a patient with a routine clinical diagnosis of disease and a patient with disease detected by screening. The shaded area represents the lead time between detection by screening and detection by routine diagnosis.

that a cancer is detectable by screening is greater for slow-growing neoplasms. If length of survival is measured, individuals with breast cancers detected by screening appear to live longer, in part because the cancers in these patients grow at a slower pace than the cancers in routinely diagnosed patients.

To overcome lead-time bias and length-biased sampling, and therefore to assess the true benefit of a screening program, it is useful to measure disease-specific mortality rates within an entire population. Individuals who are randomly assigned either to a screening program or to no screening are followed to determine whether they die from the disease of interest. Such a study was performed in the 1960s by the Health Insurance Plan (HIP) of New York. In the HIP study, women were randomly assigned to receive routine care

or to undergo a screening program comprised of yearly mammograms and breast examinations.

The results of that study on the usefulness of mammography as a screening tool appear in Figure 6–10. In the evaluation of any screening test, it is important to identify false-negative results. In the HIP study, in the screened group asymptomatic women with a positive result were referred for biopsy. At the time, there was no definitive or gold standard test such as FNA that could be performed on healthy women after a mammogram to determine whether cancers had been missed. An approximation of the number of false-negative screening tests (47 in this example) was derived by determining the number of cancers that arose between yearly screening examinations; these were designated "interval cancers." If a symptomatic cancer occurred

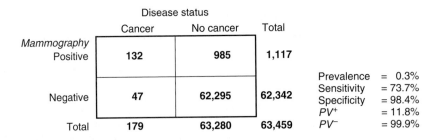

	Disease status		
	Cancer	No cancer	Total
Mammography Positive	132	985	1,117
Negative	47	62,295	62,342
Total	179	63,280	63,459

Prevalence = 0.3%
Sensitivity = 73.7%
Specificity = 98.4%
PV⁺ = 11.8%
PV⁻ = 99.9%

Figure 6–10. Results of mammographic screening in the Health Insurance Plan (HIP) of New York study. (Data reproduced, with permission, from Shapiro S et al: In: *Periodic Screening for Breast Cancer: The Health Insurance Plan Project and Its Sequelae, 1963–1986.* Johns Hopkins, 1988.)

after a screening mammogram but prior to the next mammogram, it was presumed that the first mammogram was falsely negative.

In Figure 6–10, note that mammography had an excellent specificity (98%), yet the false-positive tests still outnumbered the true-positive tests by over 7 to 1 (PV^+ = 12%). This means that among women with positive mammograms who were referred for surgical biopsy to obtain a definitive diagnosis, more than seven biopsies were negative for every one instance of breast cancer that was found. This high false-positive rate is related to the low prevalence of breast cancer at any single point in time in the general population. A low PV^+ is fairly typical for a screening test designed to detect the presence of a disease that affects only a small proportion of persons in the source population at a given point in time. It is important, therefore, to consider the possible anxiety, expense, and morbidity associated with false-positive results when screening initiatives are introduced into the general population.

The purpose of the HIP study was to determine if repeated use of mammography could reduce breast cancer mortality. The use of a concurrent control group allowed investigators to assess the relationship between mammographic screening and mortality from breast cancer. A random assignment of women to either screening or routine care tended to balance the screened and unscreened groups with respect to factors that might affect subsequent breast cancer mortality (see discussion of randomization in Chapter 7). Evaluation of age-specific breast cancer mortality rates, rather than length of survival, diminished the possible distorting effect of lead-time bias. After the initial screening, slow-growing tumors presumably were removed from the screened women, and the effectiveness of subsequent annual mammograms in reducing breast cancer mortality was less likely to reflect length-biased sampling. The HIP researchers concluded that mammography reduced breast cancer mortality among the screened population by 30% when compared with the control group of women who were receiving routine care. The results of this landmark study, combined with findings from investigations of similar design in other countries, established the effectiveness of screening using mammography.

A list of criteria for a successful screening program is presented in Table 6–1. A screening program for breast cancer using mammography can be assessed with these criteria. Breast cancer is an important public health problem in the United States; at some time during her lifetime, one of every nine women will be diagnosed with breast cancer. Early detection allows less extensive surgical treatment and reduces morbidity and mortality from this disease. Since the incidence of breast cancer increases steadily with age, a high-risk population can be defined as any group of women 50 years of age or older. Although screening recommendations for women under age 50 remain controversial, it is widely recommended that women aged 50 or older have a mammogram once a year. Although the test does cause some discomfort, most women find the procedure acceptable. There is an extremely small risk of developing breast cancer associated with the radiation received during mammography. This risk is negligible, however, when compared with an average woman's baseline risk of developing the disease. Finally, mammography is a relatively sensitive and specific test.

SUMMARY

In this chapter, the principles of evaluating and interpreting diagnostic tests were introduced, using the diagnosis of breast cancer as an example. The process of reaching a diagnosis can be represented as a weighing of probabilities. When a particular diagnosis is excluded or ruled out, the probability that the disease is present is close to 0. When a particular diagnosis is confirmed, the probability that the disease is present is close to 100%. The challenge for the clinician is to collect information that will allow successive improvements in

Table 6–1. Criteria for a successful screening program.

Basis for Criteria	Criteria
Effect of morbidity and mortality on population	Morbidity or mortality of the disease must be a sufficient concern to public health.
	A high-risk population must exist.
	Effective early intervention must be known to reduce morbidity or mortality.
Screening test	The screening test should be sensitive and specific.
	The screening test must be acceptable to the target population.
	Minimal risk should be associated with the screening test.
	Diagnostic work-up for a positive test result must have acceptable morbidity given the number of false-positive results.

probability, until the presence of a disease is either confirmed or excluded.

All clinical information is subject to error. Accounting for the various errors that can arise in diagnostic testing allows the physician to select tests and interpret the results of those tests appropriately. One type of error is referred to as a **false-negative** result because the test fails to detect a disease when it is present. A test is said to be **sensitive** when the percentage of false-negative errors is low. A second type of error is referred to as a **false-positive** result because the test indicates that a disease is present when in fact it is not. A test with a low percentage of false-positive results is said to be **specific.**

Sensitivity and specificity are characteristics of a diagnostic test. It is useful to consider two other measures, **positive predictive value** (PV^+) and **negative predictive value** (PV^-), which are used to interpret the results of a diagnostic test. PV^+ is the percentage of persons with a positive test result who actually have the disease of interest. PV^- is the percentage of persons with a negative test result who do not have the disease of interest. Both positive and negative predictive values are heavily influenced by either the pretest probability that the patient has the disease of interest, or by the prevalence of the disease in the particular population that is tested.

In some situations, a test result has only one of two possible outcomes: positive or negative. In other circumstances, however, multiple levels of outcome or even a continuous range of values can occur. For multilevel or continuous outcome test results, a dividing line or **cutoff point** can be chosen to separate findings considered to be positive or negative. The choice of a cutoff value affects the sensitivity and specificity of a test, and consequently the positive and negative predictive values as well. Raising the threshold for considering a result to be positive typically will lead to a gain in specificity (fewer false-positive results) but a loss of sensitivity (more false-negative results or missed cases). On the other hand, lowering the threshold for considering a result to be positive typically will reduce the level of false-negative results (raise sensitivity) and increase the likelihood of false-positive results (lower specificity).

The performance of diagnostic tests also can be assessed by the use of likelihood ratios. The **likelihood ratio for a positive test** (LR^+) is the probability of a positive test result for a person with the disease of interest divided by the probability of a positive test result for a person without the disease of interest. Values of the LR^+ of 10 or greater are consistent with a test that provides considerable diagnostic value. The **likelihood ratio for a negative test result** (LR^-) is the probability of a negative test result for a person with the disease of interest divided by the probability of a negative test result for a person without the disease of interest. Values of the LR^- of 0.1 or smaller are consistent with a test that provides considerable diagnostic value. When combined with a pretest estimate of disease probability, the LR^+ can be used to estimate the posttest probability of disease.

For diagnostic tests that produce results on a continuous scale of measurement, the performance of a test can be represented graphically by a **receiver operating characteristic (ROC) curve.** The area under the ROC curve serves as an overall measure of test performance, with an area of 1 indicating a perfect test and an area of 0.5 indicating a test that is unable to distinguish persons with and without the disease of interest. The respective areas under the ROC curves for two diagnostic tests for a particular disease can be used to identify the test that will provide the greater diagnostic value.

The use of tests to detect the presence of a disease at an earlier time than it would be detected through routine methods is referred to as **screening.** The evaluation of a screening test must take into account two types of distorting effects: **lead-time bias** and **length-biased sampling.** Lead-time bias can occur in a comparison of survival time. Screening detects cases in which the disease occurs earlier in the clinical course; therefore survival time may appear to be longer, even though the time of death is the same as if no screening had occurred. Lead-time bias may be minimized by evaluating mortality rates—rather than duration of survival—as the outcome. Length-biased sampling can occur when the screening test preferentially detects slowly progressive disease that is less likely to cause death or may result in a delayed death. Length-biased sampling can be reduced by repeated screening efforts, as slowly progressive forms of disease can be removed by the initial screening, and thus should not be overrepresented in later screenings.

A successful screening program will focus on a disease with appreciable health impact, for which early diagnosis and effective treatment can reduce the risk for significant morbidity and mortality. In addition, it is essential to define a high-risk population for whom (1) the test is acceptable and (2) the test can be administered with minimal risk. The false-negative, and particularly the false-positive, errors of the screening test should be relatively small, and the expense and morbidity of further evaluation of false-positive results must be acceptable. When evaluated using these criteria, screening using mammography is judged to be a very useful technique, at least for women over age 50.

STUDY QUESTIONS

A population-based evaluation was conducted in Japan of annual screening for lung cancer with low-dose computed tomography. The subjects un-

derwent baseline evaluations in 1996, with repeat annual examinations the next two years. Confirmation of a lung cancer diagnosis was based on cellular pathology. A summary of the results of all three screenings combined is provided in Table 6–2.

Questions 1–13: For each numbered question below, select the most appropriate answer from the lettered options. Each option can be used once, more than once, or not at all.

A. .004
B. .07
C. .09
D. .10
E. .44
F. 3.9
G. 4.3
H. 6.7
I. 9.5
J. 23.9
K. 93.3
L. 96.1
M. 100

1. The prevalence of disease (%)
2. Sensitivity (%)
3. Specificity (%)
4. Positive results out of all tests (%)
5. False-positives out of all persons without cancer (%)
6. False-negatives out of all cancer patients (%)
7. Negative predictive value (%)
8. Positive predictive value (%)
9. Likelihood ratio for a positive test result
10. Likelihood ratio for a negative test result
11. Pretest odds of disease
12. Posttest odds of disease
13. Posttest probability

Table 6–2. Summary of low-dose computed tomography (CT) screening for lung cancer in Japan.[a]

CT Result	Cancer Present	Cancer Absent	Total
Positive	56	532	588
Negative	4	13,194	13,198
Total	60	13,726	13,786

[a]Data from Sone S et al: Results of three-year mass screening programme for lung cancer using mobile low-dose spiral computed tomography scanner. Br J Cancer 2001;**84**:25.

REFERENCES

Clinical Reasoning

Kerlikowske K et al: Evaluation of abnormal mammography results and palpable breast abnormalities. Ann Intern Med 2003;**139**:274.

Osler W: Medical education. In: *Counsels and Ideals,* 2nd ed. Houghton Mifflin, 1921.

Sensitivity and Specificity

Bibbo M et al: Stereotaxic fine needle aspiration cytology of clinically occult malignant and premalignant breast lesions. Acta Cytol 1988;**32**:193.

Smith C et al: Fine-needle aspiration cytology in the diagnosis of primary breast cancer. Surgery 1988;**103**:178.

Positive and Negative Predictive Value

Gallagher EJ: Clinical utility of likelihood ratios. Ann Emerg Med 1998;**31**:391.

Likelihood Ratios

Gallagher EJ: Clinical utility of likelihood ratios. Ann Emerg Med 1998;**31**:391.

Pearl WS: A hierarchical outcomes approach to test assessment. Ann Emerg Med 1999;**33**:77.

ROC Curves

Choi BCK: Slopes of a receiver operating characteristic curve and likelihood ratios for a diagnostic test. Am J Epidemiol 1998;**148**:1127.

Gallagher EJ: Clinical utility of likelihood ratios. Ann Emerg Med 1998;**31**:391.

Screening Tests

MacLean CD: Principles of cancer screening. Med Clin North Am 1996;**80**:1.

FURTHER READING

Grimes DA, Schulz KF: Uses and abuses of screening tests. Lancet 2002;**359**:881.

Knottnerus JA et al: Evaluation of diagnostic procedures. BMJ 2002;**324**:477.

Shapiro S et al: Breast cancers detected—Sensitivity and specificity of screening. In: *Periodic Screening for Breast Cancer: The Health Insurance Plan Project and Its Sequelae,* 1963–1986. Johns Hopkins, 1988.

e-PIDEMIOLOGY

Further Reading

http://www.bmj.com/archive/7107/7107ed.htm
http://bmj.com/epidem/epid.a.html#pgfId=1006649
http://www.pitt.edu/~super1/lecture/lec8751/index.htm

Sensitivity and Specificity

http://www.pitt.edu/~super1/lecture/lec0342/index.htm

Positive and Negative Predictive Value

http://www.bmj.com/archive/7107/7107ed.htm

Likelihood Ratios

http://gim.unmc.edu/dxtests/introduc.htm

ROC Curves

http://www.pitt.edu/~super1/lecture/lec3671/index.htm

Screening Tests

http://www.pitt.edu/~super1/lecture/lec0591/index.htm
http://www.pitt.edu/~super1/lecture/lec0721/index.htm
http://www.pitt.edu/~super1/lecture/lec4021/index.htm

Clinical Trials

KEY CONCEPTS

1. A clinical trial is the direct comparison of two or more treatment modalities in human groups.

2. Evidence-based medicine is the integration of current best evidence with clinical expertise, pathophysiological knowledge, and patient preferences to make health decisions.

3. The practice of evidence-based medicine is encouraged because it may lead to more consistent and objective clinical decisions.

4. A type I error occurs when a study finds a difference in effectiveness between the treatments being compared when in fact no difference exists.

5. A type II error occurs when a study fails to find a difference in treatment effectiveness between the treatments being compared when in fact a difference does exist.

6. Statistical power is the ability of a study to detect a true difference between groups being compared.

7. When treatments are assigned by randomization, probability alone determines assignment, rather than the personal preferences of either physicians or patients.

8. When patients are unaware of their treatment assignment in a clinical trial, it is referred to as a single-blinded study. In a double-blinded study, neither the patients nor the treating physicians know individual treatment assignments.

9. A ratio of either rates or risks can be used to compare the outcomes in the experimental and control groups.

10. Meta-analysis is a statistical integration of the results of several independent studies.

11. A sensitivity analysis can be used to determine whether differences across studies may be explained by characteristics of the various populations studied.

PATIENT PROFILE

An active 13-year-old middle school student complains to her parents of increasing thirst, frequency of urination, and fatigue that has persisted for a week. The following morning, the girl and her parents visit their family pediatrician. While taking the history, the physician notes the above-mentioned symptoms, as well as a decrease in the girl's academic performance over the previous week. She is consuming more than 3 liters of liquid a day and urinating approximately eight times during a 24-hour period; at least one of those times requires her to awaken from sleep. On physical examination, she is found to be afebrile, with a pulse of 80, which is slightly elevated for the patient, a normal *blood pressure lying and sitting, and a normal respiratory rate. The pediatrician notes that the girl's weight has dropped 2 kg since a visit 3 months earlier. The remainder of the physical examination is unremarkable.*

In the office, the pediatrician performs a urinalysis, which reveals a normal microscopic examination; the dipstick examination of the urine is negative for blood, white blood cells, and bilirubin, but is 4+ positive for glucose and 1+ positive for ketones. The pediatrician expresses concern to the parents that the girl may have diabetes mellitus. A complete blood count and blood chemistries are sent to a local laboratory, and the doctor arranges for the patient and her parents to see a pediatric endocrinologist within the hour.

In the endocrinologist's office, the results of the blood tests confirm that the girl has a markedly elevated blood glucose (565 mg/dL) and a slightly elevated blood urea nitrogen (24 mg/dL). Her serum bicarbonate is normal. The endocrinologist discusses the diagnosis of type I diabetes mellitus with the patient and her parents and asks them to speak with a nurse educator in the office to begin to learn about diabetes mellitus, the self-administration of insulin, dietary control, and glucose monitoring.

CLINICAL BACKGROUND

In the United States, the prevalence of diabetes mellitus is estimated to be between 2% and 4% of the population. The two basic types of diabetes mellitus are contrasted in Table 7–1. Type I diabetes is characterized by a markedly decreased or absence of production of in-

sulin, possibly due to an autoimmune destruction of the pancreatic beta cells. Without insulin to facilitate the entry of glucose into cells, plasma glucose levels rise. When the level of plasma glucose exceeds an amount that can be reabsorbed by the kidney (approximately 180 mg/dL), the resulting glucosuria obligates an osmotic diuresis. The concentration of glucose in the urine necessitates the elimination of excessive water in the urine. Excess glucose is also lost in the urine.

The resulting loss of water and calories leads to the cardinal signs of diabetes: increased urination, thirst, and appetite accompanied by weight loss and dehydration. Prior to the discovery of insulin, patients diagnosed with type I diabetes mellitus died of their disease within weeks. After the purification of insulin from animals, subcutaneous injections of insulin allowed patients with type I diabetes mellitus to survive. Today, type I diabetic patients inject synthetically manufactured human insulin. The development of machines that measure plasma glucose levels from small samples of blood and automatically adjust insulin levels has facilitated the management of diabetes. Although the discovery of insulin and the development of glucose monitoring virtually eliminated acute deaths due to insulin deficiency, persons with type I diabetes continued to suffer the long-term complications of the disease—premature atherosclerotic cardiovascular and peripheral vascular disease resulting in heart attacks, stroke, and amputations; retinopathy (ie, damage to the arterial vessels that can lead to blindness); and nephropathy (ie, damage to the microvasculature of the kidney ultimately leading to kidney failure).

During the 1980s, the cause of these long-term complications was debated within the medical community. One group argued that if blood glucose levels were controlled more tightly, a corresponding decrease in the

Table 7–1. Comparison of type I and type II diabetes.

	Type I	**Type II**
Synonym	Insulin-dependent diabetes mellitus (IDDM), juvenile onset	Non-insulin-dependent diabetes mellitus (NIDDM), adult onset
Age of onset	Usually < 30	Usually > 40
Ketosis	Common	Uncommon
Body weight	Nonobese	Obese (50–90% of patients)
Endogenous insulin secretion	Severe deficiency	Moderate deficiency
Insulin resistance	Occasional	Almost always
HLA[a] association	DR3, DR4	None
Identical twins	< 50% concordance	Almost 100% concordance
Islet cell antibodies	Frequent	Absent
Treatment with insulin	Always necessary	Usually not required

[a]HLA, human leukocyte antigen.

long-term complications of diabetes would result. Others postulated that other physiologic abnormalities associated with diabetic disease contribute to the long-term vascular complications. This debate is of critical importance to our patient, a teenager with newly diagnosed diabetes. Conventional twice-a-day injections of regular insulin in combination with a longer acting insulin would control her glucose well enough to avoid complications associated with very high blood glucose levels. However, more intensive therapy with four injections of insulin per day and more frequent monitoring of blood glucose levels would more closely approximate secretion of insulin by the normal pancreas, and theoretically might reduce the risk of long-term vascular complications. At the same time, more intensive therapy could also result in more frequent episodes of low blood glucose levels (hypoglycemia), which, although it is rare, can result in coma. The pediatric endocrinologist might also be concerned that frequent episodes of hypoglycemia would interfere with the normal growth of an adolescent.

Although there are theoretical reasons why a physician would want to maintain normal blood glucose levels in our patient, there are also hazards associated with the intensive therapy described above. To determine the safety and efficacy of new therapies, researchers must conduct a clinical trial. *A randomized, controlled clinical trial is a study design in which one treatment is compared directly with another treatment to determine which of the two treatments would be of greatest benefit.*

INTRODUCTION TO CLINICAL TRIALS

In the Patient Profile, the clinician is faced with a decision concerning treatment: which of two possible regimens to use to control blood glucose levels. Hippocrates' axiom—"First, do no harm"—is a time-honored warning to clinicians contemplating medical intervention. "One must attend in medical practice not primarily to plausible theories," Hippocrates wrote, "but to experience combined with reason." In other words, a treatment plan should be reasonable in theory but should also be tested experientially. More than 2000 years ago, Hippocrates noted that judging the benefits of a treatment should be based on the treatment's effects on patients.

In modern medicine, a randomized, controlled clinical trial of one therapy versus another is the accepted gold standard by which the usefulness of a treatment is determined. To practice modern medicine and select appropriate therapy, it is necessary to understand the design and conduct of clinical trials.

This important method of evaluating treatments utilizes two types of knowledge, both alluded to by Hippocrates: reason and experience. "Reasonable" treatment is treatment suggested by a knowledge of

basic biomedical science. For the clinical situation presented in the Patient Profile, a knowledge of the pathophysiology of diabetes mellitus and the long-term complications of this disease would indicate the need for tight control of blood glucose levels and the avoidance of any possible long-term complications of diabetes. However, as stated by Hippocrates, the clinician cannot base therapeutic decisions on theory alone; the dictates of reason must be submitted to the test of experience.

Clinicians employ two types of experience to assess a treatment regimen—their own personal experience and the written or orally conveyed experience of their colleagues. Written experience may take the form of a report of a single case, a series of cases, or a comparison of one treatment with another.

The direct comparison of two or more treatment modalities in human groups is referred to as a clinical trial. The development of the clinical trial is a product of the application of modern scientific method to clinical medicine. The purpose of the clinical trial is to provide information that will help in the selection of and use of appropriate, timely, and effective treatments.

EVIDENCE-BASED MEDICINE

The integration of current best evidence with clinical expertise, pathophysiological knowledge, and patient preferences to make health care decisions is referred to as **evidence-based medicine.** The practice of evidence-based medicine requires several skills, beginning with the ability to define precisely the question of interest concerning management of disease. The evidence-based practitioner then must be able to locate the relevant information from the medical literature and assess this information critically. Finally, the evidence obtained must be integrated into decisions about management of disease.

The use of evidence-based medicine is encouraged for several reasons:

1. It can provide an efficient framework for accessing and systematically interpreting the medical literature.
2. It can provide an objective basis for selecting a strategy for disease management, thereby enhancing clinical outcomes.
3. It can serve as a rational basis for modifying the practice of disease management by individual clinicians.
4. It can provide a coordinated plan for disease management when care is delivered by a multidisciplinary team.

5. It can identify gaps in current knowledge and thereby suggest prioritized areas for further investigation.

6. It can suggest areas in which flexibility in disease management is justified by a lack of evidence to support a particular approach.

7. It can facilitate assessment of the process of disease management, suggesting opportunities for improved quality and efficiency.

The practice of evidence-based medicine is grounded in several key assumptions. First, it is acknowledged that many aspects of clinical medicine cannot be subjected to formal testing through clinical trials. Therefore a clinician's personal experience is a useful and necessary companion to information gathered from the medical literature. Second, although knowledge of underlying pathophysiology is valuable for the formulation of plans for diagnosis and treatment, such knowledge is not sufficient in itself and can lead to ineffective strategies of disease management. Third, the critical assessment of evidence requires an appreciation of the methods used to design, collect, and analyze clinical studies. Fourth, systematic approaches to the collection and interpretation of routine clinical information facilitate more consistent and objective clinical decisions.

There are a number of barriers to the practice of evidence-based medicine. Many clinicians have limited training in formal assessment of research studies. Even if clinicians have the necessary skills, they may have little time to search and evaluate the literature. Even if time is available, there are many important issues about disease management for which there is a paucity of evidence to appraise.

Considering these obstacles, it may be surprising that evidence-based medicine has progressed so rapidly in recent years. In part, changes in the organization, financing, and delivery of health care have encouraged a greater focus on clinical outcomes and the cost effectiveness of different management strategies. In addition, easier and faster accessibility to the relevant medical literature is possible through automated searches of electronic databases. Also, the Internet has facilitated the rapid and widespread sharing of results from critical appraisals.

Although far from universally adopted, evidence-based medicine offers the promise of improved management of disease. A prerequisite to the practice of evidence-based medicine is the ability to critically assess clinical studies. The following sections focus on the basic elements of a clinical trial. At the conclusion of this chapter, the principles of combining information across clinical trials are discussed.

STATEMENT OF THE RESEARCH QUESTIONS

As in a laboratory experiment, the first step in performing a clinical trial is to formulate the major research question. This question, usually referred to as the hypothesis, is refined to determine important study parameters, for example, the types of interventions to be compared, the nature of the outcomes to be assessed, the number of subjects in each treatment group, and the eligibility requirements for enrollment.

The parameter that is measured that will provide the answer to the most important question of the clinical trial is the primary **end point.** When determining the primary end point, clinical researchers must consider the following questions:

1. Which end points are most important clinically?
2. Which end points can be measured in a reasonably unbiased manner?
3. What practical constraints exist, such as population size, financial resources of the research study, and ability to follow patients on a long-term basis?

Researchers in the United States and Canada designed a clinical trial to address the following question: *Is intensive therapy, including more frequent injections of insulin and more frequent monitoring of blood glucose levels, "superior" to standard therapy for diabetes mellitus?*

To assess treatment efficacy, more than one end point can be measured. Types of end points include measures of quality of life, length of survival, percentage of patients surviving, complication rate, and intermediate end points that are predictive of survival or quality of life (Table 7–2). In assessing "superiority" for the treatment of diabetes mellitus, possible outcome measures include the following:

1. The percentage of patients surviving at a specified time following the initiation of treatment
2. A patient's ability to maintain an active life-style

Table 7–2. Types and examples of end points used in clinical trials.

Type of End Point	Example
Quality of life	Ability to perform usual daily tasks
Survival	Percentage of patients alive 1 year after entering trial
Complications	Percentage of patients who develop serious allergic reactions
Intermediate measures	Percentage of patients who have recurrence of symptoms

3. The risk of having a major complication from treatment

4. The risk of experiencing one of the vascular events associated with diabetes mellitus

5. Measurement of hemoglobin A1-C (HgbA1C), which is an indicator of long-term blood glucose levels

6. Blood glucose levels at specific points in time.

Examples of two of these questions restated symbolically as hypotheses follow:

$$H_0 : \pi_0 = \pi_1$$

where H_0 is the so-called **null hypothesis** and π_0 and π_1 are the percentages of persons in the standard therapy or intensive therapy groups, respectively, who develop diabetic retinopathy during the 5-year period following entry into the study.

$$H_0 : \mu_0 = \mu_1$$

where μ_0 and μ_1 are the mean HgbA1C levels at 1 year following entry into the trial for persons in the standard therapy or intensive therapy groups, respectively.

Note that these hypotheses are stated in the null form—*there is no difference between the treatment groups regarding the specified end point.* The purpose of the clinical trial is to test whether the observed outcomes are consistent with these null hypotheses. If the observed data are not consistent with the null hypothesis, the null hypothesis (H_0) is rejected in favor of an alternative hypothesis (H_A) such as the following:

$$H_A : \pi_0 \neq \pi_1$$

where π_0 and π_1 again are the respective percentages of persons developing diabetic retinopathy during the 5-year period following entry into the study in the standard therapy and intensive therapy groups. This alternative hypothesis states that the two treatments will differ with respect to the development of diabetic retinopathy. Similarly, an alternative hypothesis for the HgbA1C outcome could be stated as follows:

$$H_A : \mu_0 \neq \mu_1$$

where μ_0 and μ_1 again are the respective mean HgbA1c levels for the standard therapy and intensive therapy groups. In other words, this alternative hypothesis states that the two treatments will differ with respect to mean HgbA1c levels achieved in patients after treatment.

The most important end points for any therapy for a potentially fatal disease would be survival, or survival accounting for quality of life. However, researchers in

this trial of therapy for diabetes chose diabetic retinopathy as the primary end point of the study for several reasons:

1. Death from diabetes often occurs decades after the onset of the disease. If death were the primary end point, the trial could not have been completed in a timely manner.

2. Retinopathy is a serious complication of diabetes. Vascular damage in one organ correlates with vascular damage at other sites of the body. Since vascular disease is the predominant physiologic process resulting in morbidity and mortality from the disease, the researchers felt that it was a reasonable choice as a primary end point.

3. The eye provides a unique portal through which damage to the vascular system can be visualized noninvasively. Furthermore, the measurement of the progression of retinopathy could be standardized and evaluated by taking photographs of each patient's retina at various points in time; moreover, researchers could evaluate the amount of retinal damage as documented in the photographs without knowledge of the treatment group to which each patient had been randomized.

4. Retinopathy, an intermediate end point, is thought to be predictive of two important final end points: survival and quality of life.

DETERMINATION OF SAMPLE SIZE

The number of subjects to be enrolled in a clinical trial—the sample size—must be determined in relation to the primary research end point. At the conclusion of any experiment, data are analyzed and a statistical decision is made to reject or accept the null hypothesis. This decision is based on probabilities, and unfortunately may be correct or incorrect. The relationship between the possible results of the diabetes therapy trial and the "truth" is shown in Figure 7–1. For the pur-

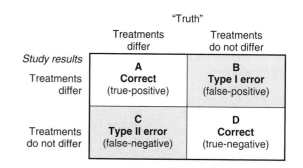

Figure 7–1. Comparison of study results and "truth."

poses of this discussion, "truth" can be thought of as the results of the intervention, if applied correctly to the entire universe of patients with the clinical condition under study. A clinical trial can be considered a sample of the "truth." Using a sample of a population, the hope is to make valid inferences about the entire population, but since only a sample can be evaluated, the risk of inaccurate conclusions exists.

In cells A and D of Figure 7–1, the results of the study agree with the "truth." In cells B and C, however, the study results do not agree with the "truth"—errors are made. These two types of error differ in their origin and implications.

If the study finds a difference in treatments, when in actuality there is no difference (cell B), a type I error is present. Under this circumstance, the *study results are falsely positive.* In the diabetes therapy trial, a type I error would have occurred if the investigators had concluded that there is a difference between treatments in the proportion of patients who developed retinopathy, when in "truth" there is no difference in those two proportions.

If the study fails to find a difference in treatments when in actuality there is a difference (cell C), a type II error is said to have occurred. Under this circumstance, *the study results are falsely negative.* In the diabetes therapy trial, a type II error would have occurred if the investigators had concluded that there is no difference between treatments in the proportion of subjects determined to have progressive retinopathy, when in fact one of the treatment regimens is associated with a reduced risk of retinopathy.

Falsely positive or falsely negative studies can occur because of faulty methodology, chance occurrences, or both. Whereas methodologic error can be minimized by careful attention to study design, errors due to chance can never be completely eliminated. Such errors, however, can be estimated. The notation used to denote the likelihood of a type I error—that the observed difference between groups is not a true difference but is due instead to chance—is the **alpha level.** Conversely, the notation used to denote the likelihood of a type II error—that the study did not find a difference when there actually is one—is the **beta level.** Researchers specify the alpha and beta levels when planning a study. The alpha level is specified commonly as 0.05, which means that the investigator is willing to accept a 5% risk of committing a type I error (falsely concluding that the groups differ when in reality they do not). The investigator must also specify beforehand the beta level, or risk of committing a type II error. Often a beta level of 0.20 is considered adequate—in other words a one in five chance of missing a true difference between the groups is allowed.

The **statistical power,** or ability of a study to detect a true difference between groups, is $(1-\beta)$. Statistical power for a study with a beta level of 0.20 would be 0.80, or 80%. Such a study would have an 80% chance of detecting a specified difference in outcome between the treatment groups.

Once the alpha and beta levels have been specified, the research team must specify another extremely important study parameter before determining sample size—the magnitude of the difference in outcome between treatment groups that the study will be designed to detect. This difference between the treatments under comparison is of great importance and should be selected on the basis of clinical information. In deciding on the level of outcome difference worthy of detection, the investigator might consider one or more of the following questions:

1. What difference in outcome would be important to clinicians treating this type of patient?

2. What difference would be meaningful to a patient who may suffer the consequences of the disease?

3. What difference in outcome would justify use of the more effective treatment in spite of greater expense or greater side effects?

Formulas for the determination of sample size and illustrative calculations are provided in Appendix B. Suffice it to say here that all three factors just mentioned (acceptable levels of type I and type II errors and the expected magnitude of difference in outcome between groups) are inversely related to the required sample size (Table 7–3). That is, if only a 1%, rather than the more commonly accepted 5%, chance of committing a type I error can be tolerated, the sample size must be increased. Similarly, a decrease in the acceptable level of type II error (enhanced statistical power) necessitates studying more subjects.

As the expected magnitude of difference in outcome (eg, proportion of subjects developing retinopathy) be-

Table 7–3. Factors that affect sample size requirements.

Factor	Effect on Sample Size Required
Decrease acceptable type I error	Increase
Decrease acceptable type II error	Increase
Decrease variability of outcome measures	Decrease
Decrease expected differences in outcome and between groups	Increase

tween treatment groups decreases, a larger sample size is required to detect the difference. In contrast, as the variability of the outcome (eg, the standard deviation of HgbA1c level) diminishes, fewer subjects are required to demonstrate a difference in outcome between the groups.

RANDOMIZATION

A central tenet of the clinical trial is that patients should be assigned to treatment groups by a method that maximizes the probability that the two groups will be similar in background characteristics that may influence either the response to therapy or the primary outcome measure.

For the modern clinical trial, the assignment to treatments is done by **randomization.** *With randomization, the determination of assignment to treatment group is based on probability alone and is not influenced by the preference of the physician or patient.*

The assignment to a treatment group for each patient is independent of (not influenced by) the assignment for all other patients. When there are two possible treatment assignments with equal sample sizes (as in the diabetes trial), each patient has a 50% chance of being assigned to either treatment. Such an assignment could be decided by a coin toss: if the coin comes up heads, the patient is assigned to standard therapy; if the coin comes up tails, the patient is assigned to intensive therapy. Of course, tossing a coin is a rather inelegant way to assign patients to treatment groups, so many investigators use more sophisticated devices, such as tables of random numbers or computer-generated random assignments. The basic design of a randomized controlled clinical trial is illustrated in Figure 7–2, using the diabetes therapy trial study as an example.

As recently as 50 years ago, the primary means of evaluating the benefit of a new treatment was to treat a series of patients with the new method and then compare the outcome with that observed in the past for a group of patients who received the standard therapy. The patients who received the standard therapy are called **nonconcurrent** or **historical controls.** Consider how such a study might have been performed to address the question concerning treatment of diabetes. If researchers wanted to test the hypothesis concerning the clinical efficacy of intensive therapy (experimental treatment) versus standard therapy (or control treatment), a group of patients would be given intensive therapy and the proportion of patients who develop retinopathy in a specified period of time would then be

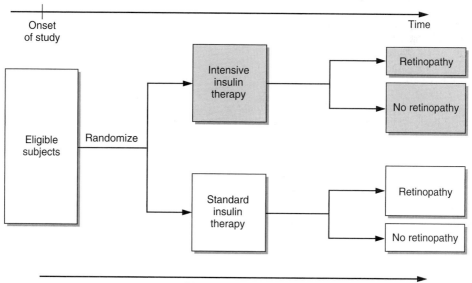

Figure 7–2. Schematic diagram of the design of a randomized controlled clinical trial comparing standard therapy with intensive insulin therapy for the treatment of diabetes mellitus. Shaded areas correspond to patients randomized to intensive insulin therapy.

compared with the proportion of patients who develop retinopathy among a group of patients treated at an earlier time with standard insulin therapy (Figure 7–3). There are several inherent problems with this approach:

1. The diagnostic criteria for progression of retinopathy may change over time.

2. The techniques used to measure retinopathy may change over the time period of the study.

3. Additional treatment modalities, such as advances in knowledge regarding dietary control, could become available over time and for ethical reasons would have to be employed on the patients during the second part of the study.

4. Most importantly, the patients who presented with diabetes during the time when patients were being treated with standard insulin therapy may not have been similar in prognostic characteristics (sex, age, socioeconomic status) to the patients who present during the intensive treatment period.

If concurrent controls are necessary to compare treatment groups, a basic question arises: *How should patients be assigned to each treatment group?*

Physicians or patients could choose which treatment a patient will be given. This technique, however, is seriously flawed. Although health care providers strive to be objective decision makers, they are empathetic to the needs of their patients and often have opinions concerning the efficacy of a treatment prior to the results of clinical trials. Patients—who of course have a direct personal interest in any treatment result—would very likely choose a treatment based on their assessment or expectation of its efficacy.

To avoid unfair comparisons that may result from these preferences of patients and physicians, the assignment to treatment group should therefore be determined by chance, independently of the wishes of clinicians and patients. *The purpose of randomization is to achieve "equality" of baseline characteristics of treatment groups, so that the comparison of treatments is considered fair.* To assess the equality of the treatment groups, demographic and prognostic factors may be compared between groups. If patients have been randomly allocated, it is expected that the groups will be similar in demographic and prognostic features.

A comparison of treatment groups after randomization from the diabetes therapy trial is given in Table 7–4. Note that two groups of patients were studied in this trial. The primary prevention group was defined by its complete lack of retinopathy at entry into the trial. The secondary prevention group included patients who already had signs of diabetic retinopathy at time of entry into the trial. The separation of the trial participants into groups is a technique known as **stratification.** The researchers chose to stratify by the presence or absence of retinopathy because they felt that this variable was of great importance in assessing the effect of treatment. By stratifying, the researchers ensured that they would have randomization within each of these two important but different groups.

As can be seen in Table 7–4, the two treatment groups are remarkably similar with regard to age, sex, duration of disease, insulin dose, glycosylated hemoglobin, and mean blood glucose level, and in regard to other characteristics known to be risk factors for vascular disease for subjects in both the primary and secondary prevention groups.

If the object is to ensure that similar numbers of patients with certain important prognostic characteristics are included in each treatment group, those characteristics can be accounted for in the randomization process. Suppose researchers wanted to guarantee that at the end of the diabetes therapy study there would be equal percentages of males and females in each treatment group.

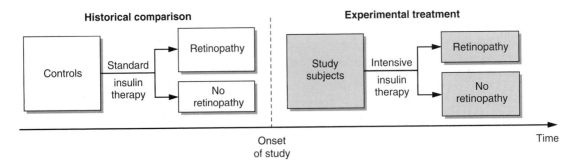

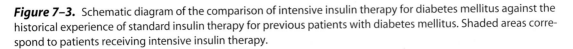

Figure 7–3. Schematic diagram of the comparison of intensive insulin therapy for diabetes mellitus against the historical experience of standard insulin therapy for previous patients with diabetes mellitus. Shaded areas correspond to patients receiving intensive insulin therapy.

Table 7–4. Distribution of baseline characteristics of patients enrolled in the diabetes therapy trial.

Characteristic	Standard Therapy (N = 378)	Intensive Therapy (N = 348)
Age (years)	26 ± 8[a]	27 ± 7
Adolescents, 13–18 years (%)	19	16
Male sex (%)	54	49
White race (%)	96	96
Duration of IDDM[b] years)	2.6 ± 1.4	2.6 ± 1.4
Insulin dose (U/kg of body weight/day)	0.62 ± 0.26	0.62 ± 0.25
Glycosylated hemoglobin (%)	8.8 ± 1.7	$8.8 \pm 6 1.6$
Mean blood glucose (mg/dL)	229 ± 80	234 ± 86
Body weight (% of ideal)	103 ± 14	103 ± 13

Adapted and reproduced, with permission, from The Diabetes Control and Complication Trial Research Group: The effect of intensive treatment of diabetes on the development and progression of long-term complications in insulin-dependent diabetes mellitus. N Engl J Med 1993;**329**:977.
[a]Plus–minus values are means ± standard deviation.
[b]IDDM, insulin-dependent diabetes mellitus.

The order in which the two treatments were assigned to groups of four patients of the same sex could be random; the first four male patients would be assigned to either the standard or the intensive therapy group and the next four males would be assigned to the other group. Females would be assigned in the same manner. At the end of the study there would be an equal number of male and female patients in each treatment group. Assignment of patients in this manner is termed **block randomization.** *The purpose of randomization in blocks of patients is to protect against imbalanced treatment assignment (due to "luck of the draw") with respect to prognostically important patient subgroups.*

THE PLACEBO EFFECT AND BLINDING

In the year 1801, Haygarth reported the results of what may have been the first **placebo-controlled trial.** A popular treatment for many diseases at that time was to apply metal rods, known as Perkins tractors, to the body and thus relieve symptoms through a supposed electromagnetic influence of the metal. Haygarth treated five patients with imitation wooden tractors and found that four gained relief. The following day, he used the metal tractors on the same five patients and obtained identical results: relief in four of the five subjects. In describing the results of his experiment, Haygarth quoted James Lind, who is credited with performing the first clinical trial: "An important lesson in physic is here to be learnt, viz., the wonderful and powerful influence of the passions of the mind on the state and disorders of the body. This is too often overlooked in the cure of diseases."

The influence of treatment of any kind on the perceptions patients have about their illness cannot be forgotten when designing a clinical trial. This concept is most important when the outcome measure is subjective. The patient's desires may also influence decisions made by clinicians subsequent to the initial randomization in a clinical trial. An additional factor that could potentially lead to differential treatment of groups within a trial is the clinician's decision-making process during a clinical trial. For example, will a clinician who has certain beliefs concerning a treatment's efficacy be likely to discontinue a therapy believed to be inferior in favor of the alternative therapy?

To account for the placebo effect and to reduce the introduction of bias due to the conceptions of patients and clinicians, studies may be conducted in a **blinded** fashion (Table 7–5). *"Blinding" means that the treatment assignment is not known to certain persons.* In a **single-blinded study,** the treatment assignment is unknown to the patients; in a **double-blinded study,** the treatment assignment is unknown to both the patients and their treating physicians. In a double-blinded study, the treatment assignment is revealed to the patient and physician only if there are serious or unexpected side effects or when the study is completed.

Table 7–5. Summary of various types of blinding to assignment of treatment in clinical trials.

Blinding	Knowledge of Treatment Assignment	
	Patient	Investigator
None	Yes	Yes
Single	No	Yes
Double	No	No

In the diabetes therapy trial, neither patients nor their physicians were blinded to their treatment group. Blinding was not possible because the patients and physicians are intimately involved in regulation of insulin dose on either arm of the trial. The researchers did blind the physicians who evaluated the photographs of the retina when assessing subjects for retinopathy. This was done to eliminate the possibility of **observation bias.**

Although blinding of both the patients and the treating physicians is desirable, there are trials, such as the diabetes therapy trial, that cannot be conducted in a blinded fashion because the treatments are so obviously different that it is not feasible to keep the assignment secret. Whenever possible, however, blinding should be employed, because lack of blinding could influence perceptions of outcome and reduce the confidence in study results.

ETHICAL ISSUES CONCERNING CLINICAL TRIALS

The investigator who contemplates entering a patient into a randomized clinical trial is faced with several ethical dilemmas. First, is the method of the randomized clinical trial ethically acceptable? One of the most important ethical tenets in medicine is that the patient's welfare is of primary concern, and a caregiver should prescribe the optimal treatment for a patient. It could be argued that even if a clinician has only a hunch or feeling that one treatment is superior, the patient should be offered that treatment. Therefore randomization between two treatments might be considered to be unethical. Given the seriousness and possible side effects of medical interventions, however, the axiom "first, do no harm" must always be borne in mind. The history of medicine is replete with examples of treatments now known to be either of no benefit or actually harmful. The clinical trial is considered to be the best method available to determine the benefits and potential harm of treatment regimens.

If the clinical trial method is accepted as appropriate, a decision must be made concerning how to perform trials as ethically as possible. The following is a list of guidelines for medical professionals who are conducting clinical trials:

1. None of the treatment options included in a randomized trial should be known to be inferior to another treatment option based on previous randomized studies, and if a standard treatment regimen exists, it should be used as the control.

2. The trial should address a question that is of clinical importance and seek to answer the question in a way that will be useful for future patients.

3. Patients should be told that they are part of a clinical experiment and should be informed in understandable language about all treatment options, the risks and benefits of participation, and the nature of randomization. The patient who then agrees to participate is said to have given informed consent, which implies that the patient freely chooses to be included in the trial.

4. The investigators undertaking the trial should be able to recruit in a timely manner the number of patients needed to meet the required sample size.

EVALUATION OF CLINICAL TRIALS

Relatively few physicians design clinical trials, and a limited number enter patients into clinical trials—but all clinicians read published accounts of clinical trials and use the results to guide the treatment of patients. A checklist of questions to help the physician interpret and evaluate clinical trials appears in Table 7–6.

Design Issues

The null hypothesis—and what would constitute a meaningful difference in outcome—should be stated in the methods section of a reported clinical trial. In the diabetes therapy trial, the primary outcome and the difference that was considered meaningful were clearly stated prior to beginning the trial. Trials should be designed to test one specific hypothesis or only a few hypotheses, and these should be evident to the reader.

The characteristics of the study population are particularly important when assessing the relevance of a specific trial to an individual practitioner's patients. In the diabetes therapy trial, the eligibility and exclusion criteria are clearly stated, as summarized in Table 7–7. Summary data about sex, age, and medical histories of the participants appear in Table 7–4. The combination of the entry criteria and the demographic characteristics of the study's entrants provides the reader with an adequate description of the study group. With this information, the reader is better able to judge whether the results of this study are applicable to a particular patient. Patients are often excluded from a trial for pragmatic reasons, such as inability to comply with treatment or lack of fluency in the language of the investigators. These exclusions, however, may limit the ability to generalize study findings to other patient groups.

Once randomized to a particular treatment regimen, a patient may adhere (comply) or elect not to follow the prescribed regimen. Possible reasons for noncompliance are listed in Table 7–8. The investigator cannot force participants to comply, since such coercion would vio-

Table 7–6. Checklist for evaluating clinical trials.

1. What was the null hypothesis?
  a. What was the outcome of interest:
  b. What was thought to be a meaningful difference in outcome?
2. Which group was being tested?
  a. How was the study population for the trial selected? (1) Exclusion criteria or (2) random versus volunteer
  b. What were the demographic and health characteristics of the group?
3. How many subjects were entered in the study?
  a. Was the size decided prior to the onset of the study?
4. How were the experimental and control groups selected?
  a. Were they selected in a way to ensure equal distribution of known risk factors?
5. Were the treatment regimens described adequately?
  a. If appropriate, was there a nontreated group?
  b. If the control is "standard therapy," was the treatment reasonable?
6. Was this a blinded study?
  a. Did the patients know which treatment they received?
  b. Did the physicians know which treatment patients received?
  c. Did the persons measuring outcome know if patients were in the control or experimental group?
7. What were the results?
  a. Were the treatment groups similar with regard to known prognostic factors?
  b. Were side effects recorded and reported?
  c. Who was included in the final results?
  d. Who was lost to follow-up? Did they differ from those who completed the study?
  e. During analysis, were patients kept in their originally assigned groups?
  f. Were enough of the data presented so that the conclusions can be justified?
  g. Were known risk factors accounted for in the analysis?
  h. Were confidence intervals reported?
  i. If the results were negative, was statistical power addressed?
8. Were the results biologically plausible and consistent with previous literature?
  a. If not, was this addressed?

late the rights of subjects to participate of their own free choice.

There are several possible ways, however, to increase compliance in a clinical trial (Table 7–9). The investigator may be able to select subjects who can be expected to be compliant. Motivation to participate is likely to be enhanced if the patients perceive themselves to be at high risk of an adverse health consequence. In the diabetes therapy trial, all enrolled subjects had an illness that put them at risk for the long-term vascular complications of diabetes. Also, participants are apt to be motivated to comply if the treatments offered may reduce the need for painful or debilitating therapy. In the diabetes therapy trial, for instance, patients may

Table 7–7. Summary of enrollment criteria for subjects in the primary prevention group of the diabetes therapy trial.

Patient Characteristic	Enrolled Subjects
Age	13–39 years
Diagnosis	Insulin-dependent diabetes mellitus
Duration of disease	1–5 years
Past medical conditions	Absence of hypertension, hypercholesterolemia, and diabetic complications or medical conditions
Complications of diabetes	No retinopathy, urinary albumin excretion of < 40 mg per 24 hours

Adapted and reproduced, with permission, from The Diabetes Control and Complications Trial Research Group: The effect of intensive treatment of diabetes on the development and progression of long-term complications in insulin-dependent diabetes mellitus. N Engl J Med 1993;**329**:977.

Table 7–8. Possible reasons for noncompliance in a randomized clinical trial.

Misunderstanding of instructions
Inconvenience of participation
Side effects of treatment
Cost of participation
Forgetfulness
Disappointment with results
Preference for another treatment

---

have hoped that more intensive therapy, or participation in a clinical trial with stringent guidelines for treatment, would help reduce the long-term complications of disease.

In nonurgent situations, the investigator may be able to assess probable compliance before randomization is performed. To monitor compliance the investigator may ask eligible participants to take either an active or an inert medication. This pretest interval is referred to as a "run-in" test period. Individuals who show a likelihood of compliance are randomized to the treatments of interest, and those likely to be noncompliant are excluded from the trial. Other strategies to increase compliance include providing incentives for participation or maintaining frequent contact with subjects. Compliance also is likely to be enhanced by keeping the duration of the intervention as brief as possible.

Regardless of how carefully a clinical trial is designed, it is likely that some subjects will not adhere to the treatment regimen. The extent to which participants actually comply can be assessed by various approaches. Personal reports by subjects and family members provide a simple but possibly unreliable basis on which to determine compliance. In drug studies, a traditional approach to assessing compliance is to count the number of unused pills at regular intervals. However, because pills can disappear for reasons other than ingestion by the subject, pill counts provide suggestive but not definitive evidence of compliance. The most conclusive evidence of compliance with a drug regimen is likely to be obtained by measurement of the drug (or a metabolite) in the subject's blood or urine. However, even this type of biological assay has limited utility, with the most obvious constraints being cost, inconvenience to subjects, and the difficulty of collecting specimens from some individuals. Moreover, long-term compliance typically cannot be assessed by measurements of such specimens, as the presence of most drugs is detectable in blood or urine for no more than a few days. The diabetes therapy trial was fortunate to be able to measure glycosylated hemoglobin, a long-term measure of blood glucose control, as a secondary end point. Although measurement of glycosylated hemoglobin levels is not a direct measure of compliance, among the two treatment groups it provided an independent measure of effect of treatment that was expected to differ if the treatments did differentially affect subjects' plasma glucose levels.

Despite the difficulties inherent in assessing compliance, it is important to estimate the extent to which subjects adhere to the assigned regimens. The ability of a study to identify a true effect of treatment (statistical power) may be diminished if a substantial proportion of the participants do not comply with the assigned treatment. That is, the observed difference in outcomes between the study groups may be reduced because of noncompliance. Accordingly, it may be necessary to include a larger initial sample size to compensate for the loss of discriminatory power. As will be emphasized later in this chapter, it is important to include all randomized patients in the main analysis of a clinical trial. Therefore, every effort should be made to determine the outcomes of both compliant and noncompliant subjects.

Analysis of Results

Loss of some patients to follow-up is likely to occur in any clinical trial. The greater the number of patients who are lost and the less information available about them, the less confidence can be placed in the results of the trial. In the analysis of results from a clinical trial,

Table 7–9. Strategies to enhance compliance with treatment assignment in randomized clinical trials.

Select motivated persons
Pretest ability and willingness of participants to comply
Provide simple and lucid instructions to subjects
Offer incentives to comply (eg, no charge for therapeutic intervention and associated examinations)
Provide positive reinforcements to subjects for adherence to treatment regimen
Maintain frequent contact with participants and remind them about importance of adherence to the regimen
Measure adherence through pill counts or sampling of biological specimens
Limit duration of intervention

---

patients should be left in the treatment group originally assigned by the study (intention to treat) even if they received one of the other treatments after the original treatment regimen failed. In the diabetes therapy study 95 women assigned to the standard therapy group received more intensive therapy during a pregnancy. In the analysis, these women remained in the standard therapy group. In another smaller subgroup of patients, researchers discontinued intensive therapy and resumed standard therapy. However, these patients remained in the intensive therapy group during analyses. This may seem counterintuitive, as these patients actually received some of both treatment regimens. The purpose of this trial, however, was to help clinicians determine the best treatment at the time of initial presentation for entry into the trial. Subsequent treatment decisions may include the alternative treatment, but those subsequent decisions have no bearing on the original clinical question posed by the trial and thus are not pertinent to group assignment. Design of the diabetes therapy trial with consideration of intention to treat is illustrated schematically in Figure 7–4.

All participants who are randomized should be included in the analysis of a clinical trial. Selective removal of subjects from the comparison of outcomes, even if it seems justified for pragmatic reasons, may lead to erroneous conclusions. Consider, for example,

the question of whether to include noncompliers in the analysis. Because these individuals did not receive the assigned treatments as intended, it may seem illogical to leave them in the analysis. It has been shown, however, that noncompliers tend to have worse outcomes than compliers, regardless of their treatment assignment. If the treatment assignment affects the level of compliance, then excluding noncompliance from the analysis can produce a misleading result.

Removal of noncompliers from the analysis may also limit the ability to generalize study findings to clinical practice. In recommending treatment to a particular patient, the physician must consider the possibility that the treatment will not be completed as intended. The essential question of a clinical trial is whether a treatment should be offered at a particular point in time. Therefore the relevant information on treatment benefit is the outcome among all patients who were offered the treatment, rather than just those who completed it.

A well-reported clinical trial should contain enough of the primary data to enable the reader (1) to compare the main outcome measure between the treatment groups and (2) to perform basic statistical tests to determine whether it is reasonable to exclude chance variation as a cause of observed differences between the compared groups. For the clinical trial, it is useful to review three very common types of comparisons: the compari-

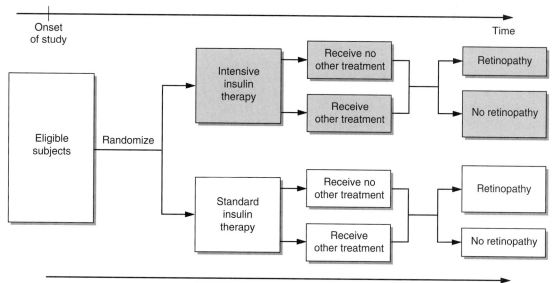

Figure 7–4. Schematic diagram of the design of a randomized controlled clinical trial comparing standard insulin therapy with intensive insulin therapy for the treatment of diabetes mellitus with analysis by intention to treat. Shaded areas correspond to patients randomized to intensive insulin therapy.

son of two risks, the comparison of time to an event (survival analysis), and the comparison of two means.

Many outcomes from a clinical trial are yes/no outcomes (eg, death or no death, cure or no cure, recurrence or no recurrence) and therefore can be displayed in simple tabular format. Whether a patient developed retinopathy in the primary prevention group in the diabetes therapy trial is presented in Table 7–10.

The incidence rate of developing retinopathy in each arm of the primary treatment group was determined by dividing the number of subjects who developed retinopathy by the number of person-years of follow-up. **Person-years** are calculated by summing the years that each subject is in the study prior to the development of retinopathy. This allows all subjects to be included in the results of a study, regardless of how long each subject was enrolled. This issue is common to the clinical trial, as recruitment of subjects into a trial often occurs over several years. The incidence rate (*IR*) of retinopathy for the standard therapy group was calculated to be 4.7 per 100 patient-years of follow-up, and 1.2 per 100 patient-years of follow-up for the intensive therapy group. There are several ways to compare these two rates.

One way to compare the rates is to calculate the percentage of incidence of retinopathy that would be avoided if intensive therapy were used instead of standard therapy. This percentage is known as the **percentage rate reduction** and is calculated as follows:

$$\text{Percentage rate reduction} = \frac{IR_{(standard)} - IR_{(experimental)}}{IR_{(standard)}} \times 100$$

If the percentage rate reduction = 0, there is no reduction in incidence rate attributable to the new therapy, and the treatments are judged to be equivalent.

Table 7–10. Results of the diabetes therapy trial concerning the risk of developing retinopathy.

	Treatment		
Retinopathy	**Standard Therapy**	**Intensive Therapy**	**Total**
Yes	91	23	114
No	287	325	612
Total	378	348	726

Adapted and reproduced, with permission, from The Diabetes Control and Complications Trial Research Group: The effect of intensive treatment of diabetes on the development and progression of long-term complications in insulin-dependent diabetes mellitus. N Engl J Med 1993;**329:**977.

The further the percentage rate reduction is from zero, the greater the difference between the two groups. For the diabetes therapy trial, the percentage of retinopathy that could have been prevented by patients using intensive therapy rather than standard therapy is calculated as follows:

$$\text{Percentage rate reduction} = \frac{4.7 - 1.2}{4.7} \times 100$$
$$= 74\%$$

That is, almost three fourths of the retinopathy that occurred in the standard therapy group could have been avoided if those patients had been treated with intensive therapy. The value of 74% is known as a **point estimate** because it is the single value along the scale from 0 to 100% that is most consistent with the results of the trial.

A useful method to gauge the precision of any point estimate is to calculate the 95% confidence intervals for the estimate. If the clinical trial were repeated many times, the values falling between the upper and lower bounds of the 95% confidence interval would include the true point estimate value 95% of the time. If the 95% confidence interval of the percentage risk reduction includes 0, the data are consistent with the null hypothesis, and the difference between the groups is not statistically significant at an alpha level of 0.05. If the 95% confidence interval does not include 0, the difference is statistically different at an alpha level of 0.05.

The approximate 95% confidence interval (*CI*) for the percentage rate reduction in the diabetes therapy trial calculated above is 60–83%. Since the interval does not include 0, this decreased rate is considered statistically significant at an alpha level of 0.05. This means that given the observed data, if the trial were repeated often, 95% of the time the percentage rate reduction would fall between 60% and 83%. The 95% confidence interval for the percentage rate reduction for retinopathy is illustrated schematically in Figure 7–5.

Another method of comparing two rates is by forming a ratio of the rates, the so-called **rate ratio** (*RR*). For other situations, in which risks rather than rates of events are estimated, the risks of end points can be measured for the experimental and control groups, then contrasted by dividing the risk of adverse events for the experimental group by the risk of adverse events for the control group; this is the risk ratio or **relative risk.** If the *RR* = 1.0, the rate (or risk) of the outcome of interest in the two treatment groups is exactly equal. The farther the ratio is from 1.0, the greater the difference in rate (or risk) between the two groups. For this trial, the rate of retinopathy in the intensive therapy group compared with the standard therapy group would be calculated as follows:

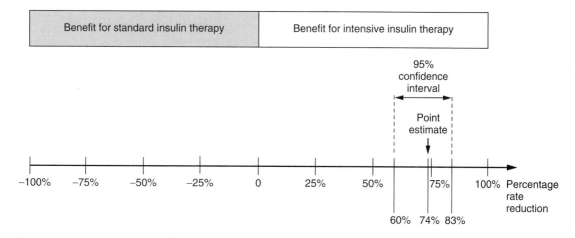

Figure 7–5. The point estimate and corresponding approximate 95% confidence interval for the percentage rate reduction in the diabetes therapy trial.

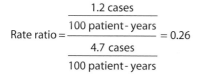

$$\text{Rate ratio} = \frac{\dfrac{1.2 \text{ cases}}{100 \text{ patient-years}}}{\dfrac{4.7 \text{ cases}}{100 \text{ patient-years}}} = 0.26$$

That is, the rate of developing retinopathy in the intensive treatment group is about one quarter that of the standard therapy group. The value of 0.26 is another example of a point estimate, because it is the single value along the rate ratio scale most consistent with the observed data. Similar to the percentage rate reduction, 95% confidence limits for the *RR* point estimate can also be calculated. If the 95% confidence interval includes the null value of 1.0, there is no statistical differ-

ence between rates in the two groups, and the null hypothesis would be accepted. If the 95% confidence interval does not include 1.0, the difference in rates between the two groups would be considered statistically significant at the 5% level. The point estimate and 95% confidence interval for the rate ratio of retinopathy in the diabetes therapy trial is illustrated schematically in Figure 7–6. Note that the point estimate of the *RR* does not lie at the midpoint of the 95% confidence interval. The asymmetry of the confidence interval occurs because the distribution of possible values of the *RR* is skewed toward the right (ie, all the values corresponding to a benefit for intensive therapy are compressed into the range of zero to 1, whereas the values corresponding to a benefit for standard therapy are spread from 1 to positive infinity).

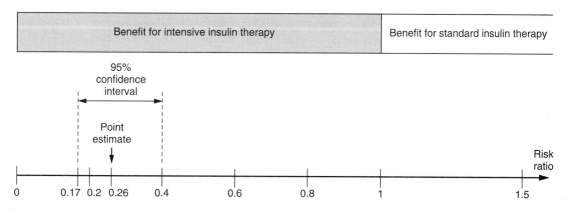

Figure 7–6. The point estimate and corresponding approximate 95% confidence interval for the rate ratio of retinopathy in the diabetes therapy trial.

The *RR* is a simple, easily understood method to evaluate results of clinical trials. For time-to-event data, however, survival analysis has several advantages over the **RR**. The survival curve, as described in Chapter 2, is a graphic presentation of time-to-event data. Since it graphically depicts events as they occur over time, the survival curve provides information on the rapidity with which events occur. Furthermore, the survival curve can make use of data from patients who are followed for varying lengths of time. For the diabetes therapy trial, the cumulative risk of retinopathy was plotted over time (Figure 7–7). Although this figure is not a display of survival (life versus death), it does represent "survival" without the occurrence of the event of interest, in this case retinopathy. A patient who is followed for only 3 years provides useful information on risk of developing retinopathy for that period of time, but would provide no information pertinent to a comparison beyond 3 years. Survival analysis also allows the median survival duration (eg, time to retinopathy development) as well as the percentage of survivors (eg, persons without retinopathy) to be estimated at any time along the curve.

Time since first treatment is depicted along the horizontal axis, and the percentage of patients with retinopathy is displayed on the vertical axis. At the time of initial treatment (years = 0), 0% of the patients in each group have developed retinopathy (100% have survived without retinopathy). As time from treatment progresses, the percentage of patients who are diagnosed with retinopathy increases, although more rapidly in the control group. At the end of 9 years of follow-up, 14% of the patients treated with intensive therapy have been diagnosed with retinopathy compared with 55% of the standard therapy subjects.

The survival curves could be used to estimate the relative risk of being diagnosed with retinopathy at any point in time. For example, the intensive to conventional group relative risk of retinopathy at 5 years is as follows:

$$\text{Relative risk} = \frac{6}{15} = 0.4$$

This relative risk indicates that the intensive therapy subjects have about 60% less risk than the conventional therapy subjects of developing retinopathy within 5 years. Alternatively, the median time to development of retinopathy for the two groups can be estimated and contrasted. The median time is the point at which half of an initial study group remains free of the occurrence of interest. In this example, the estimated median time to development of retinopathy for the standard therapy group is 8.5 years. The median time to development of retinopathy for the intensive therapy group has not been reached after 9 years of follow-up. That is, patients treated with intensive therapy are developing retinopathy at a slower rate than patients treated with standard therapy.

Several tests of significance can be used to compare survival curves (see Dawson and Trapp, 2004). As is demonstrated by the diabetes trial data, although this type of analysis is called survival analysis, it is not limited to the analysis of deaths. Any event that occurs over time (time to disease recurrence, time to return to work, etc) can be compared in this fashion.

Another comparison frequently used in clinical trials is the comparison of means. In the diabetes therapy trial, blood glucose levels were measured at the onset of the study and at regular intervals thereafter. In Table 7–4, one of the baseline characteristics compared between the standard therapy and intensive therapy groups is mean blood glucose level. It is possible to distribute patients into several discrete categories based on blood glucose level (eg, < 140, 140–179, 180–239, 240 or greater), but that would involve a loss of useful information about the actual observed glucose measurements. Instead, the mean or average blood glucose level

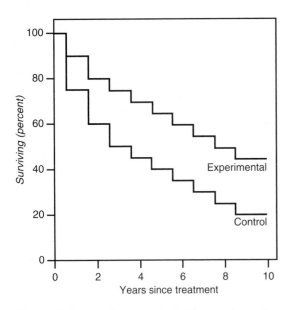

Figure 7–7. Cumulative survival without retinopathy in patients with insulin-dependent diabetes mellitus who receive intensive insulin or standard insulin therapy. (Adapted and reproduced, with permission, from the Diabetes Control and Complications Trial Research Group: The effect of intensive treatment of diabetes on the development and progression of long-term complications in insulin-dependent diabetes mellitus. N Engl J Med 1993;**329**:981.)

can be compared. The null and alternative hypotheses for this comparison would be stated as follows:

$$H_0 : \mu_1 = \mu_2$$
$$H_A : \mu_1 \neq \mu_2$$

A test of the equality of two means can be accomplished by performing a t test as follows:

$$t = \frac{\bar{x}_1 - \bar{x}_2}{\left(s_p \sqrt{\dfrac{1}{n_1} + \dfrac{1}{n_2}} \right)}$$

where x_1 and x_2 are the observed mean blood glucose levels of the standard and intensive treatment groups, respectively, s_p is an estimate of the pooled variance of the two means, and n_1 and n_2 are the sample sizes for each group. To illustrate the use of a t test, the observed mean blood glucose levels in patients treated with intensive and conventional therapy can be compared as follows:

$$t = \frac{231 - 155}{\left(44.8 \sqrt{\dfrac{1}{378} + \dfrac{1}{348}} \right)} = 22.8$$

A t statistic of 22.8 for this sample size corresponds to a p value of < 0.0005. In other words, there is less than a 0.05% chance that a difference in means as large as that observed with these sample sizes could have occurred by sampling variability alone. Accordingly, the null hypothesis of no difference between the means is rejected. If a study concludes that no difference exists between treatment regimens, the amount of difference the authors thought was important should be specified, as well as the likelihood that the study did not find a difference due to chance alone. The likelihood that a negative result is due to chance is the beta error; 1 minus the beta error $(1 - \beta)$ is the statistical power (see Sample Size Determination).

Meta-analysis

In the preceding section, the analysis of a single clinical trial was discussed. Rarely is a single study capable of providing the definitive answer to a clinical question. The diabetes therapy trial discussed in this chapter is one of the most important contributions to the evidence on the value of intensive treatment in reducing the complications of diabetes mellitus. The strengths of the study included its comparatively large sample size and long duration of follow-up. The substantial reduction in the risk of complications with intensive therapy

suggests that a clinically meaningful benefit can be obtained and it was shown that this was unlikely to have occurred by chance alone.

However, the tight eligibility requirements for this study produced a study population that was relatively young, healthy, and had few minority participants. Whether these results apply to patients who are older, sicker, or members of minority groups cannot be determined from this study. To assess whether the results of this clinical trial are applicable to patients who did not meet the eligibility requirements of this study, it is useful to consider whether other clinical trials have been conducted on this topic. If other clinical trials exist, they may have included patients with characteristics different from those in this investigation. Treatment effects then can be compared across these studies. If the results of the various studies show a consistent pattern of results, then it is possible to be more confident that the benefits of intensive therapy are not confined to a narrow subset of patients.

One approach to considering the results of multiple studies is referred to as **meta-analysis.** The term meta-analysis refers to *a statistical analysis that combines or integrates the results of several independent clinical trials.* A meta-analysis may be thought of as a special type of **systematic review.** A systematic review is *any type of synthesis of evidence on a topic that has been prepared using strategies to minimize errors.* When the results of individual studies in a systematic review are not combined statistically, the product may be described as a qualitative systematic review. A meta-analysis, on the other hand, is a systematic review in which the results of two or more studies are combined statistically.

A well-conducted meta-analysis offers several advantages over other types of reviews. First, a meta-analysis allows the direct presentation of the data on which the summary conclusions are made. Accordingly, the results of a meta-analysis are likely to be more data driven and objective than in other types of reviews. Second, the statistical summation in a meta-analysis produces a quantitative outcome measure and leads to precise estimates of effect. Third, if outcomes vary across studies, it may be possible to develop explanations for the pattern of variation in results, thereby gaining greater insight into the clinical question.

In essence, a meta-analysis is a study of other studies. As with any other type of investigation, a meta-analysis should be planned in advance and should follow a research protocol. The research plan should specify the hypotheses, the sampling strategy, the inclusion criteria, the data to be collected, and the approach to analysis of the information. At each of these steps, strategic decisions must be made that will impact the final product.

To illustrate this point, consider the seemingly straightforward issue of selecting the studies for inclusion. If interest is centered on clinical trials concerning intensive therapy for diabetes mellitus, a search of the published literature on this topic seems to be the logical sampling strategy. Because not all studies are published, the published literature may not yield a fair representation of all available information on the topic. It has been shown that studies with statistically significant findings are more likely to be published than studies with negative results. Also, studies sponsored by governments or nonprofit organizations are more likely to be published than those sponsored by the private sector (presumably because of the desire to protect proprietary information). Additional sampling distortion can result from the fact that papers published in certain influential journals are more likely to be cited, and therefore are easier to identify than works published elsewhere. Also, some studies result in multiple publications, which makes them easier to detect. In some instances, it may not even be possible for the meta-analyst to determine that two separate published papers arise from the same source clinical trial population. For pragmatic reasons, a meta-analysis may be confined to English language publications, which selects for more widely read journals and may result in an overrepresentation of studies with positive results.

Thus, the published literature on a topic may selectively exclude information that would affect the ultimate conclusion. This potential source of error is sometimes referred to as **publication bias.** Attempts can be made to identify and include unpublished studies in a meta-analysis, but there are obvious difficulties in locating such information and securing access to it. One approach to finding unpublished studies is to search for relevant investigations in a registry of clinical trials. Since studies are registered before they are completed, their inclusion in a registry is less likely to be influenced by whether the results were positive. If both published and unpublished studies are included, it is possible to analyze the results separately. An apparent difference in results between published and unpublished studies suggests the possibility of a publication bias.

Once the universe of clinical trials on a topic is identified, the meta-analyst must decide which specific studies to include in the study. This process is analogous to the need to establish eligibility criteria for enrolling patients in a clinical trial. For a meta-analysis, the decision about whether to include a particular study typically is based on (1) an assessment of its quality and (2) the ability to combine it with other studies based on respective patient populations, treatment regimens, and outcomes. Judging quality can be a subjective process, so it is advisable to limit inclusion criteria to basic features of a well-designed clinical trial. Examples of such inclusion criteria might include

1. Proper randomization of treatment assignments
2. Blinded assessment of outcome
3. Analysis based on the intention-to-treat principle.

Once the eligible source studies are selected, a standard abstract form should be used to extract key information. Independent abstraction of information by two reviewers is a useful practice to help reduce errors in data collection. Blinding of the abstractors to the identity of the original investigators, their affiliations, sources of support, and publication may help to reduce the potential of observation bias.

The outcome must be measured in a similar way across studies. For dichotomous outcomes (eg, the development of retinopathy or not), a rate ratio or relative risk may be the appropriate measure. For continuous outcomes (such as blood glucose level), a difference in means for the experimental and control groups may be employed. It should be noted, however, that the magnitude of a mean difference is affected by the distribution of the underlying population. For example, the mean difference in blood glucose levels between experimental and control subjects would be expected to be greater in a study population of diabetics with higher initial blood glucose levels than in a study population with lower initial levels. Accordingly, differences are often presented in units of standard deviation, thereby adjusting for the underlying distribution of values.

At the heart of a meta-analysis is the statistical combination of results from the individual clinical trials. The simplest approach to this combination would be to calculate the arithmetic average (mean) of the individual results. The simple mean of individual results would give equal weight to each of the studies. Because studies with smaller sample sizes are more prone to the effects of chance variation than studies with larger sample sizes, it is desirable to assign less influence to the smaller studies. By calculating a **weighted average** (in contrast to a simple or unweighted average) of results, more emphasis can be placed on the most statistically precise individual trial findings.

The statistical models used to combine results fall into two broad categories. The so-called **fixed-effects model** assumes that any differences in results across individual studies are attributable entirely to random variation. In contrast, the **random-effects model** assumes that the underlying relationship in question varies across studies in addition to the influences of random variation. When the results of the individual clinical trials being summarized are similar, minimal differences between the fixed- and random-effects models will be obtained. In general, however, the random-effects model will lead to somewhat less precise summary estimates, as reflected in wider confidence intervals. When the results of the underlying clinical trials vary widely, they are said to be **heterogeneous.** Under conditions of heterogeneity, the summary estimates obtained through the fixed- and random-effects models will differ, possibly to a considerable extent. It is important, therefore, to be able to determine whether the results of individual clinical trials are heterogeneous.

One approach to addressing the question of whether the variation across individual study results can be attributed to random variation alone is to perform a statistical test for heterogeneity. A statistically significant result for a test of heterogeneity would suggest that the variation across studies is greater than can be attributed to random variation alone. In such instances, therefore, a random-effects model would be the preferred approach to summarizing the data. On the other hand, if the test of heterogeneity is not statistically significant, the level of variation observed across individual study results can be explained by random variation. In such circumstances, a fixed-effects model would be an acceptable approach to summarizing the data.

Whether the question of heterogeneity of results should be addressed only, or even primarily, by a test of statistical significance is a matter of some debate. Because the tests of heterogeneity have limited statistical power, they are prone to type II errors, that is, they may lead to false-negative conclusions about the presence of heterogeneity in the underlying data. A statistically nonsignificant result may falsely reassure the meta-analyst (and the reader) that there is no evidence of heterogeneity in the underlying data. It is recommended, therefore, that the question of heterogeneity of results across studies be explored further during the course of the meta-analysis.

Heterogeneity of findings across studies can arise for a number of reasons in addition to random variation. The characteristics of the individual patient populations may be an important contributor to differences in observed effects. As previously noted, eligibility and exclusion criteria for a particular clinical trial may impose limitations on the selection of subjects based on age, sex, race, general health status, and other characteristics. To the extent that eligibility requirements vary across studies, the source populations may differ in fundamental ways that affect their likelihood of response to the treatment under investigation.

Aspects of the design of a clinical trial, for example, whether blinding was performed, the rate of compliance with treatment, the duration of follow-up, and the completeness of follow-up, may influence the results obtained. Approaches to analysis of individual study results, such as adhering to the intention-to-treat principle, can also impact the results.

Whether a clinical trial is stopped early is likely to be related to the findings. In general, clinical trials are not terminated prematurely unless an unexpectedly large difference in outcomes is observed between the experimental and control group. Such a difference could arise because the experimental treatment is much more effective than the control treatment (placebo or standard therapy). Alternatively, the complications or side effects of treatment may be greater in one treatment group than the other, causing the investigators to terminate the clinical trial early. In either case, the results of prematurely concluded trials are likely to differ from those trials brought to the originally intended conclusion.

Given all of the potential sources of heterogeneity, it is not surprising that variation in results across the selected studies is a common occurrence in meta-analyses. At one level, this variability is disconcerting because consistency of results across studies is a useful approach to establishing that an observed treatment effect is real. The ability to reproduce findings across independent investigators, study populations, and settings increases confidence in the inferences drawn concerning the effectiveness of the experimental treatment. Heterogeneity in results, particularly if it cannot be explained, raises uncertainty in the inferences that can be drawn from a meta-analysis.

An important approach to exploring heterogeneity is referred to as **sensitivity analysis.** In this context, a sensitivity analysis is an exploration of the summary results within subsets of the studies under review. If subgroups of studies can be identified that yield consistent results, which in turn differ from the results of other subgroups, some insight may be gained concerning the overall sources of heterogeneity. For example, if a meta-analysis includes both published and unpublished clinical trials, it might be useful to summarize the results of the published studies separately from the results of the unpublished studies. A larger treatment effect in the published studies would support the suspicion of a publication bias. Analysis of results according to the sample size of clinical trials also might provide evidence of a publication bias. Large studies have greater statistical power than small studies, and therefore are better able to detect small treatment effects. Because studies with statistically significant results presumably are more likely to be published than other studies, weaker treatment effects in large trials compared with small trials is a potential indication of a publication bias. That is to say, small studies with weak effects were less likely to be published and therefore were less available for meta-analysis. Similarly, subgroup analysis may reveal a stronger treatment effect among clinical trials that were stopped early. Through these types of subgroup analyses, nonrandom patterns of variation in study results may be detected and explained. In this sense, a sensitivity analysis can reveal subgroups of studies with consistent results, and thereby provide greater insight into the true effects of the treatment under study. However, a sensitivity analysis must be interpreted with caution, as it is possible that the patterns observed might have arisen by chance. Overinterpretation of subgroup analyses can lead to erroneous conclusions.

It is also important to recognize circumstances in which a meta-analysis may not be advisable. For some questions of clinical interest, there may be an insufficient number of trials available to yield a conclusive summary. Even when a large number of trials on a topic are available, fundamental differences in their study populations, design, and outcome measures may make it unwise to attempt to combine results. Also, when there is considerable heterogeneity of treatment effect across studies that cannot be explained by a sensitivity analysis, it may be imprudent to calculate a weighted average of the individual study results.

In summary, meta-analysis is a powerful tool to help assess the cumulative evidence on the effectiveness of a particular treatment. By combining information across studies, it can lead to a statistically precise and objective estimate of the effect of interest, and it allows the consistency of findings across studies to be considered. On the other hand, the quality of the design and data of the original clinical trials, which is beyond the control of the meta-analyst, will affect the quality of the meta-analysis. Decisions made by the meta-analyst, such as which clinical trials to include and how the summary analyses are performed, will also affect the quality of the meta-analysis. Ultimately, the value of a meta-analysis will rest on its ability to help make informed treatment decisions. We will return to the topic of meta-analyses and systematic reviews in Chapter 13 in the context of discussing the interpretation of epidemiologic literature.

The Cochrane Collaboration

The Cochrane Collaboration is an international organization whose goal is to help people make well-informed decisions about health care. It addresses this goal by preparing, maintaining, and ensuring accessibility to current, rigorous systematic reviews of the benefits and risks of health care interventions. This organization was founded at a meeting in Oxford, England in late 1993. It is named in memory of Archie Cochrane (1909–1988), a physician epidemiologist who was a pioneer in the field of health services research. Cochrane was noted for his strong belief that health care decisions should be based on a critical synthesis of well-designed clinical trials of treatment effectiveness.

The Cochrane Collaboration involves six organizational units: Collaborative Review Groups, Fields, Centers, Methods Working Groups, Consumer Networks, and a Steering Committee. The core work of the organization is the preparation of systematic reviews, which are conducted by the Collaborative Review Groups. Each Review Group is comprised of individuals who share interests in particular health problems. The results of the systematic reviews are incorporated in the Cochrane Library, an electronic repository of evidence needed to make informed health care decisions. The Library was established in 1995 and is updated quarterly. It contains the following resources:

1. The Cochrane Database of Systematic Reviews—a regularly updated collection of completed systematic reviews and protocols of systematic reviews that are in progress.
2. The Database of Abstracts of Reviews of Effectiveness—an inventory of more than 2000 reviews that were completed outside of the Cochrane Collaboration.
3. The Cochrane Controlled Trials Register—a database that by 2003 contained citations for nearly 400,000 controlled trials identified by contributors to the Collaboration.
4. The Cochrane Review Methodology Database—a reference list of articles on the science of synthesizing evidence and the practical aspects of preparing systematic reviews.

Over its relatively short history, the Cochrane Collaboration has already produced a remarkable body of information. By 2003, 1837 systematic reviews were published. In spite of this impressive progress, the Collaboration faces many challenges. First, although the goal of the Collaboration is to produce reviews across the full spectrum of health care, it is dependent on the interests of persons who volunteer to prepare systematic reviews. Second, the use of such a wide range of reviewers of various backgrounds and skill levels makes it difficult to ensure a uniform high standard of work quality. Third, availability of the information in the Cochrane Library is not yet universal. Barriers to its availability include lack of knowledge about its existence and the subscription cost. However, with the progress already achieved by the Cochrane Collaboration, there is reason for optimism that this organization will play an increasingly important role in promoting well-informed health care decisions.

SUMMARY

Evidence-based medicine can be defined as the integration of current best evidence with clinical expertise, pathophysiological knowledge, and patient preferences to make health care decisions. Although there are barriers to the practice of evidence-based medicine, such as the skills and time required to appraise the literature, this approach encourages effective management of disease. It can serve to optimize health outcomes and promote cost-effective disease management.

Fundamental to the practice of evidence-based medicine is the ability to assess the design, conduct, and analysis of clinical studies critically. For the purpose of assessing the comparative benefits of alternative treatments, the randomized controlled clinical trial is the gold standard approach. Therefore the evidence-based practitioner must be thoroughly familiar with this research method.

The advantages and disadvantages of randomized controlled clinical trials, as compared with alternative study designs, are set forth in Table 7–11. The principal strength of this approach derives from assigning treatments to patients by **randomization,** thereby tending to balance the study groups with respect to both known and unknown prognostic factors.

Before enrolling patients in a clinical trial, the investigator can determine the baseline and follow-up information that will be required on all subjects. Procedures can then be put in place to enable the researchers to collect data in a fairly complete and accurate manner. The investigator can also allocate subjects to desired dose levels rather than relying on physician or patient preferences. When **blinding** of the evaluators or patients is feasible, the assessment of clinical outcomes is less likely to be influenced by knowing which treatment was used.

However, randomized controlled clinical trials are subject to certain constraints. Restrictive criteria for inclusion of subjects may produce a very homogeneous study population, which may restrict the ability to extrapolate results to patients with other characteristics. Clinical trials—particularly those involving chronic processes—may require years of follow-up to determine the outcome of treatment. A prolonged observation period leads to higher costs, increases the likelihood that patients will be lost to follow-up, and delays the time at which a treatment recommendation can be made. The use of intermediate end points, such as measurement of

blood glucose levels or glycosylated hemoglobin in the diabetes therapy trial, can help limit the length of required follow-up. Nevertheless, a definitive conclusion about treatment benefit often requires years of observation.

Large sample sizes typically are required in clinical trials when the magnitude of difference in responses between study groups is small. Furthermore, large numbers of subjects are likely to be required to demonstrate differences between study groups when there is wide variability in responses to treatment. Increasing the size of the study population not only raises the cost of a trial, but may also lead to pragmatic difficulties in locating a sufficiently large pool of eligible patients.

Ethical concerns may arise in a clinical trial if one or more of the treatment options has serious potential side effects or if early data suggest—but do not establish—a therapeutic advantage for one of the treatments. In this situation, a decision must be made about whether the trial should be continued until a definitive conclusion is reached or should be terminated early so that all patients have the opportunity to receive the apparently superior treatment. To minimize the possible influence of real or perceived conflicts of interest, an external advisory group should review these ethical questions.

An investigator cannot control the behavior of subjects enrolled in a clinical trial. Even after initial informed consent has been given to participate in a clinical trial, a subject has the right to withdraw at any time. Some subjects may elect to remain in the trial but not comply with the assigned regimen. **Noncompliance** can reduce the statistical power of a clinical trial and thereby lead to a false-negative conclusion. Accordingly, every effort must be made to achieve maximal compliance with assigned treatment without infringing on the patient's right to refuse therapy. Ultimately, treatment decisions should be based on the best evidence available concerning therapeutic benefit. The standard approach to gathering this evidence is the randomized controlled clinical trial. Although this type of investigation is labor intensive, time consuming, and

Table 7–11. Advantages and disadvantages of randomized controlled clinical trials.

Advantages	Disadvantages
Randomization tends to balance prognostic factors across study groups	Subject exclusions may limit ability to generalize findings to other patients
Detailed information can be collected on baseline and subsequent characteristics of participants	A long period of time is often required to reach a conclusion
Dose levels can be predetermined by the investigator	A large number of participants may be required
Blinding of participants can reduce distortion in assessment of outcomes	Financial costs are typically high
Assumptions of statistical tests tend to be met	Ethical concerns may arise
	Subjects may not comply with treatment assignments

expensive, it can provide the most convincing evidence of the superiority of one treatment over another. Through the use of randomized clinical trials such as the diabetes therapy study, decisions concerning patient treatment and care can be based on rigorous scientific information.

A **systematic review** is any type of synthesis of medical evidence on a topic that has been prepared using strategies to minimize errors. A particular type of systematic review is referred to as a **meta-analysis.** A meta-analysis is a statistical combination or integration of the results of several independent studies that are considered to be combinable. A meta-analysis can provide a statistically precise estimate of the treatment effect in question. It also may help to explain any observed variation in the estimated treatment effect across different studies.

Important steps in a meta-analysis include the definition of the research question of interest, the sampling of eligible studies, the abstraction of key information from the studies, the choice of an analytical strategy, and the interpretation of the results obtained. The sampling strategy including clinical trials is particularly important, as the data available for the meta-analysis will be determined by these decisions. The possible influences of a variety of factors, such as **publication bias,** must be considered when designing the process for identifying and determining the eligibility of individual clinical trials.

In calculating the summary measure of treatment effect in a meta-analysis, the individual study results typically are weighted to give the most influence to larger studies with more statistically precise estimates. Statistical summarization of results across studies typically is performed with either a **fixed-effects model** or a **random-effects model.** A fixed-effects model assumes that any variation in observed treatment effects across studies is attributable only to random variation. A random-effects model assumes that in addition to random variation, there is a different underlying effect in each clinical trial included. The two models will yield different summary measures of effect if the findings of the underlying clinical trials are **heterogeneous,** that is to say, the findings vary beyond the expected influence of chance. The pattern of heterogeneity can be explored through a **sensitivity analysis,** and thereby may lead to the identification of subgroups of studies with homogeneous effects. In so doing, the overall pattern of heterogeneity of clinical trial results may be explained by characteristics of their population groups, study features, or other characteristics.

One massive undertaking in support of the conduct and use of high-quality systematic reviews is the **Cochrane Collaboration.** This organization is dedicated to promoting well-informed health care decisions. It strives to meet this goal by preparing, maintaining, and ensuring accessibility to current, rigorous, systematic reviews of the benefits and risks of health care interventions. Established in late 1993, the Collaboration has a series of Review Groups, each of which includes individuals with a shared interest in particular health problems. These Review Groups conduct systematic reviews, which are disseminated through the Cochrane Library. In addition to the completed reviews, the Library, which is updated quarterly, includes a database of systematic reviews performed outside of the Collaboration, a register of clinical trials identified by members of the Collaboration, and a database of methodological references.

By mid-1999, the Cochrane Collaboration had completed 576 systematic reviews and had prepared protocols to conduct 538 additional reviews. Although the Collaboration intends to address all areas of health care, at present it is constrained by the interests of the volunteer reviewers. Moreover, the large number of reviewers utilized worldwide, with varying levels of skills and experience, compounds the problem of quality assurance. In spite of these challenges, the Cochrane Collaboration offers great promise in promoting health care decisions that are well informed by the best available evidence.

STUDY QUESTIONS

Questions 1–10: For each numbered question below, select the single best answer from the lettered options.

*A randomized, double-blind, placebo-controlled clinical trial is conducted to determine whether memantine, an N-methyl-D-aspartate (NMDA) antagonist, can reduce clinical deterioration in patients with Alzheimer's disease (reference: Reisberg B et al: Memantine in moderate-to-severe Alzheimer's disease. N Engl J Med 2003; **348:**1333). Among 252 patients randomized in equal numbers to memantine (20 mg per day) or a placebo, the groups were similar at baseline with respect to demographic characteristics and level of dementia. The study period was 28 weeks, with 29 experimental patients and 42 controls not completing the study. Based upon cognitive, functional, and behavioral assessments, 29% of patients treated with memantine and 10% of controls demonstrated a predefined favorable clinical response. Serious adverse events occurred among 13% of patients on memantine and 18% of controls.*

1. The similarity of treatment groups with respect to baseline characteristics most likely occurred because of
   A. Use of intention-to-treat analysis
   B. The placebo effect
   C. Use of randomization
   D. Use of blinding
   E. Use of informed consent

2. One control in ten had a clinical response. This is best explained by
   A. Use of intention-to-treat analysis
   B. The placebo effect
   C. Use of randomization
   D. Use of blinding
   E. Use of informed consent

3. Neither patients nor clinicians who evaluated them knew individual treatment assignments. This may be described as
   A. Use of intention-to-treat analysis
   B. The placebo effect
   C. Use of randomization
   D. Use of blinding
   E. Use of informed consent

4. The risk of not responding clinically among memantine patients was
   A. 0.10
   B. 0.29
   C. 0.71
   D. 0.79
   E. 0.90

5. The risk of not responding clinically among controls was
   A. 0.10
   B. 0.29
   C. 0.71
   D. 0.79
   E. 0.90

6. The risk ratio of not responding clinically among patients treated with memantine compared to the corresponding reference risk among controls was
   A. 0.10
   B. 0.29
   C. 0.71
   D. 0.79
   E. 0.90

7. The risk ratio of a serious adverse effect among patients treated with memantine compared to the corresponding reference risk among controls was
   A. 0.13
   B. 0.18
   C. 0.72
   D. 0.82
   E. 0.87

8. The results suggest that compared with controls, patients treated with memantine have
   A. Better clinical response and fewer serious adverse effects
   B. Better clinical response, but more serious adverse effects
   C. Worse clinical response, but fewer serious adverse effects
   D. Worse clinical response and more serious adverse effects
   E. The same clinical response, but fewer serious adverse effects

9. Although more controls than patients treated with memantine failed to complete the study, all patients were analyzed according to the original assignment. This is best described as
   A. Use of intention-to-treat
   B. The placebo effect
   C. Use of randomization
   D. Use of blinding
   E. Use of informed consent

10. Some patients may have enrolled with cognitive deficits great enough to impair their understanding of the purpose and risks of the study. In these instances, caregivers represented the patients in accepting the risks and benefits of the study. This process is best described as
    A. Use of intention-to-treat
    B. The placebo effect
    C. Use of randomization
    D. Use of blinding
    E. Use of informed consent

FURTHER READING

Doll R: Controlled trials: The 1948 watershed. BMJ 1998;**317:** 1217.

REFERENCES

Clinical Background

American Diabetes Association: Implications of the diabetes control and complications trial. Diabetes Care 1999;**22**(Suppl 1):S24.

Evidence-Based Medicine

Ellrodt G et al: Evidence-based disease management. JAMA 1997; **278**:1687.

Straus SE, Sackett DL: Using research findings in clinical practice. BMJ 1998;**317**:339.

Statement of the Research Questions

Diabetes Control and Complications Trial Research Group. The effect of intensive treatment of diabetes on the development and progression of long-term complications in insulin-dependent diabetes mellitus. N Engl J Med 1993;**329**:977.

Roland M, Torgerson D: What outcomes should be measured? BMJ 1998;**317**:1075.

Randomization

Krause MS, Howard KI: What random assignment does and does not do. J Clin Psychol 2003;**59**:751.

The Placebo Effect and Blinding

Haygarth J: *Of the Imagination as a Cause and as a Cure of Disorders of the Body.* R. Crutwell, 1801.

Schulz KF, Grimes DA: Blinding in randomized trials: hiding who got what. Lancet 2002;**359**:696.

Ethical Issues Concerning Clinical Trials

Tramer MR et al: When placebo controlled trials are essential and equivalence trials are inadequate. BMJ 1998;**317**:875.

Evaluation of Clinical Trials

Marcus SM: Assessing non-consent bias with parallel randomized and non-randomized clinical trials. J Clin Epidemiol 1997; **50**:823.

Storms W: Clinical trials: are these your patients? J Allergy Clin Immunol 2003;**112**:S107.

Design Issues

Diabetes Control and Complications Trial Research Group: The effect of intensive treatment of diabetes on the development and progression of long-term complications in insulin-dependent diabetes mellitus. N Engl J Med 1993;**329**:977.

Analysis of Results

Altman DG, Bland JM: Time to event (survival) data. BMJ 1998; **317**:468.

Dawson B, Trapp RG: *Basic and Clinical Biostatistics,* 4th ed. Appleton & Lange, 2004.

Diabetes Control and Complications Trial Research Group: The effect of intensive treatment of diabetes on the development and progression of long-term complications in insulin-dependent diabetes mellitus. N Engl J Med 1993;**329**:977.

Wang D et al: A primer for statistical analysis of clinical trials. Arthroscopy 2003;**19**:874.

Meta-analysis

Cook DJ, Mulrow CD, Haynes RB: Systematic reviews: Synthesis of best evidence for clinical decisions. Ann Intern Med 1997; **126**:376.

Egger M, Davey Smith G, Phillips AN: Meta-analysis: Principles and procedures. BMJ 1997;**315**:1533.

Egger M et al: Uses and abuses of meta-analysis. Clin Med 2001; **1**:78.

Greenhalgh T: Papers that summarize other papers (systematic reviews and meta-analyses). BMJ 1997;**315**:672.

Jones PW: An introduction to systematic reviews in respiratory medicine. Respir Med 2003;**97**:97.

Melander H et al: Evidence b(i)ased medicine—selective reporting from studies sponsored by pharmaceutical industry: review of studies in new drug applications. BMJ 2003;**326**:1171.

The Cochrane Collaboration

Jadad AR, Haynes RB: The Cochrane Collaboration—Advances and challenges in improving evidence-based decision making. Med Decis Making 1998;**18**:2.

e-PIDEMIOLOGY

Clinical Background

http://www.pitt.edu/~super1/lecture/lec0771/index.htm

http://www.pitt.edu/~super1/lecture/lec0781/index.htm

http://www.pitt.edu/~super1/lecture/lec10341/index.htm

Introduction to Clinical Trials

http://www.bmj.com/epidem/epid.9.shtml

http://www.pitt.edu/~super1/lecture/lec8601/index.htm

Statement of the Research Questions

http://www.pitt.edu/~super1/lecture/lec0222/014.htm

Sample Size Determination

http://www.amaassn.org/public/peer/7_13_94/pv3037x.htm

Randomization

http://www.pitt.edu/~super1/lecture/lec0222/012.htm

The Placebo Effect and Blinding

http://www.pitt.edu/~super1/lecture/lec0222/015.htm

Ethical Issues Concerning Clinical Trials

http://www.pitt.edu/~super1/lecture/lec0222/025.htm

Evaluation of Clinical Trials

http://www.bmj.com/archive/7106/7106ed.htm
http://www.pitt.edu/~super1/lecture/lec0222/022.htm

Analysis of Results

www.cche.net/usersguides/overview.asp#

Meta-analysis

http://www.bmj.com/archive/7109/7109ed2.htm
http://www.pitt.edu/~super1/lecture/lec1171/index.htm
http://www.pitt.edu/~super1/lecture/lec3221/index.htm
http://www.pitt.edu/~super1/lecture/lec7681/index.htm

The Cochrane Collaboration

http://www.cochrane.de/cc/cochrane/cdsr.htm
http://www.clchrane.de/revabstr/mainindex.htm

Cohort Studies

KEY CONCEPTS

1. Studies in which the investigator passively observes events without determining assignment of exposure are referred to as observational.

2. Cohort studies are observational studies in which the investigator determines the exposure status of subjects and then follows them for subsequent outcomes.

3. A prospective cohort study is one in which the exposure and subsequent outcome status of each subject is determined after the onset of the investigation.

4. A retrospective cohort study is one which utilizes historical information on exposure status and subsequent outcome.

5. The risk ratio or relative risk is a measure of association between the exposure and disease and is defined as the risk among the exposed divided by the risk among the unexposed.

6. A risk ratio > 1 implies that exposure increases the risk of disease, whereas a risk ratio < 1 implies that exposure decreases the risk of disease.

7. The attributable risk percentage is a measure of the proportion of the total risk among exposed persons that is related to their exposure.

PATIENT PROFILE

A pediatrician was called to the hospital to attend the delivery of a newborn. The mother, a 28-year-old primigravida, had experienced elevated blood pressure during an otherwise uncomplicated pregnancy. The labor was induced because the pregnancy had continued 2 weeks past the expected date of delivery. During labor, evidence of fetal distress was seen. When the membranes ruptured, the obstetrician noted thick greenish fluid containing meconium. At the time of delivery, the male newborn was limp and cyanotic, and had no spontaneous respiratory effort and a heart rate of only 50 beats/minute. When meconium was suctioned from his mouth and nose, the baby did not grimace, cough, or sneeze.

Vigorous efforts at resuscitation were initiated, including bag-and-mask ventilation with 100% oxygen and chest compressions, but the Apgar score at 1 minute of life was 1. The Apgar score (Table 8–1), an index of neonatal asphyxia, can range from 0 (very asphyxiated) to 10 (no asphyxia). Despite continuing resuscitation, the 5-minute Apgar score improved only to 2, with a heart rate of 110 beats/minute. The 10-minute Apgar score remained depressed at 3, and the neonate was transferred to the newborn intensive care unit. With aggressive medical management, the 3100-g neonate continued to improve without evidence of acute neurologic complications. He was discharged from the hospital on the twelfth day of life.

Table 8–1. Apgar score for evaluation of neonatal asphyxia.[a]

Sign	Score		
	0	1	2
Heart rate (beats/min)	Absent	< 100	> 100
Respiration	Absent	Slow, irregular	Regular, crying
Muscle tone	Limp	Slow flexion	Active motor
Color	Blue, pale	Body pink, extremities blue	Completely pink
Reflex response to catheter in nostril	None	Grimace	Cough, Sneeze

Adapted from Apgar V. James LS: Am J Dis Child 1962;**104**:419.
[a]The values for each of the five categories are added to yield a result from 0 to 10.

CLINICAL BACKGROUND

Perinatal asphyxia can be defined as fetal hypoxia during labor and delivery. Hypoxia in the perinatal period is believed to be a major cause of both perinatal deaths and impaired development and neurologic function among survivors. The causes of perinatal asphyxia are not completely understood, but a number of factors have been associated with hypoxia during labor and delivery, including preeclampsia or eclampsia, maternal hypotension, placental insufficiency, and prematurity. The passage of meconium and the presence of this material in the amniotic fluid indicate possible fetal distress.

The pathogenesis of perinatal asphyxia is presented in Figure 8–1. The development of severe metabolic acidosis in the fetus indicates a lack of oxygen. This is because tissues must resort to anaerobic glycolysis for energy production. The degree of hypoxia that a fetus can tolerate before cellular injury occurs is variable and depends on a variety of factors, including previous asphyxia during the pregnancy, metabolic needs versus metabolic reserves, and blood flow to vital organs.

In experimental studies on newborn primates, varying degrees of asphyxia have been induced. These studies have shown that for brain injury to occur, the fetus must be exposed to marked asphyxia for at least 25 minutes. These studies also indicate that this degree of asphyxia will probably lead to fetal death rather than survival with neurologic impairment. In general, research has shown that the immature nervous system is more resistant to hypoxic injury than the mature brain.

STUDY DESIGN

The parents of the newborn in the Patient Profile are understandably distraught by the unanticipated complications in their baby's first hours of life. Naturally, they have questions about what the future will bring. Will their son develop normal mental capacity? Will he have physical disabilities? Questions such as these from concerned parents often can be answered from the pediatrician's own clinical experience. Physicians who have seen only a few such patients, however, must consult the medical literature to respond to parental concerns.

In undertaking such a search, the pediatrician will find a variety of case reports concerning infants who have had severe perinatal asphyxia and have developed various acute and chronic medical problems. Some of these reports describe dismal outcomes, including death. However, there are also reports of instances of severe asphyxia during delivery in which the child later had normal neurologic development and excellent school performance. Thus the pediatrician may be uncertain about what to tell parents. Clearly, a broad spectrum of outcomes is possible. What the pediatrician in our example needs to find are studies that offer reliable evidence of the likelihood of each of the various possible outcomes.

The most definitive conclusions could be drawn from a **clinical trial.** This would be a study in which newborns are randomly assigned to groups with different levels of perinatal asphyxia and then followed with measurements of outcome, such as achievement of developmental milestones and school performance. This type of study has actually been performed on laboratory animals, but obviously such a study on human infants would be unethical. An investigator could not intentionally expose humans to potentially harmful conditions simply to learn about the effects on outcome.

Since intentional exposure of human newborns to asphyxia cannot be justified on ethical grounds, the investigator might resort to observing the outcomes of newborns who develop asphyxia under natural circumstances.

This type of study is characterized as **observational,** because the investigator does not determine the assignment of exposure, but instead passively observes events as they unfold. The ob-

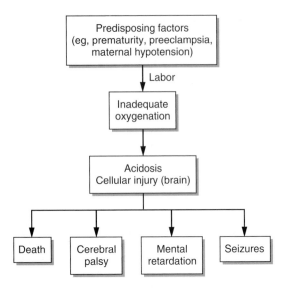

Figure 8–1. Schematic representation of the pathogenesis of perinatal asphyxia.

servational study design that is most similar to the clinical trial is a cohort study. In this type of study, as illustrated in Figure 8–2, the investigators identify a population (**cohort**) and determine their initial characteristics (exposure status). A cohort for an asphyxia study might consist of infants born with perinatal asphyxia and infants born without this condition.

The researchers then follow the cohort over time and determine the outcome in the exposed and unexposed groups. It is important to remember that in a **cohort study,** information about the risk factor (exposure) is determined prior to the observation of disease status.

A large cohort study was conducted in the United States on the utility of Apgar scores as predictors of chronic neurologic disability. In this study, investigators evaluated 49,000 infants whose Apgar scores were recorded at 1 and 5 minutes of age. For those infants who did not achieve a score of 8 or higher at 5 minutes, Apgar scores were then recorded at 10, 15, and 20 minutes. All the children were then followed to the age of 7 years. The occurrence of seizures was determined through clinical observations in the newborn nursery; interval histories were recorded at 4, 8, 12, and 18 months of age and yearly thereafter. The presence of cerebral palsy was determined by physical examination at age 7 years. A psychological and developmental assessment was also performed at age 7. The design of this study is shown in Figure 8–3.

This study demonstrated that low Apgar scores are a risk factor for the development of cerebral palsy. However, 55% of the children with cerebral palsy at age 7 had Apgar scores of 7 or higher at 1 minute, and 73% scored 7 or higher at 5 minutes. Of the 99 children

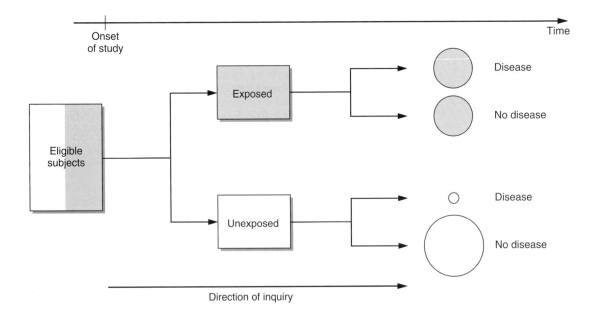

Figure 8–2. Schematic diagram of a cohort study. Shaded areas represent exposed persons, and unshaded areas represent unexposed persons.

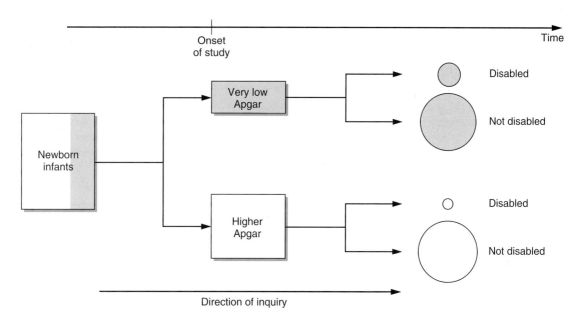

Figure 8–3. Schematic diagram of a cohort study of the relationship between perinatal asphyxia and chronic neurological disability. Shaded areas represent newborns with very low Apgar scores, and unshaded areas represent newborns with intermediate or high Apgar scores.

who survived and had Apgar scores of 0–3 at 10, 15, or 20 minutes, 12 were found to have cerebral palsy. Eleven of those 12 also had delayed mental development. Ten of those infants had seizures in the first 24 hours of life. Of the children who survived and had Apgar scores of 0–3 at 10 minutes or later, 80% were free of any major handicap at early school age.

This study of a large population of children provides the pediatrician in the Patient Profile with the kind of information needed to discuss the baby's prognosis with his parents. The study represents a range of experience that no individual practitioner could compile, even in a lifetime of practice. The pediatrician can now advise the parents that although their baby does have an increased risk of cerebral palsy and developmental delay, such an outcome occurs in only about one of eight asphyxiated neonates. Because the baby did not have a seizure in the first 24 hours of life, the prognosis may be more favorable. It should be reassuring to the parents to learn that 80% of even the most severely asphyxiated newborns were free of major neurologic handicap at early school age.

Perhaps the contributions of cohort studies can be illustrated best by the Framingham Heart Study, one of the most widely recognized and most influential studies of this type. In that investigation, the status of the residents of Framingham, Massachusetts, was determined with respect to potential risk factors for cardiovascular

disease. Beginning in 1950, a sample of 6500 individuals aged 30–59 years was chosen from a total population of approximately 10,000 people in that age group. Approximately 5100 subjects with no clinical evidence of atherosclerotic cardiovascular disease agreed to participate in the study. Each subject was examined at the beginning of the study and was reexamined every 2 years thereafter. For example, the investigators identified subjects who had elevated blood pressure, subjects who smoked, and subjects who had elevated serum cholesterol levels. The population was followed over 35 years to identify subjects who suffered a myocardial infarction, stroke, or other adverse cardiovascular event. This protocol allowed investigators to determine if an individual with hypertension, for example, was more likely to suffer a stroke than someone with normal blood pressure.

More than 250 research reports have been produced by the Framingham Heart Study investigators and their collaborators. The Framingham Heart Study is the source of much of our current knowledge about the risk factors for cardiovascular morbidity and mortality. This cohort has also been used to collect information regarding various other diseases.

Framingham was chosen as the site for the study for many reasons, but primarily because the community is stable and there is broad representation of occupations among the population. The Framingham study is limited, however, because its participants are mainly white, middle class individuals.

TIMING OF MEASUREMENTS

A cohort study is usually **prospective,** that is, exposure to the risk factor and subsequent health outcomes are observed after the beginning of the study (Figure 8–3). For example, a prospective cohort study of neonatal asphyxia and subsequent mental retardation could be started in 2000. The degree of neonatal asphyxia could be determined for births occurring through 2001, and the development of mental retardation could be assessed between 2001 and 2006, or later. An alternative name for such a cohort study is a **longitudinal study.**

Occasionally, a cohort study is **retrospective** (or historical), that is, it utilizes information on prior exposure to the risk factor and subsequent disease status. As shown in Figure 8–4, a retrospective cohort study of neonatal asphyxia and neurologic disability designed in 2001 might involve a review of the medical records of infants born in a particular hospital in 1989 to determine the level of asphyxia, followed by a review of school achievement records over

the period 1999–2000 to determine the degree of intellectual functioning. Note that exposure to risk factors and the subsequent development of the health outcome occur prior to the beginning of the retrospective cohort study.

The advantage of the retrospective cohort design is that all the events under study have already occurred, and conclusions can therefore be drawn more rapidly. In addition, the cost of a retrospective cohort study might be substantially lower for the same reason. The retrospective approach may also be the only feasible way to study the effects of exposures that no longer occur, for example, discontinued medical treatments. On the other hand, a retrospective cohort study must usually rely on existing records or subject recall; both are usually less complete and accurate than data collected in a prospective study. Attributes of prospective and retrospective cohort studies are compared in Table 8–2.

It should now be clear that a prospective cohort study often takes a long time to complete. Furthermore, to ensure that there are enough subjects to reach a valid conclusion, a cohort study (either prospective or retrospective) usually requires a fairly large number of individuals with the potential to develop the outcome

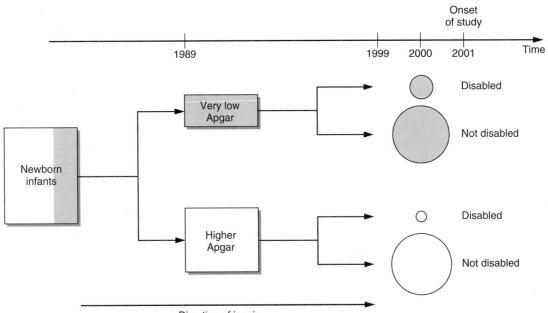

Figure 8–4. Schematic diagram of a retrospective cohort study of the relationship between perinatal asphyxia and chronic neurological disability. Shaded areas represent newborns with very low Apgar scores, and unshaded areas represent newborns with intermediate or high Apgar scores.

Table 8–2. Comparison of the attributes of retrospective and prospective cohort studies.

Attribute	Retrospective Approach	Prospective Approach
Information	Less complete and accurate	More complete and accurate
Discontinued exposures	Useful	Not useful
Emerging new exposures	Not useful	Useful
Expense	Less costly	More costly
Completion time	Shorter	Longer

of interest. For example, in the study of perinatal asphyxia, data concerning 49,000 subjects were accumulated over a 7-year period. For this reason, such studies can be expensive to complete. In fact, if the outcome of interest under study is rare, the sample size required for a cohort study may be so large that it would be impractical to undertake such a study. On the other hand, if the exposure or risk factor is rare, a well-designed cohort study may offer superior statistical power to evaluate associations between exposure and subsequent development of disease, because this type of study allows selective inclusion of exposed persons. A cohort study of perinatal asphyxia, for example, could include all newborns with Apgar scores of 0–3, but only a sample of the larger pool of newborns with higher scores.

Following subjects over a long period of time can lead to various problems. Subjects may move away or leave the study for other reasons, including death from causes other than the disease under investigation. If the losses to follow-up are substantial, and the lost subjects differ in outcome from those who remain in the study, the validity of the results can be affected seriously. It is also possible for exposure status to change during the course of the study. Obviously, birth asphyxia occurs only once. In other circumstances, however, the exposure under study may be subject to variation over time. For example, a cigarette smoker may quit, or in an occupational cohort study, employees may change jobs,

and therefore their level of exposure to an occupational hazard may change. Diagnostic methods used for the disease under study may also vary over time.

The advantages and disadvantages of cohort studies are presented in Table 8–3.

SELECTION OF SUBJECTS

Selection of subjects for a cohort study is influenced by various factors, including (1) the type of exposure under investigation, (2) the frequency of the exposure in the population, and (3) the accessibility of subjects and the likelihood of their continuing participation. Both exposed and unexposed groups must be free of the outcome of interest at the start of the study, and they must be similarly eligible to develop the outcome of interest during the course of the study. If some subjects already have the outcome of interest at the onset of the study, the temporal relationship between exposure and outcome will be obscured.

The Exposed Group

The type of exposure under investigation is critical for selection of the exposed group. Some exposures during pregnancy are common, such as gestational diabetes or hypertension. For these exposures, a general population of pregnant women could be used to construct the co-

Table 8–3. Advantages and disadvantages of cohort studies.

Advantages	Disadvantages
Direct calculation of risk ratio (relative risk)	Time consuming
May yield information on the incidence of disease	Often requires a large sample size
Clear temporal relationship between exposure and disease	Expensive
Particularly efficient for study of rare exposures	Not efficient for the study of rare diseases
Can yield information on multiple exposures	Losses to follow-up may diminish validity
Can yield information on multiple outcomes of a particular exposure	Changes over time in diagnostic methods may lead to biased results
Minimizes bias	
Strongest observational design for establishing cause and effect relationship	

hort. Other exposures, such as in vitro fertilization, are not common. In a cohort study designed to evaluate whether in vitro fertilization is a risk factor for developmental disability in the offspring, it may be necessary to sample exposed subjects from an infertility clinic rather than from among pregnant women in the general population.

Feasibility issues are also important in selecting the exposed population. The investigator should identify an accessible population that is motivated to participate in the study and unlikely to discontinue participation. The availability of historical information such as medical records may also be a factor in selecting this group. Examples of groups that have been chosen for feasibility reasons include nurses, members of health maintenance organizations, residents of stable communities, and labor union members.

The degree of exposure may differ depending on the goals of the study. For some exposures, subjects are classified into one of two groups: exposed or unexposed. In vitro fertilization is an example of this type of dichotomization. Other studies involve a range of exposure levels, for example, Apgar scores as an indicator of perinatal asphyxia. The investigator may take a graded exposure variable, such as the Apgar score, and transform it into a categorical exposure by dividing subjects into those whose score exceeds a certain designated value (eg, Apgar score of 3) and those whose score falls below that value. The value chosen to separate groups is referred to as a **cutoff point** and can be selected in various ways. For example, the cutoff point might be selected on the basis of the underlying distribution of values, such as the point that separates the 10% of subjects with the lowest Apgar scores from the remainder of the population. Alternately, a standard cutoff point can be used that is believed to have pathophysiologic implications, regardless of the underlying distribution in the population.

Thus, Apgar scores can be classified in three different ways: dichotomous (0–3 versus > 3), multiple ordered (0–3, 4–6, 7–10), or continuous (by gradations). If the exposure can be categorized into multiple levels or gradations, the investigator can determine whether a relationship exists between the dose (of the exposure) and the response. In the present context, the study may seek to determine whether the risk of chronic neurologic disability rises as the Apgar score decreases. If such a trend is observed, the argument that perinatal asphyxia is a cause of chronic neurologic disability is strengthened.

The Unexposed Group

Feasibility issues for the unexposed group are similar to those for the exposed group. The unexposed group must be accessible for entry into the study and for fol-low-up. When the purpose of a cohort study is to investigate a community, such as in the Framingham Heart Study, that community is the source of the unexposed persons. Because there may be more unexposed people in the community than are needed for the investigation, a representative sample may be taken. In the Framingham Heart Study, several risk factors were of interest, all of which were relatively prevalent in the community. In this situation, a sample of the entire community was drawn and then subdivided into exposure groups, depending on the risk factor of interest in a particular analysis. In the study of perinatal asphyxia, the unexposed group was defined as the infants with the highest Apgar scores (7–10), indicating the lowest degree of perinatal asphyxia.

For cohort studies that involve the selection of a specific exposed population, selection of an appropriate comparison population may be less clear-cut. For example, in a study of in vitro fertilization as a risk factor for congenital malformations, the comparison group might be pregnant women who are followed in other obstetric practices. If, however, pregnant women in the comparison population are not followed with a comparable level of clinical scrutiny, or if the unexposed group of pregnant women differs from the exposed group of pregnant women in other ways that might be related to congenital malformations, the study may lead to a false conclusion. The investigator may relate an observed increased risk of congenital malformation to in vitro fertilization, when in fact the elevated risk is the result of other differences between the exposed and unexposed groups. This type of problem illustrates why a randomized controlled clinical trial may be less susceptible to error than a cohort study. With randomization, factors known to be related to the development of disease—as well as other factors not yet recognized as related to the disease—tend to be balanced between the groups. This increases confidence that an observed association is in fact the result of the exposure of interest rather than the result of some other characteristic.

The underlying principle in selecting the unexposed group is that it should yield a fair comparison with the exposed group. Occasionally, the frequency of outcome occurrence in the exposed population is compared with the occurrence in the general population. This is particularly useful when members of the general population are very unlikely to be exposed to the study factor. However, the general population may not be comparable with those in the exposed group. For example, follow-up for disease occurrence may be more (or less) complete than for the exposed study group. This may lead to erroneous conclusions. Furthermore, if the exposed and unexposed groups are chosen from different time periods (a nonconcurrent study), medical care or other factors may differ between the groups in a way that makes the comparison unfair and the results invalid. Suggestions for the selection of exposed and unexposed subjects are presented in Table 8–4.

DATA COLLECTION

The investigator must collect information on both the independent variable (exposure) and the dependent variable (response) during the course of a cohort study.

Exposure

It is essential to define the exposure clearly. Some exposures are acute, one-time episodes, never repeated in a subject's lifetime (eg, asphyxia at birth). Other exposures are long term, such as cigarette smoking or the use of oral contraceptives. Exposures may also be intermittent, such as pregnancy-induced hypertension, which may occur during one pregnancy, disappear after delivery, and perhaps reappear during subsequent pregnancies. The types of exposure characteristics that should be considered are presented in Table 8–5.

A subject who originally satisfies the criteria for inclusion in a cohort study should not subsequently be excluded from the analysis because of a change in exposure status during follow-up. This type of exclusion may lead to a biased conclusion. Specifically, it is possible that a change in exposure status may indicate a change in outcome status. For example, in a study of the relationship between the use of an antinausea medication during pregnancy and subsequent risk of spontaneous abortion, the medication may be discontinued for a subject because of early signs of threatened abortion. Excluding this subject from the analysis, therefore, may result in an underestimate of the true link between use of the medication and risk of abortion. The potential for changes in exposure status has important implications for the frequency of follow-up. Frequent re-

Table 8–5. Measurements of exposure used in cohort studies.[a]

Measurements of Exposure	Examples
Intensity	Mean blood pressure level
Duration	Weeks of hypertension
Regularity	Number of affected pregnancies
Variability	Range of measured blood pressures

[a]Example: gestational hypertension.

assessment of exposure and outcome status may be required if exposure status changes over time.

The source of available information about exposure may constrain the ability of the investigator to define and measure exposure experience. If the information comes from medical records, as is sometimes necessary in a retrospective cohort study, the accuracy of exposure information may be poor. For example, there are inherent disadvantages in using Apgar scores from medical records. Sometimes the Apgar scoring system is recorded by the medical staff as part of the required paperwork after delivery, without careful timing of the observations and detailed assessment by multiple observers. The medical staff providing patient care may be distracted by other responsibilities. In the previously cited prospective cohort study of neonatal asphyxia, a specially trained independent observer who was not responsible for patient care recorded the score in a standard manner on a standardized study form at exactly 1, 5, and 10 minutes of life.

In general, objective measures of exposure or biological markers of exposure are preferred over subjective measures. For example, in a study of maternal use of illicit drugs and pregnancy outcome, one approach to exposure assessment would be to question pregnant

Table 8–4. Guidelines for selection of exposed and unexposed subjects in cohort studies.

Unexposed	Exposed	Unexposed and Exposed
Unexposed persons should be sampled from the same (or comparable) source population as the exposed group	The baseline characteristics of exposed persons should not differ systematically from those of unexposed persons, except for the exposure of interest	Both exposed and unexposed groups should be free of the disease of interest and equally susceptible to development of the disease at the beginning of the study
Multiple comparison groups of unexposed subjects chosen in different ways may reinforce the validity of findings		Equivalent information (quantity and quality) should be available on exposure and disease status in the exposed and unexposed groups
		Both groups should be accessible and available for follow-up

women about their use of illicit drugs. Self-reports of illicit drug use, however, are likely to underrepresent actual exposure. Repeated measurements of drug metabolites in urine might provide a more accurate and reliable assessment of exposure.

Clinical Response

Before the start of the study, it is imperative to determine that subjects do not have the outcome (disease) under investigation. This may be particularly difficult if the outcome is a disease that develops slowly, has an insidious onset, and is asymptomatic until its late stages. One approach to this problem is to exclude cases in which the disease emerges early in the course of the investigation, under the assumption that the biological onset of disease preceded the beginning of the study.

The degree of surveillance for disease should be similar in the exposed and unexposed groups. The frequency of examination and the duration of follow-up depend on the type of exposure and the outcome under investigation. For some diseases, the time from exposure to development of disease is short. A cohort study of the relationship between exposure to perinatal asphyxia and death within the first week of life would have a short follow-up period. Other outcomes, such as chronic neurologic disability, may require years to assess. Because the investigators were interested in performance and cognitive ability at early school age, the study of the relationship of perinatal asphyxia to neurologic development required 7 years of follow-up.

Information on outcome status may come from various sources. Some cohort studies rely on information from the records of physicians and hospitals. This would be particularly pertinent for a cohort study focusing on a population with good access to health care and standardized recordkeeping practices, such as a prepaid health plan. Other cohort studies may combine physician records with periodic examinations by the investigators. The Framingham Heart Study is an example of this type of study. Another approach to collecting information on disease is to have the subjects report whether they develop the outcome of interest. The study may also involve reviews of medical records in a subset of subjects to confirm self-reports.

If the outcome under study is death from any cause, the investigator may use information from death certificates. Death certificates may have limited utility, however, if the study focuses on a specific disease, because cause-of-death information on death certificates may be inaccurate (see Chapter 4). Obviously, in that circumstance the best information would come from autopsy reports. This approach may not be feasible, however, since most people who die are not autopsied.

If diagnostic evaluations are required by the investigator during the study, an appropriate diagnostic test for the disease must be available (see Chapter 6). This approach has limitations because diagnostic tests are not always available or feasible. To ensure a fair comparison between the exposed and unexposed groups, the accuracy and reliability of diagnosis must not differ between the groups. Thus it can be helpful if those who assess outcomes are unaware of the subjects' exposure status. The study of perinatal asphyxia relied on standard neurologic examination and psychological tests. The examiners had no access to the medical records, and thus were blind to the Apgar scores of the children. This blinded approach should facilitate an assessment of neurologic outcomes that is comparable for exposed and unexposed children.

It is possible for exposure status to alter the surveillance for disease. An example of this problem could occur in a study of neonatal asphyxia and intellectual development. Physicians are more likely to administer psychological and developmental tests to an infant who had a difficult birth with low Apgar scores; that child is therefore more likely to be diagnosed as having subtle developmental problems than another child who has not been singled out for close surveillance. This could lead to an overestimate of the relationship between neonatal asphyxia and subsequent developmental disability. This problem, however, can be avoided, as in the cited study, by ensuring that a standard diagnostic protocol is followed, regardless of exposure status.

ANALYSIS

Several different approaches can be used to analyze the results of a cohort study, as described in the following sections.

Risk Ratio

The results of a cohort study can be summarized using the format shown in Table 8–6. In that table, the letters *A–D* represent numbers of subjects in the four possible combinations of exposure and outcome status (in this instance, death).

A. Exposed persons who later die
B. Unexposed persons who later die
C. Exposed persons who do not die
D. Unexposed persons who do not die

The total number of subjects in this study is the sum of $A + B + C + D$. The total number of exposed persons is $A + C$, and the total number of unexposed persons is $B + D$.

Table 8–6. Summary of risk data from a cohort study.

Outcome[a]	Exposed	Unexposed	Total
Death	A	B	A + B
No death	C	D	C + D
Total	A + C	B + D	A + B + C + D

[a]In some studies, the outcome is development of disease rather than death.

Among exposed persons, the risk (R) of death is defined as

$$R_{(exposed)} = \frac{\text{Exposed persons who die}}{\text{All exposed persons}}$$

$$= \frac{A}{A+C}$$

As indicated in Chapter 2, risk can vary between 0 (no exposed persons die) and 1 (all exposed persons die). As in all statements of risk, some time period for the development of the outcome must be specified. For example, the outcome might be the risk of death in the first year of life. Among unexposed persons, the risk of death is defined as

$$R_{(Unexposed)} = \frac{\text{Unexposed persons who die}}{\text{All unexposed persons}}$$

$$= \frac{B}{B+D}$$

As indicated in Chapters 4 and 7, one approach to contrasting the risk in two groups is to create a ratio measure. The **risk ratio** (RR) or relative risk is

$$RR = \frac{R_{(exposed)}}{R_{(unexposed)}} = \frac{A/(A+C)}{B/(B+D)}$$

If the exposed and unexposed persons have the same risk of death, the RR is 1 (ie, the null value). That is, exposure is not related to the outcome.

If the risk among exposed persons is greater than the corresponding risk among unexposed persons, the RR is greater than 1 (ie, hazardous exposure). In contrast, if the risk among exposed persons is smaller than the corresponding risk among unexposed persons, the RR is less than 1 (ie, beneficial exposure).

The calculation of risk ratio can be illustrated from the study of perinatal asphyxia. The data in Table 8–7 relate to infants who weighed more than 2500 g at birth. Exposure is defined as an Apgar score of 0–3 at 10 minutes of life, and the comparison group of less exposed newborns had Apgar scores of 4–6 at 10 minutes. In the actual study, a third group with Apgar scores of 7–10 was included, but the data are not described here in detail.

The risk among exposed newborns is

$$R_{(exposed)} = \frac{42}{122} = 0.344 = 34.4\%$$

That is, about one of three newborns weighing more than 2500 g and having very low Apgar scores at 10 minutes died during the first year of life. The risk among "less exposed" newborns is

$$R_{(less\ exposed)} = \frac{43}{345} = 0.125 = 12.5\%$$

In other words, one in eight neonates weighing over 2500 g and having intermediate Apgar scores at 10 minutes died during the first year of life.

Without any further calculations, it should be obvious that the neonates with very low 10-minute Apgar scores had a worse prognosis than those with intermediate 10-minute Apgar scores. Quantification of the magnitude of this effect is achieved by calculating the risk ratio

$$RR = \frac{42}{122} \bigg/ \frac{43}{345} = 2.8$$

The RR of 2.8 means that newborns at this birth weight with very low 10-minute Apgar scores are al-

Table 8–7. Relationship between 10-minute Apgar scores and risk of death in the first year of life among children with birth weights of at least 2500 g.[a]

	Apgar Score 0–3	Apgar Score 4–6	Total
Death	42	43	85
No death	80	302	382
Total	122	345	467

[a]Data used, with permission, from Nelson KB, Ellenberg JH: Apgar scores as predictors of chronic neurologic disability. Pediatrics 1981;**68**:36.

most three times more likely to die in the first year of life than similar-weighing newborns with intermediate 10-minute Apgar scores. The *RR* is a measure of the strength of association between exposure and outcome. The farther the *RR* is from the null value of 1, the stronger the association. The strength of association is an important criterion in evaluating whether an observed association is likely to represent a cause-and-effect relationship. The *RR* of 2.8 is consistent with a moderate-to-strong relationship between the exposure (10-minute Apgar score) and outcome (infant death).

As discussed in Chapter 7, a sense of the statistical precision of this estimated risk ratio can be obtained by calculating **confidence intervals** around the point estimate of 2.8. Using the approximation method described in Appendix C, the 95% confidence interval for the data presented in Table 8–7 is (1.9, 4.1). That is, at the 95% level of confidence, the range of *RR* values consistent with the observed data falls between 1.9 and 4.1. Thus the data are consistent with a risk of death in infants with very low Apgar scores between roughly a doubling and a fourfold increase (Figure 8–5). As demonstrated in Chapter 7, the point estimate does not lie in the middle of the *RR* confidence interval. The asymmetry of this interval derives from the skew of the range of values of the risk ratio toward the positive direction (ie, all beneficial effects are compressed into the range 0–1, whereas hazardous effects range from 1 to positive infinity).

Since the null value is excluded from this 95% confidence interval, it can be concluded that the findings are **statistically significant.** In other words, these data are not consistent with the null hypothesis of no associ-

ation between Apgar scores and infant mortality (at the prespecified 95% level of confidence). An association as strong as that observed between Apgar scores and infant mortality, therefore, cannot be explained by chance alone.

As indicated earlier, the argument that the linkage between Apgar score and death in the first year of life is one of cause and effect is strengthened if a dose–response relationship can be demonstrated. A third group of newborns, with Apgar scores of 7–10, was therefore included in the study. Comparison of the risk of death in that group with the previous reference group, which had intermediate Apgar scores of 4–6, yields a risk ratio of 0.15, with an approximate 95% confidence interval of (0.11, 0.21). This result means that newborns with a 10-minute Apgar score of 7–10 have only about one-sixth the risk of death in the first year of life as newborns with Apgar scores of 4–6. This disparity is statistically significant, and the very narrow width of the confidence interval indicates a statistically precise estimate (because it is based on a large number of observations).

The dose–response relationship between Apgar score and the risk ratio of death in the first year of life for newborns weighing more than 2500 g is shown in Figure 8–6. The reference group against which others were compared in the preceding calculations was the group with Apgar scores of 4–6 (ie, the risk ratio for this group is defined as 1). A clear trend of decreasing risk ratio with increasing Apgar score is seen, and this trend is unlikely to have occurred by chance alone. Thus, there is strong evidence in these data for a dose–response relationship.

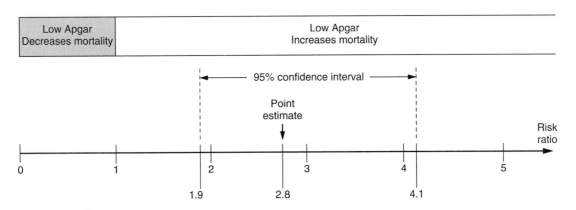

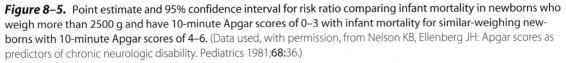

Figure 8–5. Point estimate and 95% confidence interval for risk ratio comparing infant mortality in newborns who weigh more than 2500 g and have 10-minute Apgar scores of 0–3 with infant mortality for similar-weighing newborns with 10-minute Apgar scores of 4–6. (Data used, with permission, from Nelson KB, Ellenberg JH: Apgar scores as predictors of chronic neurologic disability. Pediatrics 1981;**68**:36.)

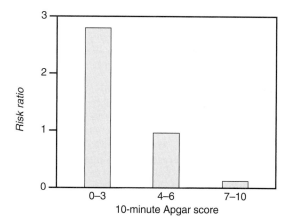

Figure 8–6. Dose–response relationship for the association between 10-minute Apgar scores and risk of death in the first year of life among newborns with a birth weight over 2500 g. (Data used, with permission, from Nelson KB, Ellenberg JH: Apgar scores as predictors of chronic neurologic disability. Pediatrics 1981;**68**:36.

Attributable Risk Percent

The risk of a specified outcome can be compared with measures other than a ratio. For example, the risk for one group can be subtracted from the risk for another group. This measure is termed the risk difference, or excess risk. Some authors use the term "attributable risk" for this measure, but that expression is discouraged here because it may be confused with other expressions. The risk difference (*RD*) is defined as

$$RD = R_{(exposed)} - R_{(Unexposed)}$$
$$= \frac{A}{A+C} - \frac{B}{B+D}$$

Using the previously cited data relating 10-minute Apgar scores (0–3 versus 4–6) to the risk of death in the first year of life, we calculate the risk difference as

$$RD = \frac{42}{122} - \frac{43}{345} = 0.344 - 0.125 = 0.219$$

That is, the risk of death in the first year of life is increased by 0.219 for newborns who weigh more than 2500 g and have a 10-minute Apgar score of 0–3, compared with similar-weighing newborns with a 10-minute Apgar score of 4–6.

Another measure of interest is the attributable risk percent (*ARP*), in which the risk difference is expressed as a percentage of the total risk experienced by the exposed group:

$$ARP = \frac{R_{(exposed)} - R_{(unexposed)}}{R_{(exposed)}} \times 100$$
$$= \frac{A/(A+C) - B/(B+D)}{A/(A+C)} \times 100$$

For the Apgar score–infant mortality data, the attributable risk percent is

$$ARP = \frac{(0.344 - 0.125)}{0.344} \times 100 = 63.7\%$$

In other words, almost two thirds of the total risk of infant mortality for newborns who weigh more than 2500 g and have 10-minute Apgar scores of 0–3 is related to an Apgar score below the 4–6 level. The attributable risk percent typically is used as an indicator of the public health impact of exposure. These data suggest that birth asphyxia is a major contributor to—but not the sole cause of—infant mortality among severely asphyxiated children.

Rate Ratio

The analyses presented thus far are based on comparisons of risk estimates across exposure groups. In a cohort study, the measured outcome may be an incidence (or mortality) rate rather than a risk. Rate data in a cohort study can be summarized using the format shown in Table 8–8. The rate ratio is derived as follows

$$\text{Rate ratio} = \frac{\text{Rate of outcome among exposed persons}}{\text{Rate of outcome among unexposed persons}}$$
$$= \frac{A/PT_{(exposed)}}{B/PT_{(unexposed)}}$$

Table 8–8. Summary format of rate data from a cohort study.

	Exposed Persons	Unexposed Persons	Total
Number of outcomes	A	B	A + B
Person-time (PT)	PT(exposed)	PT(unexposed)	PT(total)

The magnitude of the rate ratio is interpreted in the same manner as the risk ratio (< 1 = protective effect, 1 = no effect, > 1 = harmful effect of exposure). The farther away from the null value, the stronger the association between exposure and the rate of the outcome. The data collected in the study of perinatal asphyxia were not presented in a manner that allows calculation of rate ratios.

To illustrate this measure, data are drawn from the Chicago Heart Association Detection Project in Industry (Dyer et al, 1992). That investigation involved almost 40,000 men and women at 84 cooperating companies and institutions in the Chicago area. Subjects were enrolled between 1967 and 1973, screened for risk factors for cardiovascular disease, and then followed an average of 14–15 years. For white males aged 25–39 at entry, the relationship between baseline serum cholesterol level and subsequent rate of coronary heart disease (CHD) is shown in Table 8–9. The rate ratio is

$$\text{Rate ratio} = \frac{26 / 36,581}{14 / 68,239} = 3.5$$

In other words, the mortality rate from CHD among white males with borderline high cholesterol levels was about 3.5 times higher than that of white males with lower cholesterol levels. Adjustment for underlying age differences in the study groups reduced the observed rate ratio to 3.1. Comparison of mortality from CHD among white males aged 25–39 with high serum cholesterol levels (> 6.2 mmol/L [> 240 mg/dL]) with white males of the same age with normal serum cholesterol levels (< 5.1 mmol/L [< 197 mg/dL]) yielded an age-adjusted rate ratio of 5.1. Thus, a dose–response relationship was evident between baseline serum cholesterol level and subsequent CHD mortality.

SUMMARY

In this chapter, the basic approach to the design and analysis of cohort studies is presented, with illustrations drawn primarily from the literature on birth asphyxia. A cohort study is a type of observational investigation in which subjects are classified on the basis of level of exposure to a risk factor and followed to determine subsequent disease outcome. **Prospective** cohort studies are conducted by making all observations on exposure and disease status after the onset of the investigation. **Retrospective** cohort studies involve observations on exposure and disease status prior to the onset of the study. The retrospective approach offers several pragmatic advantages, but may result in less accurate and complete information on exposure and disease status.

Cohort studies are statistically efficient for the study of rare exposures because the exposed individuals can be selectively included in the study. On the other hand, cohort studies are inefficient for the investigation of slowly developing or rare diseases. The evaluation of chronic diseases through the cohort approach requires a long follow-up period and increases the chances that subjects will be lost from the study. The evaluation of rare diseases with the cohort study approach requires a large sample size and therefore is expensive and labor intensive.

There are several basic strategies to analyze cohort studies. If data are collected on the risk of developing an outcome during a specified period of time, the summary measure of effect typically is the **risk ratio,** or the risk of the outcome among exposed individuals divided by the risk of the outcome among unexposed individuals. An alternative approach to contrasting risks is the **risk difference,** which is the risk among exposed persons minus the risk among unexposed persons. If the risk difference is divided by the risk among exposed persons, a measure termed the attributable risk percent is derived. The **attributable risk percent** is an indicator of the proportion of risk that may be attributable to the exposure per se. When data in a cohort study are based on the rate of disease outcome, the standard measure of effect is the **rate ratio.**

The prospective cohort study of perinatal asphyxia cited in this chapter indicates that Apgar scores can serve as a useful predictor of subsequent risk of death and neurologic disability. An inverse dose–response relationship occurs between Apgar score level and the risk of adverse neurologic outcome. In spite of the increased risk, however, most children with low Apgar scores survive and do not manifest neurologic or developmental disability. Through proper interpretation of the results of this co-

Table 8–9. Relationship between baseline serum cholesterol level and subsequent mortality rate from coronary heart disease among white males aged 25–39 at entry into the Chicago Heart Association Study.[a]

	Cholesterol Level		
	5.2–6.2 mmol/L[b]	≤5.1 mmol/L[c]	Total
Deaths	26	14	40
Person-years	36,581	68,239	104,820

[a]Data from Dyer AR, Stamler J, Shekelle RB: Serum cholesterol and mortality from coronary heart disease in young, middle-aged, and older men and women from three Chicago epidemiologic studies. Ann Epidemiol 1992;**2**:51.
[b]201–240 mg/dL.
[c]≤197 mg/dL.

hort study, the pediatrician in the Patient Profile can inform the baby's parents that although their child faces an increased risk of certain disabilities, there is about an 80% chance that no neurologic handicaps will develop.

☑ STUDY QUESTIONS

Questions 1–5: A cohort study is conducted to evaluate the relationship between exposure to solid foods at an early age and the development of asthma. In the study, 1000 infants who had solid food introduced before 4 months of age are compared to 1000 infants who had solid food introduced after 6 months of age. The results are shown in Table 8–10. For each numbered question below, select the single best answer from the lettered options.

1. What is the risk of asthma in the group that had early introduction of solid foods?
   A. 0.10
   B. 0.15
   C. 0.20
   D. 0.25
   E. 0.35

2. What is the risk of asthma in the group that had late introduction of solid foods?
   A. 0.10
   B. 0.15
   C. 0.20
   D. 0.25
   E. 0.35

3. What is the risk ratio (early introduction of solids versus late introduction) for the occurrence of asthma?
   A. 0.05
   B. 0.50
   C. 1.0
   D. 2.0
   E. 3.0

4. The point estimate for the risk ratio in question 3 indicates that the risk of asthma associated with early introduction of solids is
   A. Decreased
   B. Increased
   C. Not affected
   D. Cannot be determined

5. The 95% confidence interval for the point estimate is 1.4 to 4.5. The correct interpretation of these results is
   A. A statistically significant association exists between early introduction of solids and increased risk for the development of asthma at the level of $p < 0.05$.
   B. A statistically significant relationship exists between early introduction of solid foods and decreased risk for the development of asthma at the level of $p < 0.05$.
   C. It can be concluded with 95% confidence that early introduction of solids is protective for development of asthma.
   D. Breast feeding is an important intervention to prevent the development of asthma.
   E. The risk of asthma is not statistically significantly different between early and late introduction of solid foods at the level of $p < 0.05$.

Questions 6–10: A cohort study is performed to evaluate the relationship between inflammation as measured by a high C-reactive protein and the occurrence of myocardial infarction among women. In the study, 500 subjects with high C-reactive protein and 500 subjects with normal C-reactive protein are studied over a 20-year period.

During the study, 50 of the women with high C-reactive protein and 15 of the women with normal C-reactive protein develop a newly diagnosed myocardial infarction.

6. The incidence rate (per 10,000 person years) for myocardial infarction among women with a high C-reactive protein is
   A. 15
   B. 25
   C. 30
   D. 50
   E. 60
   F. Incidence cannot be determined

Table 8–10. Relationship between exposure to solid foods at an early age and development of asthma.

Introduction of Solid Food	Health Status		
	Asthma	No Asthma	Total
Early	200	800	1000
Late	100	900	1000
Total	300	1700	2000

7. The incidence rate (per 10,000 person years) for a myocardial infarction for a person with normal C-reactive protein is

A. 15

B. 25

C. 30

D. 50

E. 60

F. Incidence cannot be determined

8. The incidence rate ratio for myocardial infarction is

A. 0.9

B. 1.0

C. 2.3

D. 3.3

E. 5.0

9. The risk difference is

A. 0.005

B. 0.007

C. 0.07

D. 0.05

E. 1.0

10. The attributable risk percent is

A. 25%

B. 35.5%

C. 50%

D. 70%

E. 90%

FURTHER READING

Grimes DA, Schulz KF: Cohort studies: marching towards outcomes. Lancet 2002;**359:**341.

REFERENCES

Clinical Background

Rosenbaum P: Cerebral palsy: what parents and doctors want to know. BMJ 2003;**326:**970.

Study Design

Feinleib M: The Framingham Study: Sample selection, follow-up, and methods of analysis. In: *National Cancer Institute Monograph,* No. 67. Greenwald P (editor). US Department of Health and Human Services, 1985.

Nelson KB, Ellenberg JH: Apgar scores as predictors of chronic neurologic disability. Pediatrics 1981;**68:**36.

Timing of Measurements

Greenberg RS: Prospective studies. In: *Encyclopedia of Statistical Sciences,* Vol 7. Kotz S, Johnson NL (editors). Wiley, 1986.

Greenberg RS: Retrospective studies (including case-control). In: *Encyclopedia of Statistical Sciences,* Vol 8. Kotz S, Johnson NL (editors). Wiley, 1988.

Analysis

Dyer AR, Stamler J, Shekelle RB: Serum cholesterol and mortality from coronary heart disease in young, middle-aged, and older men and women in three Chicago epidemiologic studies. Ann Epidemiol 1992;**2:**51.

e-PIDEMIOLOGY

Study Design

http://www.bmj.com/epidem/epid.7.shtml

http://www.framingham.com/heart

Timing of Measurements

http://www.pitt.edu/~super1/lecture/lec0561/index.htm

Overview

http://www.pitt.edu/~super1/lecture/lec10301/index.htm

http://www.pitt.edu/~super1/lecture/lec8581/index.htm

Case–Control Studies

KEY CONCEPTS

1. A case–control study is an observational study in which subjects are sampled based upon presence or absence of disease and then their prior exposure status is determined.

2. Case–control studies are statistically efficient and cost-effective for the study of rare diseases, and multiple risk factors can be investigated in a case–control study.

3. Newly diagnosed persons with disease are referred to as incident cases, whereas previously existing cases are referred to as prevalent cases.

4. Ideally, the controls should have a prevalence of exposure that is the same as the population of unaffected persons.

5. A population-based study is one in which cases and controls are sampled from a defined population, such as a metropolitan area.

6. A hospital-based sample of cases and controls may be convenient and inexpensive to collect, but may be biased by factors that affect the likelihood of hospitalization for cases and controls.

7. If sampling of cases, controls, or both is influenced by prior exposure history, then a selection bias may be present.

8. Confounding occurs when the apparent effect of the exposure of interest is attributable in whole or in part to some other factor.

9. Matching in a case–control study involves sampling of controls to parallel selected characteristics of cases in order to reduce the likelihood of confounding by the matched features.

10. The odds ratio is a measure of association between the exposure and disease that can be calculated in case–control studies.

PATIENT PROFILE

A 55-year-old woman was in excellent health until 2 weeks before admission, when she developed malaise, low-grade fever, cough, and generalized muscle pain. Although she took aspirin, her symptoms became worse over the next several days, in particular increased muscle pain, which made it very difficult for her to rise from a chair. She then consulted her personal physician, who performed a thorough evaluation. The patient's history was unremarkable except for insomnia over the previous year, which she treated with self-prescribed L-tryptophan. On physical examination, she had mild, diffuse muscle tenderness and a mild, erythematous maculopapular rash over much of her body. Laboratory examination was remarkable for elevations of her blood eosinophil count (2000 cells per mm^3, < 250 cells per mm^3) and mildly elevated aldolase levels. Eosinophilia-myalgia syndrome (EMS) was diagnosed.

CLINICAL BACKGROUND

In November 1989, researchers from the Centers for Disease Control and Prevention (CDC) and local health departments published the first description of EMS. This newly recognized syndrome is characterized by incapacitating myalgias (muscle pains), elevated eosinophil counts, and in some patients, arthralgias (joint pains), skin thickening, hair loss, and interstitial lung disease.

EMS was first recognized in October 1989, when astute physicians determined that three people with unexplained myalgias and eosinophilia had consumed L-tryptophan, an essential amino acid available without prescription in drug and health food stores. Prompt response by health departments quickly led to case–control studies, the results of which suggested that ingestion of L-tryptophan was the cause of EMS. L-Tryptophan–containing products were taken off the market in November 1989.

EMS occurs predominantly in women and is relatively rare. Nationwide disease surveillance conducted by the CDC led to identification of about 1500 cases of EMS, including 40 fatalities; nearly all cases occurred between mid-1988 and the end of 1989, although the actual number of cases was probably several times higher than the reported number. In 1990, after the recall of L-tryptophan, the number of reported cases fell to near zero.

Further case–control studies showed that of the people studied, nearly everyone with EMS (cases) but only about half of those without EMS (controls) had consumed L-tryptophan produced by one particular manufacturer. Further inquiry disclosed that this company had changed manufacturing conditions prior to and during the period of the epidemic. Risk of developing EMS among those consuming L-tryptophan from this manufacturer was estimated to be 20 to 40 times higher than the risk among those consuming L-tryptophan from other sources. The epidemic was attributed to contamination of the L-tryptophan during production by the implicated manufacturer. Although many contaminants have been identified chemically in L-tryptophan produced by that manufacturer, the search to identify the specific contaminant or contaminants that cause EMS has been hampered by the lack of an animal model that can reproduce the full spectrum of EMS seen in humans.

The history of EMS illustrates the importance of astute clinical observations and the value of a rapid public health response, which led to the timely recall of L-tryptophan and the prevention of an even larger outbreak of disease. The initial study, as well as most of the subsequent investigations, linking consumption of L-tryptophan with the occurrence of EMS were based on a case–control design. In this chapter, case–control studies are described in detail.

INTRODUCTION

As with cohort studies, case–control investigations typically are designed to assess the association between occurrence of disease and an exposure suspected of causing (or preventing) that disease. In many situations, however, a case–control study is more efficient than a cohort study because a smaller sample size is required.

The primary feature that distinguishes a case–control study from a cohort study is selection of subjects based on their disease status. The investigator selects cases from among those persons who have the disease of interest and controls from among those who do not. In a well-designed case–control study, cases are selected from a clearly defined population, sometimes called the **source population,** and controls are selected from the same population that yielded the cases. The histories of prior exposure for both cases and controls are examined to assess relationships between exposure and disease. The basic design of a case–control study is shown in Figure 9–1.

The approach to the design of a case–control study can be illustrated by one study, conducted in Minnesota (Belongia et al, 1990), designed to assess the association between the use of L-tryptophan and the risk of developing EMS. In this study, investigators contacted physicians in an attempt to identify all cases of EMS in the metropolitan area of Minneapolis–St. Paul. To select controls, they randomly called selected telephone numbers in the same area. Researchers interviewed subjects and asked about potential risk factors and about their use of L-tryptophan. They asked cases about use of L-tryptophan immediately prior to onset of illness, and asked controls about recent use. For each subject who reported use of L-tryptophan, the investigators obtained the brand of L-tryptophan and lot number, so that the manufacturer could be traced. L-Tryptophan was taken significantly more frequently by cases than by controls—61 of 63 case subjects (97%)—but only 101 of 5188 control subjects (2%). Because previous studies had already demonstrated a strong association between developing EMS and use of L-tryptophan in general, the main contribution of this study was the finding that risk was strongly associated with use of L-tryptophan from a particular manufacturer. Among subjects who used L-tryptophan and for whom the manufacturer could be determined, 29 of 30 cases (97%) but only 5 of 9 controls (56%) had used L-tryptophan from the implicated manufacturer. The design of this study is illustrated schematically in Figure 9–2.

This investigation illustrates several important features of case–control studies. First, the design provides an efficient means to study rare diseases such as EMS. Case–control studies tend

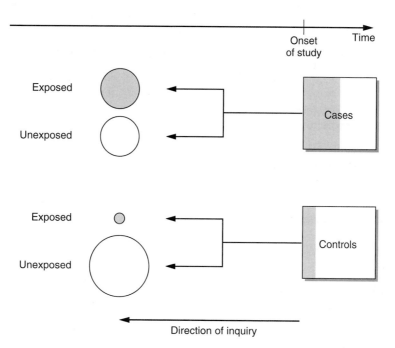

Figure 9–1. Schematic diagram of the design of a case–control study. Shaded areas represent subjects who were exposed to the risk factor of interest.

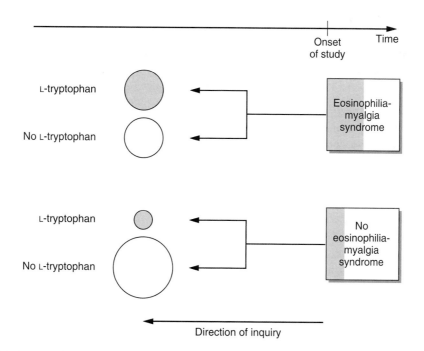

Figure 9–2. Schematic diagram of a case–control study of use of L-tryptophan and subsequent risk of developing eosinophilia-myalgia syndrome (EMS).

to be more feasible than other types of epidemiologic investigations, such as cohort studies, because fewer subjects are required. The smaller sample size is accompanied by a reduction in cost. Second, case–control studies allow researchers to investigate several risk factors. In this example, the investigators evaluated L-tryptophan and other factors as possible causes of EMS. Third, as with other nonexperimental or observational studies, a single case–control investigation does not "prove" causality, but it can provide suggestive evidence of a causal relationship that warrants intervention by public health officials to reduce exposure to the implicated risk factor. In this context, the removal of L-tryptophan-containing products from the market resulted in the virtual elimination of reported cases of EMS, although anecdotal reports of EMS-like illness still rarely occur in the apparent absence of L-tryptophan usage. These rare reports raise the speculative possibility that a contaminant that could cause EMS-like illness might still be present in some over-the-counter supplement or other source.

DESIGN OF CASE–CONTROL STUDIES

In this section, several aspects of case–control design are discussed, including sources of cases, sources of controls, and collection of information.

Cases

One of the first steps in a case–control study is to identify and select cases—a step that also determines the source population. Case identification should be complete, and the source population—the population from which cases arise—should be well defined. For example, cases might be sampled at random from all patients who are diagnosed with EMS during the study period and who reside within a certain geographic region, such as a state of the United States, or from all cases that occur among subscribers to a health maintenance organization. The source population consists of state residents in the first instance, and subscribers to the health maintenance organization in the second instance. In the previously cited study of EMS, the source population consisted of residents of the metropolitan area of Minneapolis–St. Paul, Minnesota. These cases may be identified by a surveillance system or by reviewing hospital records, other medical records, or death certificates available through institutional or population-based disease registries.

In some situations, complete identification of cases in a well-defined source population may be too time consuming or otherwise infeasible. If so, a common alternative involves use of a "convenience sample." Cases might be sampled from patients admitted to particular hospitals or from those seen in certain clinics. Although such cases can often be identified easily, the underlying source population may not be well defined, thus making it difficult to generalize results confidently.

The investigator typically studies newly diagnosed or **incident cases,** although it is sometimes necessary to include previously existing or **prevalent cases.** Prevalent cases should be excluded primarily because the exposure may affect the prognosis or the duration of the illness. When this effect occurs, the exposure status of existing prevalent cases tends to differ from that of all cases. For example, suppose that prior use of L-tryptophan either prevents death or prolongs the duration of EMS. Prevalent cases of EMS might then have a higher reported use of L-tryptophan than would all cases with this disease. Consequently, a case–control comparison of use of L-tryptophan would tend to be distorted by an inflated estimate of use for cases. The general principle involved is that the likelihood of a case being included in the study must not depend on whether that case was exposed to the risk factor of interest.

Another important step in designing a case–control study is to specify the definition of a case. The criteria should minimize the likelihood that an affected person (true case) is missed (ie, the criteria must be **sensitive**) or that a nonaffected person is falsely classified as a case (ie, the criteria must be **specific**). In general, there is a trade-off between the desire to include all cases (particularly when the disease is extremely rare, as is EMS) and the desire to prevent dilution of the case group with nonaffected persons. Moreover, restrictive criteria may require information that is unavailable for some subjects, making it impossible for such subjects to be classified fully. In practice, inclusion criteria are chosen to minimize misclassification yet promote feasibility. For example, in the previously cited study of EMS in Minneapolis–St. Paul, cases met specific criteria including the following: elevated eosinophil counts, myalgia or muscle weakness, and residence in the study area.

Controls

The next key step in a case–control study is to identify and select controls. Ideally, controls are chosen at random from the source population. If the source population is a state, city, or other well-defined area, controls in that area might be contacted by dialing telephone numbers at random (random-digit dialing), by visiting residences, by mailing letters soliciting participation, or by other means. An important goal is to select controls so that participation does not depend on exposure.

That is to say, the sample of controls should have the same prevalence of exposure as the source population of unaffected persons. If participation does depend on exposure, the case–control comparison may be distorted. In the previously cited study of EMS, the investigators selected controls by random-digit dialing in the Minneapolis–St. Paul area (the source population). Because the population of Minneapolis–St. Paul has fairly complete telephone coverage, this approach to selecting controls is unlikely to be influenced by use of L-tryptophan (the exposure) or, among users, by the manufacturer of L-tryptophan. Accordingly, within the control group selected by random-digit dialing, the manufacturer of L-tryptophan should be comparable among users to that of the source population.

Determination of Exposure

Once cases and controls are selected, the next step is to obtain as accurate information as possible about each individual's prior exposure to the risk factor of interest, as well as to other exposures. The information concerning other exposures is used to determine whether association of disease with a risk factor is due to the exposure of interest or to other characteristics of exposed persons. Because factors cannot affect risk after the disease occurs, the timing of exposures is critical. With slowly developing diseases that lack early evidence of involvement, establishing the temporal sequence of exposure and onset of disease can be difficult or impossible.

Interviews and questionnaires are the most common means of determining a subject's exposure history. Interviews can be conducted in person or by telephone. To ensure that information from cases and controls is obtained in the same manner, interviews should be standardized, monitored, and conducted by trained interviewers. Interviews are useful for collecting data because (1) questions may cover a wide range of potential risk factors, (2) costs are relatively low, and (3) information can be obtained on exposures that occurred years prior to the onset of illness. Occasionally, there is concern that cases and controls may recall exposures differently, perhaps distorting case–control comparisons. For example, cases—perhaps in an attempt to explain their illnesses—may overreport exposures. This is of particular concern when there has been a great deal of publicity about the association between the exposure and the disease of interest. For instance, after the association of L-tryptophan with EMS was first identified and publicized, knowledge of this association could have affected the reported exposures of cases in subsequent investigations.

To minimize problems associated with subject recall, attempts can be made to verify exposures through other methods. In the context of the association between use of L-tryptophan and development of EMS, for example, the interviewer might request that the subject produce the L-tryptophan package. By inspecting the package, the interviewer can confirm that it was opened (and therefore the product presumably was used); the manufacturer and the lot number can also be identified.

Information concerning risk factors may also be obtained from medical, occupational, or other records. These methods of obtaining information are not based on self-reporting and consequently should avoid the reporting bias that may occur when information is obtained through interviews. However, the amount of information found in records is often limited, so that all of the data of interest may not be available. Furthermore, this information may not be recorded in a standardized manner, leading to variability in subject classification.

An objective means of characterizing exposure is through the use of a biological marker, such as measurement of an agent—an indicator of an agent—in blood or other specimens. However, there are several difficulties inherent in the use of biological markers. First, obtaining the specimens can involve an invasive procedure that discourages subject participation. Second, many exposures do not have known biological markers. Third, even if a marker exists, it may be transient and thus not present when the measurement is taken. For example, levels of L-tryptophan in blood would reflect only relatively recent exposure and would decline rapidly after exposure is stopped. Finally, the disease state may alter metabolism, thereby distorting case–control comparisons.

The type of case–control study described in the Minneapolis–St. Paul investigation of use of L-tryptophan and development of EMS, in which newly diagnosed cases and controls are sampled from a source population, is used quite commonly. It is often called a **population-based** study because cases and controls are sampled from a defined population, in this instance, by virtue of place of residence.

HOSPITAL-BASED CASE–CONTROL STUDIES

Other types of case–control studies differ from the population-based study primarily in the way the samples of cases and controls are selected. Variations include the use of prevalent rather than incident cases and sampling of controls from a readily available, convenient group such as hospital inpatients. The **hospital-based** case–control study is used so often that it merits mention. In this type of study, the investigator typically selects cases from persons with the disease of interest who are admitted to a particular hospital or hospitals; controls are selected from persons admitted with other conditions but with no evidence of the disease of interest.

The researcher then obtains information from cases and controls, often by interviewing them in the hospital.

The hospital-based approach can be illustrated by a case–control study of Reye's syndrome, a condition characterized by acute encephalopathy associated with fatty degeneration of the liver. This illness occurs almost exclusively in children and typically follows a viral illness. To study the association between Reye's syndrome and use of various medications during an antecedent viral illness, researchers in this study selected cases from children admitted with Reye's syndrome to any of a preselected group of referral hospitals. Investigators selected controls from children admitted to these same hospitals with an antecedent illness, presumably of viral origin. Parents were interviewed to assess prior exposure to aspirin. Twenty-six of the 27 cases—but only 6 of the 22 hospitalized controls—had been exposed to a salicylate-containing medication. In nearly every instance, the salicylate was aspirin.

The hospital-based case–control study can be very convenient, as cases and controls are found in the same institutions. Moreover, potential subjects, if not too ill, may be particularly willing to participate. For example, they may have more time than would normally be available. Within a hospital-based case–control study, factors that might influence hospitalization at a particular facility, such as socioeconomic status, tend to be balanced between cases and controls. Although hospital-based studies can be convenient, they also are susceptible to distorted results. First, cases and controls in a hospital-based study may not arise from a single, well-defined population—in contrast to the population-based case–control studies described previously. This could happen, for example, if referral patterns to particular hospitals varied across different diagnoses. Moreover, controls in a hospital-based case–control study are in a hospital because they are ill, and the condition or conditions for which they are hospitalized may be associated with—and even caused by—the exposure of interest. If so, the exposure histories of controls may differ from those of nonaffected persons in the source population, and a distorted case–control comparison may result. Several selection criteria for hospital-

based controls may help to reduce this type of distortion; those criteria are listed in Table 9–1.

These difficulties probably account for a decline in popularity of hospital-based case–control studies. Despite these problems, however, hospital-based case–control studies are still performed. Typically, they are easier and quicker to conduct than population-based studies, because cases and controls are identified efficiently. Consequently, hospital-based case–control studies may be less expensive. Furthermore, the collection of information on exposure from medical records and biological markers is easier in the hospital environment. Subjects in the hospital are more accessible for interview than persons in the community. As already noted, hospital-based controls may be more cooperative with investigators because they are ill and may want to advance medical knowledge.

Despite these differences in approach and the subtle differences in interpretation that may result, the basic case–control design remains intact. Cases are selected from those with the disease of interest and controls from those without that disease. The relative strengths of population-based and hospital-based case–control studies are summarized in Table 9–2. In brief, the hospital-based approach offers logistical advantages, whereas the population-based approach tends to characterize more accurately the history of prior exposure of the source population.

SELECTION BIAS

Bias is a systematic error in a study that distorts the results and limits the validity of conclusions. Bias will be discussed in more detail in Chapter 10. Bias can occur for a variety of reasons, most of which can affect any type of study. One form—selection bias—poses a particular threat to case–control studies. This form of bias, as suggested by its name, reflects systematic errors that arise from the way in which subjects are selected.

If selection of cases, controls, or both is influenced by prior exposure, this bias may be present. In particular, if the prior exposure of the cases studied differs from that of all cases arising from the source population—or if prior exposure of

Table 9–1. Approaches to sampling of controls in hospital-based case-control studies.

Selection Criteria for Hospital-Based Controls	
To Do	**To Avoid**
Select controls from various diagnostic groups so no particular risk factors will be overrepresented	Do not select patients who have multiple concurrent conditions
Select controls from patients with acute conditions so earlier exposures could not have been influenced by the condition	Do not select patients with diagnoses known to be related to the risk factor of interest

CASE–CONTROL STUDIES / 153

Table 9–2. Relative strengths of population-based and hospital-based case-control studies.

Population-Based	Hospital-Based
Source population is better defined	Subjects are more accessible
Easier to make certain that cases and controls derive from the same source population	Subjects tend to be more cooperative
Exposure histories of controls more likely to reflect those of persons without the disease of interest	Background characteristics of cases and controls may be balanced
	Easier to collect exposure information from medical records and biological specimens

controls differs from that of persons in the source population without the disease of interest—selection bias may be present. The particular susceptibility of case–control studies to selection bias arises because of the need to obtain two samples: a sample of cases and a sample of controls. Unless each sample is obtained without regard to exposure, results may be biased.

The development of selection bias is illustrated schematically in Figure 9–3. The shaded figures represent persons who were exposed and the unshaded figures represent persons who were not exposed. In the source population, one third of persons with the disease of interest were exposed. Among the cases included in the study, however, two thirds were exposed. That is to say, exposed persons with disease were more likely than unexposed persons with disease to be selected for the study. In this illustration, an opposite sampling pattern is displayed for persons without disease. In this group, exposed persons were less likely to be selected for study

than were unexposed persons. Obviously, in this study, comparison of exposure histories of sampled cases with controls would yield a result different from that achieved by contrasting exposure of persons with and without the disease of interest in the source population.

There are at least three ways in which this type of bias could arise in case–control studies of EMS:

1. Preferential diagnosis of exposed cases may lead to selection bias. After the initial publicity concerning the suspected association of EMS with use of L-tryptophan, physicians may have been more inclined to suspect the diagnosis of EMS among those who were known to have used L-tryptophan. If so, subjects with EMS who did not take L-tryptophan could have been underrepresented within the case group, thus leading to selection bias.

2. Low participation may lead to selection bias. For example, eligible subjects may refuse to participate, or physicians may advise their patients not to participate. If prior use of L-tryptophan among those who did not participate differed from prior use among participants, selection bias must be suspected.

3. Errors in sampling controls from the source population can also create selection bias. For example, if sampled controls had a condition such as insomnia that would make them more likely than other people to use L-tryptophan, selection bias could occur.

Studies of EMS and use of L-tryptophan raise an interesting point concerning susceptibility of different studies to selection bias due to preferential diagnosis of exposed cases. Selection bias could have affected any case–control study of the association between development of EMS and *any* use of L-tryptophan that was conducted after the extensive media publicity. Nearly all the published case–control studies, however, were designed to investigate the association between risk of developing EMS and the manufacturing *source* of the L-tryptophan. These studies were less susceptible to selection bias. For example, consider the possibility that preferential diag-

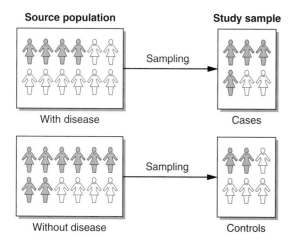

Figure 9–3. Schematic diagram of the origin of selection bias in a case–control study. The shaded figures represent persons who were exposed, and the unshaded figures indicate persons who were unexposed.

nosis of EMS in exposed cases led to underrepresention of unexposed subjects in the case series. This type of problem was unlikely in the studies concerning the source of L-tryptophan because most physicians would not have known the source, nor would they have been aware of the link between a particular manufacturer and risk of L-tryptophan. Thus preferential diagnosis of EMS in exposed cases (those who used L-tryptophan from the implicated manufacturer) should not have occurred to any significant extent, and this group should not have been overrepresented in the case group.

MATCHING

Confounding is a distortion of results that occurs when the apparent effects of the exposure of interest are attributable entirely or in part to the effects of an extraneous variable. Confounding is likely to occur when persons exposed to the risk factor of interest differ from nonexposed persons with respect to the prevalence of other risk factors for the disease of interest. Confounding is discussed in more detail in Chapter 10.

In this chapter, several possible ways to control confounding are presented, including matched sampling.

Matching is a popular approach to control confounding in case–control studies. Its popularity reflects the belief that matching cases and controls forces these groups to be similar with respect to important risk factors, and thereby makes case–control comparisons less subject to confounding. This perception about matching is valid, provided the appropriate matched analysis is conducted.

The first step in matching is to identify a case. Investigators then select from the source population one or more potential controls who have the same values that the case has for each matching factor. The process of matching by race and sex is illustrated schematically in Figure 9–4. To match on a continuous variable such as age, it is typically necessary to form categories, such as 5-year intervals (years 10–14, 15–19, 20–24, etc). In a study with matching on race, sex, and age in 5-year intervals, a 17-year-old African-American female case would be matched to an African-American female control aged 15–19 from the source population. As in an unmatched study, these controls would come from the defined source population. More than one control can be matched to each case, but the ratio of controls to cases rarely exceeds 4:1 because additional controls beyond this ratio add relatively little to the statistical power of the study.

The use of matching is common in clinical studies, particularly when the disease of interest is extremely rare, as is EMS. In this situation, there are a small number of potential cases and a large number of potential

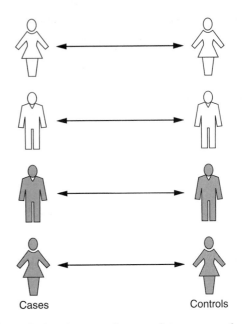

Figure 9–4. Schematic diagram of the process of matching controls to cases by race and sex.

controls. Matching can increase the statistical efficiency of case–control comparisons and thus achieve a particular level of statistical power with a smaller sample size. The matching protocol often simplifies decisions about how to sample controls. In addition, matching tends to ensure that case–control differences in the risk factor of interest cannot be explained by reference to the matched variables.

However, these advantages of matching must be weighed against a number of disadvantages. As indicated in Table 9–3, matching can be time consuming and therefore expensive. Any potential cases or controls that cannot be matched must be discarded, which can be viewed as a wasteful process. Any variable that is matched in a study cannot be evaluated as a risk factor in that investigation. Finally, matching on ordinal or continuous variables may result in categories that are too broad to remove completely the effects of the matched variables from the exposure–disease relationship.

Another investigation of development of EMS and use of L-tryptophan conducted by researchers in Minnesota illustrates the use of a matched case–control study design (CDC, 1989). In that study, researchers contacted area physicians to identify people with unexplained eosinophilia and severe myalgia. They also required that a muscle biopsy, if done, show eosinophilic perimyositis or perivasculitis. For each case, they identified a control who matched the case on age, sex, and telephone exchange. They interviewed subjects and

Table 9–3. Advantages and disadvantages of matching in case-control studies.

Advantages	Disadvantages
May increase the precision of case-control comparisons and thus allow a smaller study	May be time-consuming and expensive to perform
The sampling process is easy to understand and explain	Some potential cases and controls may be excluded because matches cannot be made
If analyzed correctly, provides reassurance that matched variables cannot explain case-control differences in the risk factor of interest	The matched variables cannot be evaluated as risk factors in the study population
	For continuous or ordinal variables, matching categories may be too broad, and residual case-control differences in these variables may persist

asked about prior use of L-tryptophan, prior use of selected other medications, and diet. For each of the 12 case–control pairs, the case had consumed L-tryptophan prior to onset of illness, but none of the matched controls had consumed L-tryptophan. Results of this study indicated a strong association between ingestion of L-tryptophan and risk of developing EMS.

ANALYSIS

The type of analysis employed in a case–control study depends on whether subjects were sampled in an unmatched or in a matched approach. These two analytic strategies are described in the following sections.

Unmatched Design

The data obtained in an unmatched case–control study can be summarized as indicated in Table 9–4. For simplicity, only two levels of exposure are discussed here, although the basic methods can be expanded to include multiple levels of exposure. Each subject can be classified into one of four basic groups defined by disease and prior exposure status:

A. Cases who were exposed
B. Cases who were not exposed
C. Controls who were exposed
D. Controls who were not exposed.

The format of Table 9–4 should appear familiar, since it resembles that of Table 8–6. Although the summary tables for cohort and case–control studies appear similar, it is important to remember that the underlying approaches to sampling differ, and the analysis must account for these differences. In a cohort study, sampling is based on exposure status, and the investigator thus determines the total numbers of exposed ($A + C$) and unexposed subjects ($B + D$) included in the study. Then risk of disease development can be estimated separately for exposed and unexposed groups, and these two risks can be compared in a risk ratio (RR).

A case–control study, on the other hand, begins with sampling of persons with the disease of interest and individuals without the disease ($A + B$ and $C + D$, respectively). With this approach, the proportion of persons in the study who have the disease is no longer determined by the risk of developing the disease in the source population, but rather by the choice of the investigator. That is, a disease that occurs infrequently in the source population can be oversampled, so that affected individuals constitute a large proportion of the study sample. This ability to oversample affected individuals is the reason case–control studies are statistically efficient for the study of rare diseases.

In a case–control study the investigator determines the ratio of persons with the disease to persons without it, and thus the proportion of study subjects who have the disease does not provide an estimate of the risk of developing the disease. As shown in the following section, however, an indirect estimate of the incidence rate ratio can still be obtained in a case–control study.

Odds Ratio

With the notation introduced in Table 9–4, the probability that a case was exposed previously is estimated by

Table 9–4. Summary of data collected in an unmatched case-control study.

	Exposed	Unexposed	Total
Case	A	B	A + B
Controls	C	D	C + D
Total	A + C	B + D	A + B + C + D

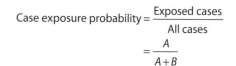

$$\text{Case exposure probability} = \frac{\text{Exposed cases}}{\text{All cases}}$$
$$= \frac{A}{A+B}$$

The odds of exposure for cases represent the probability that a case was exposed divided by the probability that a case was not exposed. The odds then are estimated by

$$\text{Odds of case exposure} = \frac{\text{Exposed cases}}{\text{All cases}} \Big/ \frac{\text{Unexposed cases}}{\text{All cases}}$$

$$= \frac{A}{A+B} \Big/ \frac{B}{A+B} = \frac{A}{B}$$

Similarly, the odds of exposure among controls are estimated by

$$\text{Odds of control exposure} = \frac{C}{D}$$

The odds of exposure for cases divided by the odds of exposure for controls are expressed as the **odds ratio** (*OR*). Substituting from the preceding equations, the *OR* is estimated by

$$\text{Odds ratio} = \frac{\text{Odds of case exposure}}{\text{Odds of control exposure}}$$

$$= \frac{A}{B} \Big/ \frac{C}{D} = \frac{A \times D}{B \times C}$$

The *OR* is sometimes termed the exposure odds ratio or the cross-product of Table 9–4, because it results from dividing the product of entries on one diagonal of this table by the product of entries on the cross-diagonal.

When incident cases and controls are sampled from the same source population (with selection independent of prior exposure), the exposure **OR** provides a valid estimate of the incidence rate ratio (see Appendix D). In other words, if properly designed, a case–control study can yield a measure of association between exposure and disease that approximates the incidence rate ratio.

The calculation of the *OR* can be illustrated by data from a case–control study of EMS in which risk associated with use of particular brands of L-tryptophan was studied. Among those who took L-tryptophan, 22 of 58 cases took one particular retail lot (lot A), compared with 7 of 93 controls, as summarized in Table 9–5. The *OR* for these data is as follows

$$\text{Odds ratio} = \frac{A \times D}{B \times C} = \frac{23 \times 86}{36 \times 7} = 7.5$$

In other words, the odds for use of lot A for patients with EMS were over seven times greater than the odds for use of lot A among controls in this study. To the extent that the *OR* provides a valid estimate of the incidence rate ratio, it could be concluded from this inves-

Table 9–5. Summary of data from the study of eosinophilia-myalgia syndrome (EMS) and use of Lot A.

	Use Lot A	Use Other Lot	Total
Cases	22	36	58
Controls	7	86	93
Total	29	122	151

tigation that use of Lot A increased the likelihood of developing EMS more than sevenfold.

As with the risk ratio, a 95% confidence interval around the point estimate of the *OR* can be calculated. A formula to calculate an approximate 95% confidence interval is given in Appendix E. With the data presented in Table 9–5, the approximate 95% confidence interval for the *OR* is 2.9 to 19.1. That is, the data from this study are consistent with a moderately to strongly positive association between the use of a particular lot of L-tryptophan and the development of EMS. This association is unlikely to have occurred by chance alone, since the null value of the *OR* (null value = 1) is well outside the 95% confidence interval. The point estimate and confidence interval for this odds ratio are illustrated in Figure 9–5.

Matched Design

In a matched case–control study, the analysis must account for the matched sampling scheme. When one control is matched to each case, summary data can be presented in the format shown in Table 9–6. An extension of this basic format can be employed for situations in which the ratio of controls to cases differs from 1:1. Although there are four cells in Table 9–6, the entries into this format are quite different from what we find in previous tables. Each entry into Table 9–6 represents not one subject but two (a matched case–control pair). That is, each case–control pair can be classified into one of the four basic combinations of exposure status:

W—Both case and control exposed
X—Case exposed but control unexposed
Y—Case unexposed but control exposed
Z—Both case and control unexposed.

Case–control pairs that are entered into cells *W* and *Z* are referred to as **concordant pairs,** because in these pairs, the exposure status of cases and controls is the same. Case–control pairs that are entered into cells *X* and *Y,* in contrast, are referred to as **discordant pairs** because in these pairs, the exposure status of cases and controls differs.

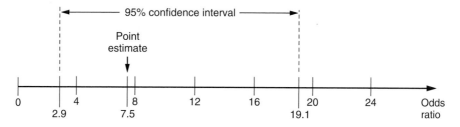

Figure 9–5. Point estimate and 95% confidence interval for odds ratio comparing patients who used lot A L-tryptophan with eosinophilia-myalgia syndrome (EMS) and controls

The *OR* for a pair-matched case–control study is given by a simple ratio:

$$\text{Odds ratio} = \frac{X}{Y}$$

This odds ratio can be interpreted in the same manner as the *OR* for unmatched studies.

To illustrate the calculation of the *OR* from a matched study, the results of a hypothetical matched study with 200 matched case–control pairs are shown in Table 9–7. The *OR* from this study is as follows:

$$\text{Odds ratio} = \frac{X}{Y} = \frac{57}{5} = 11.4$$

A 95% confidence interval around the point estimate of the matched *OR* can be calculated. A formula to calculate an approximate 95% confidence interval is given in Appendix E. With the data presented in Table 9–7, the approximate 95% confidence interval for the *OR* is 4.6 to 28.3. That is, the data from the hypothetical matched case–control study are consistent with a strong to a very strong positive association between the use of L-tryptophan and the development of EMS. This association is highly unlikely to have occurred by

chance, as the null value of the *OR* (null value = 1) is far outside the 95% confidence interval.

To further illustrate analysis of matched case–control studies, consider again the matched case–control study of L-tryptophan conducted by the researchers in Minnesota (CDC, 1989). The results of that study, summarized in Table 9–8, indicate that for every case–control pair, the case but not the control had taken L-tryptophan. Therefore, the *OR* from this study is as follows:

$$\text{Odds ratio} = \frac{X}{Y} = \frac{12}{0}$$

This odds ratio is undefined or infinite, since the denominator is zero. This suggests a very strong association between use of L-tryptophan and risk of developing EMS. The 95% confidence interval for the odds ratio is 2.8 to infinity. It is highly unlikely that this association occurred by chance, as the null value of the *OR* (null value = 1) is well outside the 95% confidence interval. (In this example, the small number of case–control pairs in the *Y* category violates the large sample assumptions of the approximate confidence interval formula in Appendix E. Therefore, a more complicated exact formula was used to estimate this 95% confidence interval.)

Table 9–6. Summary data format for a matched case-control study with one control per case.

	Control Exposed	Control Unexposed	Total
Case exposed	W	X	W + X
Case unexposed	Y	Z	Y + Z
Total	W + Y	X + Z	W + X + Y + Z

Table 9–7. Summary data from a hypothetical matched case-control study of use of L-tryptophan and risk of developing eosinophilia-myalgia syndrome (EMS).

	Control Exposed	Control Unexposed	Total
Case exposed	132	57	189
Case unexposed	5	6	11
Total	137	63	200

Table 9–8. Results of a matched case-control study of use of L-tryptophan and risk of developing eosinophilia-myalgia syndrome (EMS).

	Control Exposed	Control Unexposed	Total
Case exposed	0	12	12
Case unexposed	0	0	0
Total	0	12	12

SUMMARY

In this chapter, the basic approach to the design and analysis of case–control studies is presented, with illustrations drawn primarily from the literature on the relationship between the use of contaminated L-tryptophan and the risk of developing EMS. A case–control study is a type of observational investigation in which subjects are enrolled on the basis of the presence or absence of a particular disease (eg, EMS) and are then evaluated to determine their history of prior exposure to risk factors of interest (eg, use of L-tryptophan).

The advantages and disadvantages of the case–control approach are summarized in Table 9–9. The advantages of this design are primarily logistical. In particular, rare diseases (EMS is an example) and those with long latency periods can be studied efficiently. The sample size required for a case–control study tends to be smaller than would be needed for an alternative design, such as a cohort study. As a result, the expense of conducting a case–control study may be substantially less than the cost of conducting a cohort study. Furthermore, reliance on historical information allows rapid completion of a case–control study. The ability to reach a prompt conclusion is particularly important if the disease of interest is potentially life-threatening, as is EMS, because future cases might be prevented if preventive action is taken to limit exposure to a suspected risk factor.

The disadvantages of case–control studies relate primarily to their susceptibility to systematic errors. Because cases and controls are sampled separately, it is possible that these groups may not arise from the same source population. Bias can be introduced into the study results if exposure status is associated with the likelihood of including cases or controls into the study. Reliance on subject recall of earlier exposures or the use of historical records can lead to imprecise or inaccurate classification of exposure.

The decision to conduct a case–control study typically is motivated by a desire to explore the relationship between prior exposure to a specific risk factor and the likelihood of developing a particular disease. Ideally, the cases and the controls should derive from a single well-defined source population, such as a state or metropolitan area (a **population-based** sampling scheme). An attempt may be made to identify all newly diagnosed cases (**incident cases**) within the source population, particularly when the disease is rare or the source population is modest in size. Cases may be identified from hospital records, surveillance systems, death certificates, or other sources. Careful criteria for the presence of disease must be established to minimize false inclusions or exclusions.

Controls typically are sampled from the population that gave rise to the cases. Occasionally, for purposes of convenience, **hospital-based samples** of cases and controls are selected. The hospital-based approach tends to have the advantages of accessibility to the subjects and cooperative study participants. On the other hand, cases and controls may derive from dissimilar source populations in a hospital-based study, and prior exposure status might influence the likelihood of inclusion in this type of investigation.

Matching of controls to cases on the basis of known risk factors for the disease of interest is a common practice in case–control studies. The intent of matching is usually to decrease the possibility of **confounding,** or mixing of the effect of exposure to the risk factor of interest with the effects of exposure to other risk factors. Matching can increase the statistical precision of esti-

Table 9–9. Advantages and disadvantages of case-control studies.

Advantages	Disadvantages
Efficient for the study of rare diseases	Risk of disease cannot be estimated directly
Efficient for the study of chronic diseases	Not efficient for the study of rare exposure
Tend to require a smaller sample size than other designs	More susceptible to selection bias than alternative designs
Less expansive than alternative designs	Information on exposure may be less accurate than that available
May be completed more rapidly than alternative designs	in alternative designs

mates and thereby allow a smaller sample size. On the other hand, matching can be time consuming, and subjects who are not successfully matched must be discarded from the analysis.

The process of selection of subjects in a case–control study precludes the estimation of risks (or rates), and the risk ratio therefore cannot be calculated directly from case–control data. An indirect estimate of the risk ratio, however, can be calculated in a case–control study. This measure is referred to as the **odds ratio** and is defined as the odds of exposure among cases divided by the odds of exposure among controls. The approach to calculating the odds ratio depends on whether cases and controls were sampled in an unmatched or matched fashion. In either instance, a point estimate and 95% confidence interval for the odds ratio can be calculated as a measure of association between prior exposure to the risk factor and occurrence of disease.

A number of case–control studies of EMS are discussed. In those studies, cases and controls were sampled using various approaches. The most consistent risk factor that emerged from the studies was the prior use of L-tryptophan produced by one manufacturer. The strength of the association between prior use of L-tryptophan from the implicated manufacturer and development of EMS, the dose–response, and the consistency of results across studies—as well as other considerations such as biological plausibility—suggest the possibility that a cause-and-effect relationship exists between the exposure in question and the occurrence of disease. The decline in the incidence of reported cases of EMS after withdrawal from the market of L-tryptophan–containing products further supports this explanation.

STUDY QUESTIONS

Questions 1–4: For each numbered situation below, select the best descriptor from the following lettered options. Each option can be used once, more than once, or not at all.

A. Publication bias

B. Confounding

C. Interviewer bias

D. Misclassification

E. Cohort effect

F. Selection bias

1. In a case–control study of nosocomial urinary tract infection and catheter care among patients with a Foley catheter, information about catheter care is obtained by interviewing patients about 6 months after discharge from the hospital.

2. In the study cited in question 1, cases are sampled from patients who had been on a surgical ward and controls who had been on a medical ward.

3. In the study cited in question 1, patients who had a bladder infection are more likely to remember the number of times the catheter had been changed.

4. In the study cited in question 1, the interviewer probes more deeply when questioning patients who had had a bladder infection because she did not want to "miss anything."

Questions 5–7: For each numbered situation below, select the most appropriate advantage that best applies to the case–control design from the following lettered options. Each option can be used once, more than once, or not at all.

A. The study can be conducted at nominal expense

B. Efficient for the study of rare diseases

C. Efficient for the study of rare exposures

D. The incidence rate in the population can be estimated directly

E. The temporal relationship between exposure and disease is clearly defined

F. The ability to conduct an assessment quickly

5. Assessing risk factors for an epidemic of a newly recognized condition with rapid onset of liver disease in several communities.

6. Assessing risk factors for adrenal insufficiency (Addison's disease).

7. Assessing risk factors for a long-standing high rate of infant mortality in a developing country.

Questions 8–11: For each numbered measure below, select the most appropriate calculation from the following lettered options. Each option can be used once, more than once, or not at all.

A. 70/150

B. 20/230

C. 20/150

D. $(80 \times 280)/(20 \times 70)$

E. 70/80

F. $(70 \times 130)/(80 \times 20)$

F. Cannot be calculated with available information

8. The odds of exposure among cases in an unmatched case–control study of risk factors for adenocarcinoma of the esophagus, in which chronic heartburn was found in 70 of 150 cases and 20 of 150 controls.

9. The prevalence of exposure among cases in the study described in question 8.

10. The odds ratio for exposure in the unmatched case–control study described in question 8.

11. The risk of disease among the exposed for the case–control study described in question 8.

Questions 12–14: For each numbered situation below, select the best descriptor from the following lettered options. Each option can be used once, more than once, or not at all.

A. Concordant pair

B. Discordant pair

C. Not applicable

D. Cannot be determined from the information provided

E. More efficient than other case–control designs

12. In a pair-matched case–control study of cell phone usage while driving as a risk factor for automobile accidents, a male driver was using his cell phone when the accident occurred and his matched control was not using a cell phone at the corresponding time.

13. A pair-matched case–control study to assess post-menopausal hormone replacement as a risk factor for atherosclerotic coronary heart disease, patients were matched with controls on age, race, years since menopause, area of residence, and age at menarche.

14. In an unmatched case–control study of risk factors for deep vein thrombosis, a patient with deep vein thrombosis had traveled in an airplane, and a control of similar age had not.

FURTHER READING

Schulz KF, Grimes DA: Case–control studies: research in reverse. Lancet 2002;**359**:431.

REFERENCES

Clauw DJ, Pincus T: The eosinophilia-myalgia syndrome: What we know, what we think we know, and what we need to know. J Rheumatol 1996;**23**(Suppl 46):2.

Clinical Background

CDC: Eosinophilia-myalgia syndrome and L-tryptophan-containing products—New Mexico, Minnesota, Oregon, and New York, 1989. MMWR 1989;**38**:785.

Kilbourne EM et al: Tryptophan produced by Showa Denko and epidemic eosinophilia-myalgia syndrome. J Rheumatol 1996;**23**(Suppl 46):81.

Mori Y et al: Scleroderma-like cutaneous syndromes. Curr Rheumatol Reports 2002;**4**:113.

Swygert LA et al: Eosinophilia-myalgia syndrome. Results of national surveillance. JAMA 1990;**264**:1698.

Introduction

Belongia EA et al: An investigation of the cause of the eosinophilia-myalgia syndrome associated with tryptophan use. N Engl J Med 1990;**323**:357.

Design of Case–Control Studies

Cummings P, Koepsell TD, Weiss NS: Studying injuries with case–control methods in the emergency department. Ann Emerg Med 1998;**31**:99.

Essebag V et al: The nested case–control study in cardiology. Am Heart J 2003;**146**:581.

Hospital-Based Case–Control Studies

Cummings P, Koepsell TD, Weiss NS: Studying injuries with case–control methods in the emergency department. Ann Emerg Med 1998;**31**:99.

Hurwitz ES et al: Public Health Service study of Reye's syndrome and medications. JAMA 1987;**257**:1905.

Selection Bias

Horwitz RI, Daniels SR: Bias or biology: Evaluating the epidemiologic studies of L-tryptophan and the eosinophilia-myalgia syndrome. J Rheumatol 1996;**23**(Suppl 46):60.

Matching

Gold EB: Case–control studies and their application to endocrinology. Endocrinol Metab Clin North Am 1997;**26**(No. 1):1.

Analysis

CDC: Eosinophilia-myalgia syndrome and L-tryptophan-containing products—New Mexico, Minnesota, Oregon, and New York, 1989. MMWR 1989;**38**:785.

Hertzman PA et al: Association of the eosinophilia-myalgia syndrome with the ingestion of tryptophan. N Engl J Med 1990;**322**:869.

Slutsker L et al: Eosinophilia-myalgia syndrome associated with exposure to tryptophan from a single manufacturer. JAMA 1990;**264**:213.

e-PIDEMIOLOGY

Further Reading

http://www.nemsn.org/

Clinical Background

http://www.nemsn.org/

Design of Case–Control Studies

http://www.bmj.com/epidem/epid.8.shtml
http://www/pitt.edu/~super1/lecture/lec10281/index.htm
http://www.pitt.edu/~super1/lecture/lec8591/index.htm

Variability and Bias

PATIENT PROFILE

A 45-year-old man began working as a production supervisor, and his employer required that he undergo a complete medical examination. His physician learned that the patient's father had died of myocardial infarction at age 65. On physical examination, the patient was moderately obese, and his blood pressure was 140/86. The remainder of the examination revealed no notable abnormalities. The patient's total serum cholesterol level (nonfasting) was 242 mg/dL.

According to the guidelines of the National Cholesterol Education Program (NCEP), a total serum cholesterol concentration greater than 240 mg/dL is an indication for possible pharmacologic lowering of serum cholesterol. A value of 200–239 mg/dL is considered borderline and should trigger

dietary intervention, and a value less than 200 mg/dL is considered normal.

Based on the initial cholesterol results, the physician asked the patient to return in 2 weeks for further testing. On repeat measurement, the total serum cholesterol concentration was 198 mg/dL on a fasting lipid profile. Table 10–1 lists several different factors that could explain the observed variability in measured total serum cholesterol level. The source of this variability in the measured total cholesterol level had important implications for how the physician treated this patient.

VARIABILITY IN MEDICAL RESEARCH

Difficulties in the interpretation of test results of individual patients are magnified when groups of patients are studied. The sources of variability in test results and

162

errors in medical research are discussed in this chapter. Appreciation of these issues is important for the interpretation and appropriate application of research findings in the clinical setting.

Variability in measurements can be either random or systematic. A schematic representation of random and systematic variation is shown in Figure 10–1. The shots at the targets in both *A* and *B* are centered around the middle, but in *A* the shots are less scattered and have less variability, or more **precision.** In targets *C* and *D* the scatter is similar, but in target *D* the cluster of shots is off center. This might occur, for example, if the sight of the gun were bent. The precision is comparable, but the result in *D* is systematically off target or **biased.** The results in target *C* are accurate, or valid. It is important to consider the accuracy and precision of any measurements made in the medical setting. In clinical medicine and medical research, variability can occur at a number of different levels (eg, at the level of the individual or the population) (Table 10–1). At each level, the variability inherent in the method of measurement is important.

Variability Within the Individual

The first level of concern is variability in the true value of a person's characteristics over time. This was a source of concern for the clinician in the Patient Profile. Some

Table 10–1. Levels of variability.

Levels	Features
Individual	Individual variability
	Measurement variability
Population	Genetic variability between individuals
	Environmental variability
	Measurement variability
Sample	Manner of sampling
	Size of sample
	Measurement variability

potential sources of individual variability are listed in Table 10–2. Variation can occur because of biological changes in an individual over time. These changes may (1) occur on a minute-to-minute basis (eg, heart rate), (2) follow a regular diurnal pattern (eg, body temperature), or (3) progress with normal development (eg, height or weight).

When the variation within a subject is large, a single measurement may not adequately represent the "true" status of that individual. By repeating a test, the physician may obtain a better understanding of the true value and its variability. This may also provide the clinician with information about variability or error due to the measurement technique. In the Patient Profile, different results were obtained when the total serum cholesterol level was measured a second time—when the patient was fasting. It is unlikely, however, that the fasting state alone could cause such a drop in total serum cholesterol concentration. Furthermore, it is unlikely that the patient could have made the kind of dietary or other alterations in 2 weeks that would lead to the observed change in total serum cholesterol level.

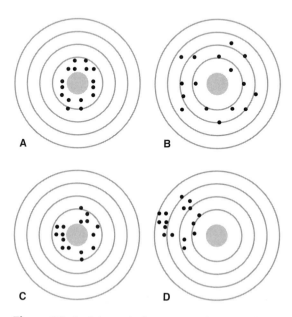

Figure 10–1. Schematic illustrations of increased random error (target **B** versus target **A**) and systematic error (target **D** versus target **C**).

Variability Related to Measurement

Laboratory measurements of total serum cholesterol level are notorious for both variability and error. To determine which value—198 mg/dL or 242 mg/dL—is closer to the truth, the physician in the Patient Profile would need to know whether both measurements were obtained in the same laboratory. For example, the first result may have been obtained from a desktop analyzer in the physician's office, whereas the lipid profile may have been measured in a standardized laboratory. In reality, the physician may not be able to discern readily which value is closer to the truth. This is one reason that programs with guidelines that support cutoff points for clinical decision making, such as the NCEP, often recommend that elevated values be confirmed by repeated measurements over time before treatment is instituted.

Table 10–2. Potential sources of variability in measurements of individuals.

Sources of Variability	Features
Individual characteristics	Diurnal variation
	Changes related to factors such as age, diet, and exercise
	Environmental factors such as season or temperature
Measurement characteristics	Poor calibration of the instrument
	Inherent lack of precision of the instrument
	Misreading or misrecording information from the instrument by the technician

Variations Within Populations

Just as there is variation in individuals, there is also variability in populations, which can be considered the cumulative variability of individuals. Because populations are made up of individuals with different genetic constitutions who are subject to different environmental influences, populations often exhibit more variation than individuals. Physicians use knowledge about variability in populations to define what is "normal" and "abnormal." The physician in the Patient Profile could refer to population survey data to learn that for 45-year-old males, a total serum cholesterol level of 200 mg/dL is close to the 50th percentile, and a concentration of 240 mg/dL is equivalent to the 75th percentile. Accordingly, the patient generally falls in the upper half of the population distribution of total serum cholesterol values. Assuming that the measurement is correct, this could be a result of genetic factors, environmental factors, or both.

Variability in Research Studies

It is worthwhile to ask how the clinician would know that a total serum cholesterol value in the upper end of the population distribution is disadvantageous. Are these values really unhealthy? Answers may be found in studies that have linked the level of total serum cholesterol with an increased risk of cardiovascular mortality. In cohort studies such as the Framingham Heart Study, groups of subjects were followed and compared according to their different levels of total serum cholesterol and the associated frequency of death from myocardial infarction or stroke. In these investigations, a higher level of total serum cholesterol was associated with an increased risk of death from cardiovascular disease.

When investigators perform such studies, they cannot usually study the entire population. Instead they study subsets or samples of the population. This introduces another source of variability—sampling variability—that is important in medical research. Using a single sample of subjects to represent the population is

analogous to using a single measurement to characterize an individual. Repeated samples from the population will give different estimates of the true population values. Sampling variability is illustrated in Figure 10–2. In the source population of 20 persons, there are five individuals (25%) with total serum cholesterol values above 240 mg/dL. In the three different samples of five subjects drawn from the source population by chance, the proportion of individuals with total serum cholesterol values above 240 mg/dL ranges from 0 to 40%.

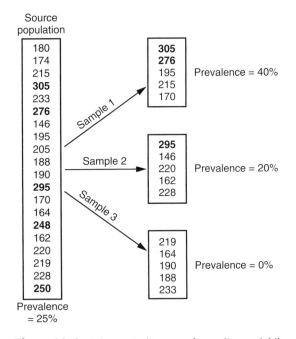

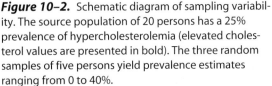

Figure 10–2. Schematic diagram of sampling variability. The source population of 20 persons has a 25% prevalence of hypercholesterolemia (elevated cholesterol values are presented in bold). The three random samples of five persons yield prevalence estimates ranging from 0 to 40%.

Each of these small samples presents a different picture of the source population. A larger sample size would result in less variability and would more likely represent the source population.

Variability can be important in other ways when two groups are compared in a study. The goal of such studies often is to determine whether a measurable difference exists between the groups. When a research paper reports no statistically significant difference between groups, the reader must ask the following question: Was there actually no difference between the two treatments, or was the estimate of effect so imprecise that the investigator could not distinguish differences between the two groups (ie, a type II error)?

A graphic display of the results of two hypothetical studies of the same question is presented in Figure 10–3. In each study, the investigators attempted to determine whether a cholesterol-lowering drug had a favorable effect on the risk of developing myocardial infarction. The

measure of effect that was estimated in each study was the risk ratio. Each study compared a group of patients randomly allocated to receive the cholesterol-lowering drug with a group chosen to receive dietary modification alone. The researchers reached different conclusions. In the study with the smaller sample, the report indicated that the drug had no beneficial effect on reducing the risk of developing myocardial infarction, when compared with diet therapy. In the study with the larger sample, the investigators concluded that the drug decreased the risk of developing myocardial infarction, when compared with dietary management.

As shown in Figure 10–3, Study A had a small sample size, which resulted in imprecise estimates (ie, wide confidence intervals) of the risk of developing myocardial infarction in the two groups. Consequently, the two estimates overlapped, and the statistical test was not capable of distinguishing between the effects of the two treatments. The investigators concluded that there was no difference in risk of developing myocardial infarction between patients who received the cholesterol-lowering drug and those who received dietary therapy. In Study B, the investigator used a larger sample size yielding the same point estimates of risk in the two groups but with much greater precision (ie, narrower confidence intervals) in the estimate of the effects of the drug. With this gain in precision, the statistical test was able to distinguish between the two groups, and the investigator was able to infer correctly that the cholesterol-lowering drug was superior to dietary therapy. Generally, the larger the sample size, the more precise the estimate of effect and the smaller the detectable differences between groups. In studies with very large sample sizes, small differences between groups may be judged to be statistically significant but have little biological or clinical meaning. For example, a study of 20,000 subjects might have concluded that a 1% difference in risk of developing myocardial infarction was statistically significant. It is unlikely, however, that a difference in risk this small would justify prolonged use of the cholesterol-lowering agent.

VALIDITY

The concept of validity concerns the degree to which a measurement or study reaches a correct conclusion. A measurement or study may lead to an incorrect (invalid) conclusion because of the effects of **bias.** The variability seen with bias is systematic or nonrandom and distorts the estimated effect. In Figure 10–1, the amount of bias can be determined by the degree to which the shots are off target in D. Unfortunately, in medical research the truth (bull's-eye) may not be known, or there may be no "gold standard" for

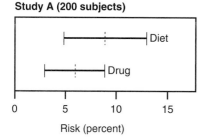

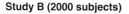

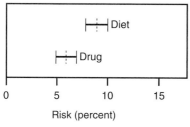

Figure 10–3. The effect of sample size on precision of risk estimates. Point estimates are shown as dashed vertical lines and 95% confidence intervals are shown as solid horizontal lines. In both studies, the 5-year risk of developing myocardial infarction was 9% among persons receiving dietary therapy and 6% among persons treated with a cholesterol-lowering drug. In the larger study, however, the 95% confidence intervals are narrower, and the difference in risk between treatment groups is statistically significant.

comparison. Consequently, the degree of bias often is difficult to determine. Two different types of validity, internal validity and external validity, are described in this chapter.

Internal Validity

Internal validity is the extent to which the results of an investigation accurately reflect the true situation of the study population. If the results are not valid in the study population, there is little reason to suspect that those results will apply to other populations. Internal validity is defined by the boundaries of the study itself. Therefore, a study is internally valid if it provides a true estimate of effect, given the limits of the population studied. Measures that can be used to improve internal validity often involve restricting the type of subjects and the environment in which the study is performed. These measures decrease the impact of factors extraneous to the question of interest.

External Validity

A result obtained in a tightly controlled environment, however, may not be applicable to more general situations. *External validity is the extent to which the results of a study are applicable to other populations.* External validity addresses the following question: Do these results apply to other patients, such as patients who are older, sicker, or less economically advantaged than subjects in the study?

External validity often is of particular interest to clinicians who must decide if a research finding is applicable to their clinical practice. Determining whether the results of a study can be generalized involves a judgment regarding the following:

1. The type of subjects included in the investigation
2. The type of patients seen by the clinician
3. Whether there are clinically meaningful differences between the study population and other populations.

An example of the kind of difficulty that can occur when study results are generalized is the criticism that too many clinical studies focus on white males. One such study is the Lipid Research Clinics-Primary Prevention Trial, which demonstrated a significant reduction in cardiovascular mortality for white men aged 35–59 years with hypercholesterolemia who were placed on a cholesterol-lowering diet and medication. Do the results also apply to women? Do they apply to men of different ages, races, or with different, but still abnormal, serum cholesterol levels? These questions led to the suggestion that federally funded research should include women, minorities, and children in the study populations.

Bias

Bias is a systematic error in a study that leads to a distortion of the results. Bias, a threat to validity, can occur in any research, but is of particular concern in observational studies because the lack of randomization increases the chance that study groups will differ with respect to important characteristics. Bias often is subdivided into different categories, based on how bias enters the study. The most common classification divides bias into three categories:

1. Selection bias
2. Information bias
3. Confounding.

Although these categories overlap, this classification is useful because it provides the reader with a systematic approach to evaluate bias. It should be remembered that with the exception of confounding, which can be quantitated, the evaluation of bias is subjective and involves a judgment regarding the likelihood of (1) the presence of bias and (2) its direction and potential magnitude of effect on the results. Even though the magnitude of bias cannot be quantified, often its influence on the results of a study can be inferred. It is important to discern whether the suspected bias is likely to make an association appear stronger or weaker than it really is. Overestimation of a risk ratio for a protective exposure and a separate hazardous exposure is demonstrated schematically in Figure 10–4. Underestimation of a risk ratio for a protective exposure and a hazardous exposure is shown in Figure 10–5.

Selection Bias

A variety of procedures can be used to select subjects for a study. Usually, it is not possible to include all individuals with a particular disease or exposure in a study, so a sample of subjects must be chosen. The procedures used for the selection of subjects depend on a number of factors, including

1. The design of the investigation
2. The setting of the study
3. The disease and exposure of interest.

Often subjects are selected in a manner that is convenient for the investigator. Under optimal circumstances, the method for inclusion of subjects leads to a valid comparison that, in turn, yields correct information regarding a disease process or treatment.

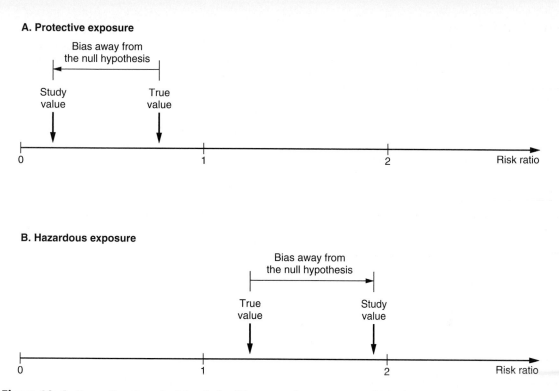

Figure 10–4. Overestimation of a risk ratio for (**A**) a protective exposure and (**B**) a hazardous exposure.

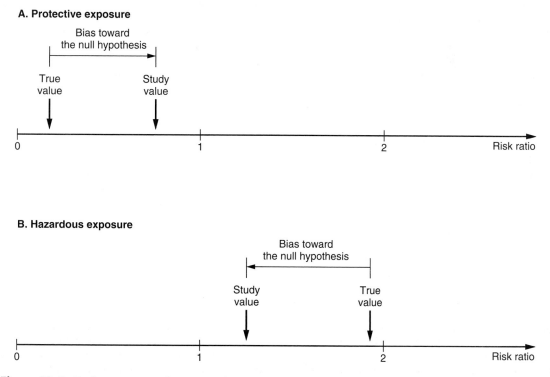

Figure 10–5. Underestimation of a risk ratio for (**A**) a protective exposure and (**B**) a hazardous exposure.

The selection process itself, however, may increase or decrease the chance that a relationship between the exposure and disease of interest will be detected, creating a **selection bias.** A schematic diagram of the steps involved in recruiting and maintaining a study population is shown in Figure 10–6. From this diagram, it is easy to see that selection factors could lead to biased results at several different steps in the process.

Some aspects of the selection of subjects lead primarily to problems with the generalization (extrapolation) of the results (ie, external validity). Subjects must agree to participate in a study, and this causes one of the most common problems. Volunteers for a study may differ from individuals who do not volunteer in various characteristics such as age, race, economic status, education level, and sex. Moreover, volunteers may be healthier than those who decline to participate. A study of a population limited to individuals who are employed may also make it difficult to generalize the results, because people who work are generally healthier than those who do not. A comparison of health outcomes between workers and the general population may show that the workers have a more favorable outcome simply because they are healthy enough to be employed (the "healthy worker" effect).

Referral of patients to clinical facilities can also lead to distorted study conclusions. Selective referral patterns can be seen in the study of children with febrile seizures. Febrile seizures are brief, generalized seizures that occur in conjunction with elevation in temperature in children aged 6 months to 6 years. There is some disagreement about whether these febrile convulsions are predictive of future seizures and other unfavorable neurologic sequelae. Ellenberg and Nelson (1980) compared the results of a number of studies on the long-term outcome of patients with febrile seizures. Studies of geographically defined populations in which affected children were followed, regardless of whether medical care was sought, consistently revealed a relatively low rate of unfavorable sequelae. Clinic-based studies tended to report a high frequency of adverse outcomes. Accordingly, it was concluded that clinic-based studies selectively included children at the more severe end of the clinical spectrum. The inferences that might be drawn regarding the prognosis of a child with febrile seizures might be very different based on whether a clinic-based or a population-based sample was studied.

Other aspects of the selection process can diminish internal validity. *In a clinical trial or cohort study, the major potential selection bias is loss to follow-up.* Once subjects are enrolled in the study, they may decide to discontinue participation. Certain types of subjects are more likely than others to drop out of a study. Furthermore, during the course of the study some subjects may die from causes other than the outcome of interest. At first glance, these losses may not appear to be related to selection because the subject already was enrolled in the study. If the lost subjects differ, however, in their risk of the outcome of interest, biased estimates of risk may be obtained.

If the unrecognized early manifestations of the disease of interest cause exposed persons to leave the study more or less frequently than unexposed persons, a distorted conclusion might be reached. For example, in a randomized controlled trial of the effects of using a cholesterol-lowering drug versus diet therapy on prevention of myocardial infarctions, bias might be introduced if drug-treated patients with coronary insufficiency were more likely to develop side effects from treatment and withdrew from participation, whereas patients with coronary insufficiency receiving dietary therapy remained in the study.

Selection bias is of particular importance in case–control studies (see Chapter 9) in which the investigator must select two study groups, cases and controls, in a setting in which the exposure has already occurred. For example, it must be decided whether to use existing (prevalent) cases who are available at the time of study, regardless of the duration of their disease, or to limit eligibility to newly diagnosed (incident) cases. If the risk

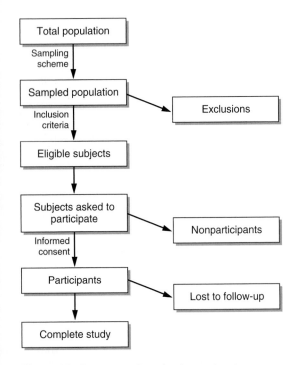

Figure 10–6. Steps in the selection and maintenance of subjects in a study.

factor of interest also is a prognostic factor, the use of prevalent cases can lead to a biased conclusion. Consider, for example, a case–control study of total serum cholesterol level as a risk factor for developing myocardial infarction. Suppose that of patients who have a myocardial infarction those with very high total serum cholesterol levels are more likely to die suddenly than those with lower serum cholesterol levels. Under these circumstances, a comparison of patients surviving myocardial infarction with controls will underestimate the true association between elevation in total serum cholesterol level and risk of developing myocardial infarction.

Another potential type of selection bias can occur when a case–control study involves subjects who are hospitalized. Patients with two medical conditions are more likely to be hospitalized than those with a single disease. Thus, a hospital-based case–control study might find a link between two diseases or between an exposure and a disease when there is no association between them in the general population. This type of bias, often called Berkson's bias, was demonstrated in a study that showed that respiratory and bone diseases were associated in a sample of hospitalized patients but not in the general population. Thus, in a hospital-based study, an exposure such as cigarette smoking, which is correlated with respiratory disease, may also appear to occur together with bone disease because those diseases are related in hospitalized patients.

Information Bias

Information (or misclassification) bias can occur when there is random or systematic inaccuracy in measurement. This can be visualized best in epidemiologic studies that involve dichotomous exposure and disease variables, such as elevated total serum cholesterol and myocardial infarction. Subjects are classified according to whether they have had high total serum cholesterol levels and whether they have had a myocardial infarction. The investigator either can be correct or incorrect, resulting in true-positive and true-negative findings, as well as false-positive and false-negative classifications of subjects with respect to either exposure or disease.

If the errors in classification of exposure or disease status are independent of the level of the other variable, then the misclassification is termed **nondifferential.** Nondifferential misclassification may occur in a case–control study if the subject's memory of exposure status is unrelated to whether the subject has the disease of interest. An example of nondifferential misclassification is sometimes referred to as unacceptability bias. Subjects may answer a question about the exposure with a socially acceptable but sometimes inaccurate response, regardless of whether they have the disease of interest. Consider a case–control study of myocardial infarction in which the exposure of interest is prior intake of foods high in saturated fats. Regardless of disease status, respondents may underreport intake of foods with high fat content because they think low-fat diets are more acceptable to the investigator. In most instances, when nondifferential misclassification occurs, it blurs differences between the study groups, making it more difficult for the investigator to detect a real association between the exposure and the disease. This is often referred to as a bias toward the null hypothesis or toward no association.

Differential misclassification occurs when the misclassification of one variable depends on the status of the other. In a case–control study, this type of misclassification could occur if the information on exposure status depends on whether the subject has the disease. If a case with a myocardial infarction is more likely to overestimate the level of dietary fat intake than a control subject, a biased result may occur. In this instance, the bias would lead to an overestimate of the relationship between dietary fat intake and risk of developing myocardial infarction.

The difference between nondifferential and differential misclassification can be demonstrated by examining the data in Figure 10–7. Consider a case–control study of the relationship between high-fat diets and risk of developing myocardial infarction in which the true odds ratio (*OR*) is 2.3. With nondifferential misclassification, the subjects did not recall the amount of fatty foods eaten, but the errors in recall did not depend on whether they had a myocardial infarction. In this situation, 20% of both cases and controls who ate high-fat diets underreported fat intake. The resulting *OR* of 2.0 was an underestimate of the true *OR*. On the other hand, if all the patients who had a myocardial infarction correctly recalled their dietary fat exposure status, but only 80% of the exposed controls correctly reported their exposure, then differential misclassification would occur. This type of misclassification can result in either an underestimate or overestimate of the true *OR*. In this example, the investigator overestimated the *OR*.

Two common types of differential information bias are often referred to as **recall bias** and **interviewer bias.** Recall bias results from differential ability of subjects to remember previous activities and exposures. Patients who have a serious disease may search their memory for an exposure in an attempt to explain or to understand why they acquired the illness. Control subjects, who do not have the disease, may be less likely to remember an exposure because it has less meaning and is less important for them.

When interviewers are employed to determine exposures in case–control studies, results may be influenced

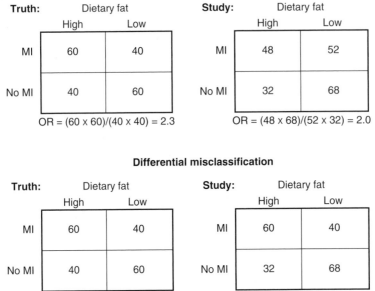

Nondifferential misclassification

Truth: Dietary fat — High / Low

	High	Low
MI	60	40
No MI	40	60

OR = (60 x 60)/(40 x 40) = 2.3

Study: Dietary fat — High / Low

	High	Low
MI	48	52
No MI	32	68

OR = (48 x 68)/(52 x 32) = 2.0

Differential misclassification

Truth: Dietary fat — High / Low

	High	Low
MI	60	40
No MI	40	60

OR = (60 x 60)/(40 x 40) = 2.3

Study: Dietary fat — High / Low

	High	Low
MI	60	40
No MI	32	68

OR = (60 x 68)/(40 x 32) = 3.2

Figure 10–7. Illustration of nondifferential and differential misclassification of exposure to high-fat diets in a case–control study of myocardial infarction (MI). (OR = odds ratio.)

by how the interviewers collect information. If they are aware of the research hypothesis, the interviewers intentionally or unintentionally may influence the responses of the subjects. They may probe more deeply for responses from cases than from controls. If a dietary exposure is examined, the interviewers may ask certain subjects specific questions about particular food items. Interviewers may also give the subjects subtle clues by tone of voice or body language that suggest a preference for certain responses. Generally, it is desirable to blind the interviewers to the research hypothesis under investigation. In a case–control study, however, it may be difficult to blind the interviewers to the disease status of cases and controls. Nevertheless, if the interviewers are not aware of the exposure of primary interest, biased data collection still can be minimized.

As a way to reduce misclassification and to improve accuracy of study measurements, investigators increasingly are using **biological markers.** As shown in Table 10–3, these markers can measure many facets of disease and exposure—or the relationship between the two. For example, biological markers can measure

Table 10–3. Uses of biological markers in epidemiology.

Application of Marker	Example
To measure susceptibility	Those with high aryl hydrocarbon hydroxylase activity have higher risk of bladder cancer
To measure internal dose	Those with high serum carotene levels may have lower risk of lung cancer
To measure biologically effective dose	Those with greater amounts of effective dose of polycyclic aromatic hydrocarbon-DNA adducts have experienced greater exposure and interaction of their DNA to these carcinogenic hydrocarbons[a]
To measure biological effect	Higher levels of the *ras* oncogene product may be a preclinical marker of early carcinogenic resopnse[a]

[a]Perera F et al: Biologic markers in risk assessment for environmental carcinogens. Environ Health Persp 1991;**90**:247.

1. Susceptibility (biological markers can be used to identify subjects with particularly high risk due to a particular biological predisposition)
2. Internal dose (biological markers can be used to measure the amount of a chemical or other exposure in the body)
3. Biologically effective dose (biological markers can be used to measure the amount of a substance that reaches the target sites)
4. Biological effect (biological markers can be used to quantify a deleterious effect of a particular exposure).

Biological markers are used in most substantive areas of investigation, including nutritional, cardiovascular, reproductive, cancer, and infectious disease epidemiology. Use of biological markers is important in observational studies for several reasons. These markers are important methodologically because they can serve to reduce misclassification by allowing more accurate assessment of exposure or disease status. Furthermore, they may allow the investigator to define more homogeneous disease categories or to identify susceptible subjects, so that the study can focus on specific subgroups. Finally, biological markers can help provide insight into the underlying disease process and pathogenesis.

The use of levels of serum dioxin to measure exposure of men who worked with the herbicide Agent Orange during the Vietnam War illustrates the use of a biological marker to measure internal dose. After the Vietnam War, concern arose about wartime exposures of servicemen to Agent Orange, in part because of its contamination with the highly toxic trace contaminant known as 2,3,7,8-tetrachlorodibenzo-p-dioxin (TCDD). Because of this concern, Air Force researchers began epidemiologic studies to assess the health effects among Air Force veterans associated with exposure to Agent Orange and TCDD. Researchers initially used job descriptions to classify exposure to TCDD. Later, after laboratory techniques became available to measure minute concentrations of TCDD within the blood, the researchers discovered that classification of exposure based on job descriptions was associated with substantial misclassification. In subsequent studies, the more accurate serum TCDD measurements were used to assess exposures.

Despite the importance of biological markers and the possibility that their use may reduce information bias, they do not eliminate the possibility of systematic errors. Although it may be diminished by employing a biological marker, misclassification remains a possibility. For example, marker instability and inter- or intraindividual variability can contribute to measurement errors. Moreover, if required biological specimens are collected after disease occurrence, as often happens in case–control studies, the presence of disease in cases may affect the biological marker. This possibility can make the biological marker particularly susceptible to differential misclassification and measurement error. Bias can even be created if the investigator adjusts inappropriately for a factor that is caused by the exposure of interest and is associated with the outcome.

Case–control studies of the relationship of β-carotene and cancer illustrate the potential for residual information bias. β-carotene is a fat-soluble antioxidant found in many fruits and vegetables. It acts as a provitamin (vitamin A), protects against development of cancer in animals, and may reduce the risk of developing cancer in humans. In a case–control study of serum levels of this antioxidant, differential misclassification could create or accentuate a protective effect, if cases with advanced cancer had altered nutritional status and a resulting lowering of β-carotene levels. Although these biases are somewhat speculative, the potential for bias in case–control studies is evident.

Thus, use of biological markers offers many advantages, particularly an improved assessment of exposure and a more homogeneous definition of disease. Nevertheless, because use of these markers does not eliminate the possibility of information bias, caution in interpretation is still warranted.

Confounding

Confounding refers to the mixing of the effect of an extraneous variable with the effects of the exposure and disease of interest. Confounding can be demonstrated by the following hypothetical example. Suppose investigators undertake a case–control study of the association between high total serum cholesterol level and risk of developing myocardial infarction. From the results of other studies, the researchers know that the risk of myocardial infarction is associated with obesity, and that total cholesterol levels also correlate with obesity (see Figure 10–8). Suppose that in our hypothetical case–control study, 36 of 60 patients with myocardial infarction (60%) are found to have high total serum cholesterol levels, and only 24 of 60 controls (40%) are discovered to have elevated serum cholesterol levels. This would suggest that elevated total serum cholesterol levels are associated with an increased risk of developing myocardial infarction.

When the observed association is examined separately in obese and nonobese persons, however, a different conclusion is reached. Among obese persons, 34 of 40 patients with myocardial infarction (85%) and 18 of 20 controls (90%) are found to have elevated total serum cholesterol levels. Among nonobese persons, 2 of 20 patients with myocardial infarction (10%) and 6 of 40 controls (15%) have high total serum cholesterol

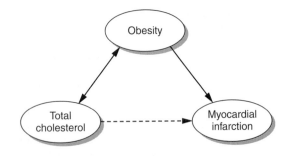

Figure 10–8. Schematic diagram of the relationship between total serum cholesterol level and risk of developing myocardial infarction, with confounding by obesity.

levels. Thus in the case of both obese and nonobese individuals, elevated total serum cholesterol levels are more common in controls than in patients with myocardial infarction. Keep in mind that in the hypothetical study, obesity was associated with myocardial infarction, since 52 of 60 obese subjects (87%) had elevated total serum cholesterol levels, and only 8 of 60 nonobese persons (13%) had high total serum cholesterol levels. Clearly, in this hypothetical example, the results are confounded by the extraneous variable, obesity. The results are illustrated in Figure 10–9.

For a variable—in this case, obesity—to be considered a potential confounder, it must satisfy two conditions:

1. Association with the disease of interest in the absence of exposure
2. Association with the exposure but not as a result of being exposed.

Because it can be evaluated in the analysis of results, confounding differs from selection bias and information bias. The presence of confounding is demonstrated by a change in the apparent strength of association between the exposure and the disease of interest when the effects of extraneous variables are taken into account. Confounding, which is not an all-or-none property of an extraneous variable, may occur to different degrees in different studies.

Generally, the list of potential confounders in a study is limited to established risk factors for the disease of interest. There are two accepted methods for dealing with potential confounders. The first is to consider them in the design of the study by matching on the potential confounder or by restricting the sample to limited levels of the potential confounder. The other method is to evaluate confounding in the analysis by stratification, as demonstrated schematically in Figure 10–9, or by using multivariate analysis techniques such as multiple logistic regression.

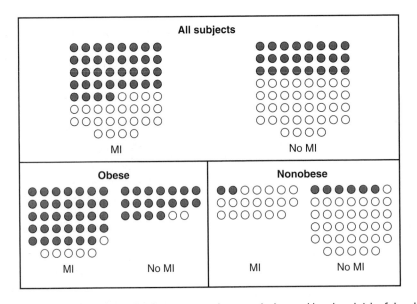

Figure 10–9. Illustration of the relationship between total serum cholesterol level and risk of developing myocardial infarction (MI), with confounding by obesity. Shaded circles represent persons with elevated total serum cholesterol levels and unshaded circles represent persons with normal total serum cholesterol levels.

The goal of any epidemiologic study is to provide a valid conclusion. To accomplish this objective, complete attention must be given to all aspects of the study, from inception to design and data collection, and finally to analysis and reporting of results. It is important to remember that bias can be introduced at any of these stages, leading to erroneous results. Thus it is useful to look carefully for potential sources of bias and to consider their possible impact. Clinicians must judge whether results can be generalized to their particular practice. Understanding the potential problems with measurement and bias in medical research improves the ability of physicians to decide on appropriate preventive and therapeutic strategies.

SUMMARY

In this chapter, the topics of variability and systematic errors in epidemiologic measurements are discussed, with illustrative examples that focus primarily on the relationship between total serum cholesterol level and the risk of developing myocardial infarction. A distinction is drawn between random variation, which is inversely related to precision in measurement, and nonrandom or systematic error, which is related to a distortion in measurement.

Variability can arise from (1) the subjects under study, (2) differences between individuals, (3) the approach used to sample subjects, or (4) the measurement process itself. Variability related to sampling is likely to diminish as the sample size increases. With extremely large sample sizes, a very small difference in outcome between study groups can be statistically significant. Whether the magnitude of this difference is sufficient to warrant a change in clinical practice is a separate, but equally important, question.

Validity concerns the extent to which the findings of a study reflect truth. **Internal validity** relates to the accuracy of study findings for the persons who are investigated. **External validity** concerns the extent to which study findings accurately apply to persons who are not studied.

Bias is defined as lack of validity. Conventionally, bias is classified into three major types: **selection bias, information (misclassification) bias,** and **confounding.** Selection bias refers to the introduction of systematic errors into study results through the manner in which study subjects are selected. Information bias results in systematic errors in study findings that originate in the approach to collecting information. Two kinds of information bias can exist. **Nondifferential misclassification** occurs when errors in the information about one variable are unrelated to the status of another variable. **Differential misclassification,** on the other hand,

occurs when errors in the information about one variable are affected by the status of another variable.

Confounding is concerned with the mixing of the primary effect of interest with the effects of one or more extraneous factors. In experimental studies, the problem of confounding is reduced by randomization, which tends to balance the study groups with respect to both known and unknown determinants of the outcome. In observational research, however, study groups may differ appreciably in factors that are (1) related to the risk of disease among unexposed persons and (2) are also associated with the exposure of interest, but not as a result of being exposed. The influence of these potential confounders can be addressed in the study design (eg, through matching or restrictive inclusion criteria) or in the analysis (eg, through stratification or regression techniques). Only known confounders can be addressed in observational research.

No study is immune from the possibility of bias. The investigator must therefore consider potential sources of bias when sampling subjects, collecting information, analyzing results, and interpreting findings. With planning and forethought, it is possible to anticipate and avoid certain types of error and thus conduct a study that leads to a convincing and valid conclusion.

STUDY QUESTIONS

Questions 1–4: For each numbered study described below, from the lettered options select the type of bias or error that would most likely result.

1. *In a case–control study of the relationship of dietary intake of fruits and vegetables and the risk of developing hypertension, the control subjects are sampled from participants at a health fair.*

   A. *Selection bias*

   B. *Nondifferential misclassification*

   C. *Confounding*

   D. *Ecologic fallacy*

   E. *Random error*

2. *In a case–control study of inflammation and the development of coronary heart disease, 20-year-old stored frozen blood specimens are used to measure C-reactive protein in cases and controls. There is concern that during storage the specimens have deteriorated, yielding lower levels than when they were first obtained.*

   A. *Selection bias*

   B. *Nondifferential misclassification*

   C. *Confounding*

D. Ecologic fallacy

E. Random error

3. In a cohort study of hormone replacement therapy and the risk of developing atherosclerotic coronary artery disease, high socioeconomic status is associated with both use of hormone replacement therapy and risk of developing coronary artery disease.

A. Selection bias

B. Nondifferential misclassification

C. Confounding

D. Ecologic fallacy

E. Random error

4. In a case–control study of alcohol consumption and the risk of hepatocellular carcinoma, both cases and controls underreport exposure to alcohol.

A. Selection bias

B. Nondifferential misclassification

C. Confounding

D. Ecologic fallacy

E. Random error

Questions 5–8: For each numbered situation below, select the most likely effect on the study findings from the lettered options.

5. In a cohort study of the effect of obesity on the development of left ventricular hypertrophy, the investigator reviewing the echocardiogram is blinded to whether the subject is obese or not.

A. Overestimation

B. Underestimation

C. No effect

D. Cannot be determined

6. In a cohort study of obesity and the risk of development of type 2 diabetes, the loss to follow-up is 35% among the obese subjects and 15% among the nonobese subjects.

A. Overestimation

B. Underestimation

C. No effect

D. Cannot be determined

7. In a case–control study of the relationship of stressful life events and the occurrence of coronary artery disease, patients with coronary artery disease are more likely to report past stressful events than are the healthy controls.

A. Overestimation

B. Underestimation

C. No effect

D. Cannot be determined

8. Prevalent patients with histories of myocardial infarctions are enrolled in a case–control study of inflammation as measured by C-reactive protein as a risk factor for developing myocardial infarction. Among patients who have had a myocardial infarction, higher C-reactive protein is associated with a higher case fatality rate.

A. Overestimation

B. Underestimation

C. No effect

D. Cannot be determined

Questions 9–10: For each numbered situation below, select the most appropriate study design from the lettered options.

9. Individuals with hypertension are randomized to a diuretic, a calcium channel blocker, a β-blocker, and an angiotensin-converting enzyme inhibitor in order to evaluate relative safety and efficacy.

A. Case–control study

B. Cohort study

C. Clinical trial

D. Ecologic study

E. Cross-sectional study

10. The ability to assign by chance the type of antihypertensive agent used reduces the likelihood of confounding of diet and physical activity in a study of treatment of blood pressure elevation.

A. Case–control study

B. Cohort study

C. Clinical trial

D. Ecologic study

E. Cross-sectional study

FURTHER READING

Grimes DA, Schulz KF: Bias and causal associations in observational research. Lancet 2002;**359**:248.

Hartman JM et al: Tutorials in clinical research: part IV: recognizing and controlling bias. Laryngoscope 2002;**112**:23.

REFERENCES

Patient Profile

Cleeman JI, Lenfant C: The National Cholesterol Education Program. JAMA 1998;**280**:2099.

National Heart, Lung and Blood Institute: *Recommendations for Improving Cholesterol Measurements: A Report from the Laboratory Standardization Panel of the National Cholesterol Education Program.* US Department of Health and Human Services. NIH Publication No. 90-2964, 1990.

Variability Related to Measurement

Report of the National Cholesterol Education Program Expert Panel on detection, evaluation and treatment of high blood cholesterol in adults. Arch Intern Med 1988;**148:**36.

External Validity

Altman DG, Bland JM: Generalization and extrapolation. BMJ 1998;**317:**409.

Knottnerus A, Dinant GJ: Medicine based evidence, a prerequisite for evidence based medicine. BMJ 1997;**315:**1109.

Lipid Research Clinic Program: The Lipid Research Clinic's Coronary Primary Prevention Trial results. 1. Reduction in incidence of coronary heart disease. JAMA 1984;**251:**351.

Selection Bias

Ellenberg JH, Nelson KB: Sample selection and the natural history of disease: Studies of febrile seizures. JAMA 1980;**243:**1337.

Roberts RS, Spitzer WO, Delmore T et al: Empirical demonstration of Berkson's bias. J Chronic Dis 1978;**31:**119.

Information Bias

Coates RJ et al: Cancer risk in relation to serum copper levels. Cancer Res 1989;**49:**4353.

Hulka BS, Wilcosky TC, Griffith JD: *Biologic Markers in Epidemiology.* Oxford University Press, 1990.

Perera F et al: Biologic markers in risk assessment for environmental carcinogens. Environ Health Perspect 1991;**90:**247.

Confounding

Weinberg CR: Toward a clearer definition of confounding. Am J Epidemiol 1993;**137:**1.

e-PIDEMIOLOGY

Patient Profile

http://www.nhlbi.nih.gov/guidelines/cholesterol/atp3full.pdf

Variability in Medical Research

http://www.bmj.com/epidem/epid.4.shtml

Validity

http://www.usd.edu/~dstevens/ctrial.htm#ERROR
http://www.pitt.edu/~super1/lecture/lec6211/index.htm

Bias

http://www.pitt.edu/~super1/lecture/lec8361/index.htm

Epidemiologic Studies of Genetics   11

KEY CONCEPTS

1. Familial aggregation of a disease is suggested when the recurrence risk among relatives of affected persons exceeds that among relatives of unaffected persons.

2. In studies of twins, greater concordance for disease among monozygotic twins as compared with dizygotic twins suggests genetically determined susceptibility.

3. If subjects with a high degree of inbreeding have an elevated risk of disease, an autosomal recessive pattern of inheritance may be suggested.

4. Co-segregation refers to the tendency of alleles that are situated closely together on the chromosomes to be inherited together.

5. Linkage of a marker gene (with a known location in the genome) and a disease susceptibility gene can suggest the particular chromosome involved and where on the chromosome the susceptibility gene is likely to be located.

6. Segregation analysis of pedigrees is a complex statistical technique used to determine whether a disease has, at least in part, a genetic origin, and if so, the likely pattern of inheritance.

PATIENT PROFILE

A 70-year-old retired car salesman is brought by his spouse of 50 years to their family physician for evaluation of "forgetfulness." Over the previous several years, the patient has had increasing difficulty remembering recent events and has become lost when driving, even near his home. More recently, he has often forgotten names and has asked the same questions several times in succession. He is not taking any medications, nor is there any history of alcoholism, use of recreational drugs, exposure to toxins, high blood pressure, or stroke. The patient's family history is unremarkable, except for a similar course of progressive memory loss and cognitive disability in his mother and in the oldest of his three siblings.

The patient appears well nourished, without evidence of systemic illness. On mental status examination, the patient does not know the year, cannot remember any of three objects 5 minutes after learning them, and cannot count backward from 100 by 7. Neurologic examination is otherwise normal. After magnetic resonance imaging and further tests to rule out specific, treatable causes of dementia, a diagnosis of Alzheimer's disease is made.

CLINICAL BACKGROUND

Dementia is characterized by impaired short- and long-term memory, along with disturbances of other cognitive functions (eg, language or visuospatial function). For a diagnosis of dementia to be made, the patient's loss of cognitive abilities must be of sufficient magnitude to interfere with the individual's performance of social or occupational activities. More than 60 different clinical disorders are associated with dementia, and Alzheimer's disease is the most common cause of dementia in many populations. This disease was first reported in 1907 by Alois Alzheimer, who described morphological changes in the brain of a patient who died with progressive dementia. The clinical diagnosis of Alzheimer's disease is made by excluding other possible causes of dementia, among which vascular disorders predominate.

The "gold standard" for arriving at a diagnosis of Alzheimer's disease is a histologic examination of brain tissue. Patients with pathologic confirmation of disease are characterized as having "definite Alzheimer's disease." Clinical diagnosis typically is rendered on the basis of the composite findings of (1) a careful history, (2) physical, neurologic, and psychiatric examinations, and (3) laboratory and radiologic assessments. Patients who satisfy the clinical criteria, but do not have pathologic confirmation of disease, are characterized as having "probable Alzheimer's disease." When optimally applied, the standardized clinical diagnostic criteria for Alzheimer's disease can yield a positive predictive value of 85% or higher, when compared with eventual findings at autopsy.

Although signs and symptoms of Alzheimer's disease vary among patients, the onset of this disorder is typically insidious, and cognitive function deteriorates continually over time. This form of dementia is rarely seen in patients under age 60, but thereafter the incidence rises markedly with age. Patients usually present with difficulties in new learning. With advancing disease over several years, patients also develop difficulty with attention, orientation, reasoning, and emotions.

Diagnostic imaging of the brain reveals generalized atrophy of the cerebral cortex with enlargement of the ventricles. On postmortem examination, brains of patients with this disease are atrophied, particularly in the neocortex. Microscopic examination of the gray matter can reveal a loss of nerve cells and synapses, with abnormally staining neurons, neurofibrillary tangles, and neuritic plaques with a protein fragment, β-amyloid, at their core. β-Amyloid is an abnormal breakdown product of amyloid precursor protein, which is routinely produced by many cells, including neurons. A variety of neurochemical deficits occur in conjunction with Alzheimer's disease, the most prominent being a loss of cholinergic neurons as reflected by a decrease in choline acetyltransferase activity.

The etiology of Alzheimer's disease and its associated morphologic and biochemical abnormalities is unknown. Research to date has emphasized genetic predisposition as well as environmental risk factors such as head trauma and exposure to aluminum, but findings have been inconsistent. Recent studies in genetics and genetic epidemiology point to several genes that appear to play a role in the etiology of Alzheimer's disease. For patients with early onset of disease (before 65 years of age), it has been estimated that as much as 50% of the disease occurrence may be explained by mutations of genes on chromosomes 1, 14, and 21. The gene on chromosome 21 codes for amyloid precursor protein, which has an autosomal dominant pattern of inheritance. The gene on chromosome 14 is referred to as presenilin 1 and the gene on chromosome 1 is referred to as presenilin 2. Both of the presenilin genes have an autosomal dominant pattern of inheritance. A fourth gene, found on chromosome 19 and referred to as apolipoprotein E (Apo E), codes for a protein involved in transport of cholesterol during neuronal growth and after injury. Apo E is associated with late-onset disease (after 65 years of age), with the e4 allele conferring increased susceptibility to developing Alzheimer's disease. Some evidence is emerging that genetic risk and environmental factors may interact. For example, head injury may be a risk factor for late-onset Alzheimer's disease, but perhaps only among those with the e4 allele of Apo E.

The prognosis for patients with Alzheimer's disease varies widely, and among other factors, is dependent on age and severity of illness at diagnosis. For very elderly patients, Alzheimer's disease may not impact on longevity, but does impair the quality of life. Death usually is not attributable to Alzheimer's disease per se, but rather to other conditions that arise during the course of illness. Presently, no specific treatments prevent, arrest, or reverse the clinical progression of the illness. For patients with Alzheimer's disease, some symptomatic relief can be achieved by addressing the neurochemical deficits. For example, cholinesterase inhibitors have been shown to slow the loss of cognitive function in at least subsets of patients with Alzheimer's disease. Recent studies have demonstrated that disease progression also can be slowed by an antagonist to N-methyl-D-aspartate (NMDA), which reduces the flow of potentially damaging calcium into neurons. Other approaches under exploration for slowing the progression of illness include the use of nonsteroidal anti-inflammatory agents, antioxidants, and estrogen.

INTRODUCTION

Researchers often use epidemiologic techniques to study genetic risk factors and interactions between genetic susceptibility and environmental factors, an application known as **genetic epidemiology.** The field of genetic epidemiology concerns the study of hereditary and environmental determinants of disease in human populations. This application of epidemiology is growing rapidly, in parallel with gains in knowledge about the human genome. As illustrated by the Patient Profile, we can apply knowledge of genetic susceptibilities to identify high-risk individuals and groups. For diseases in which screening tests and effective preventive or therapeutic regimens are available, knowledge of inherited risks can be used to enhance early detection and to encourage programs aimed at prevention.

Genetic epidemiology involves principles from the field of genetics as well as epidemiology. In particular, the design, conduct, and interpretation of studies in genetic epidemiology involve the same principles that apply to other kinds of epidemiologic research. For example, most research in genetic epidemiology involves a cohort or case–control design; but such a study differs from other epidemiologic studies primarily in that one of the "exposures" is a genetic factor.

In genetic applications, as in other areas of inquiry, early investigation of disease etiology often involves study of the descriptive epidemiology of the disease. Results of descriptive studies provide information about disease frequency and public health importance. Such findings may suggest an etiologic role of specific genetic, environmental, or other risk factors, and further investigation may evaluate a putative role for inherited susceptibility. Since a hereditary predisposition would give rise to clusters of disease within families, the epidemiologist may conduct studies to ascertain the degree of familial aggregation. If results of such studies document familial aggregation and suggest that genetic factors contribute to disease occurrence, subsequent investigation might involve assessing the association of risk of disease with specific markers, for example, a particular gene or gene product. Thus, genetic epidemiologic study of disease etiology frequently proceeds from

1. General descriptive studies, as part of an initial search for clues about etiology
2. Studies of familial aggregation, as part of a search for evidence of clustering within families
3. Epidemiologic studies designed to assess risk associated with specific genetic factors. An additional step in the investigation, one that is more an application of population genetics than of epidemiology, may involve more complex methods of genetic analysis that look for evidence of genetic etiology within pedigrees.

The basic types of investigation used in genetic epidemiology are shown in Table 11–1, along with a description of the goals of such studies and some illustrative applications. These various approaches are characterized in greater detail in the following sections of this chapter. The text is organized in a sequence that parallels the order in which these investigations might be conducted to characterize the etiology of a disease. First descriptive studies are performed, followed by research on familial aggregation, then exploration of specific genetic traits. For completeness of presentation, complex genetic analyses are mentioned briefly at the conclusion of the chapter, although these methods are often considered part of the domain of population genetics. Throughout the chapter, illustrative examples are drawn from the literature on Alzheimer's disease.

DESCRIPTIVE EPIDEMIOLOGIC STUDIES

The health researcher can use descriptive studies to shed light on the public health importance of an illness and on possible roles of genetic and environmental fac-

Table 11–1. Types of studies used to elucidate genetic influences on the risk of disease occurrence in human populations.

Type of Study	Goal	Example
Descriptive studies	Study nonspecific factors, eg, age, sex, ethnicity	Higher occurrence of classic hemophilia in males
Studies of familial aggregation	Study recurrence risks, familial aggregation, influence of inbreeding	Higher risk of breast cancer among daughters of women with breast cancer
Studies of specific genetic factors	Study risk associated with specific genetic factors, eg, enzymes or DNA sequences	Higher risk of insulin-dependent diabetes among those with certain human leukocyte antigens (HLAs)
Complex genetic analyses	Study pattern of risks within pedigrees	Higher risk of Alzheimer's disease in relative who shares alleles with a case

tors in occurrence of disease. In particular, basic characteristics of person, time, and place—as discussed in Chapter 3—can provide clues to possible genetic and environmental risk factors.

Personal characteristics associated with variations in incidence can provide important information. Higher occurrence among certain ethnic or racial groups can suggest life-style, environmental, or possibly genetic risk factors. Higher occurrence of a disease among males can suggest hormonal risk factors, life-style factors, or an X-linked genetic disease. For example, the rare occurrence among females of classic hemophilia, a deficiency of functional clotting factor VIII—coupled with the 50% risk among male offspring born to certain female carriers of this disease—points to an X-linked recessive inheritance.

Geographic and temporal variation in disease occurrence can also provide important information. In particular, environmental factors that vary in parallel with disease rates may play a causal role. For example, within the United States the north-to-south gradient of increasing mortality from malignant melanoma, a potentially lethal form of skin cancer, parallels the north-to-south gradient of rising exposure to ultraviolet radiation (UVR). This pattern supports the role of UVR as a cause of malignant melanoma. Genetic factors, if they vary in parallel with disease occurrence, also may be important.

Studies of migrants can provide information about the relative roles of genetic and environmental factors (see Chapter 3). For example, the incidence of prostate cancer is much lower in Japan than in the United States. First-generation migrants from Japan to the United States also have relatively low incidence rates, but the rates increase successively in subsequent generations. Epidemiologists interpret this pattern as supporting a causal role for environmental exposures that change as successive generations acculturate to the life-style patterns of the adopted country. If occurrence of prostate cancer was influenced only by genetics, one would not expect to find a dramatic change in risk of disease within a few generations.

Of course, discovery that nongenetic factors play an important role does not preclude the contribution of genetic factors, and conversely, discovery that genetic factors play an important role does not preclude a contribution from nongenetic factors. A very brief overview of the epidemiology and pathophysiology of phenylketonuria illustrates the importance of both genetic and environmental factors in this disease. Phenylketonuria is an autosomal recessive disorder in which those who inherit two recessive genes have altered metabolism of phenylalanine, and consequently develop mental retardation. However, special diets low in phenylalanine can prevent mental retardation, if instituted early. This strongly suggests that genetic susceptibility and diet act jointly to cause mental retardation in this disorder.

Example 1. To investigate the descriptive epidemiology of Alzheimer's disease, researchers in East Boston conducted a survey of people aged 65 and over. After testing the memory and evaluating the neurologic condition of survey participants, the researchers estimated that about 10% of participants aged 65 or over probably had Alzheimer's disease. The prevalence increased with age to a high of nearly 50% among those over age 85. Moreover, more than 80% of the cases of moderate-to-severe cognitive impairment in this population were due to Alzheimer's disease. These results point out the overall high prevalence of Alzheimer's disease, its increasing prevalence with age, and its growing public health importance as the population ages. Other aspects of the descriptive epidemiology of Alzheimer's disease, such as the low incidence in Native Americans, suggest that genetic differences by ethnicity may affect risk of developing Alzheimer's disease.

EPIDEMIOLOGIC STUDIES OF FAMILIAL AGGREGATION

Epidemiologists expect to see disease aggregate in families if susceptibility is in part genetically determined. However, disease also can aggregate in families because nongenetic risk factors cluster among relatives. A key measure of clustering or aggregation in families is the recurrence risk, that is, the risk of disease experienced by relatives of a subject with disease.

Clustering or familial aggregation is suggested if the **recurrence risk** among relatives of a person with a disease exceeds that among relatives of a comparison subject without that disease. Put another way, clustering is suggested if a value > 1 is found for the risk ratio that compares recurrence risk among those with an affected relative with recurrence risk among those without an affected family member.

To study and quantify familial aggregation, epidemiologists often use cohort studies (Chapter 8) or case–control studies (Chapter 9). To study familial aggregation with a cohort design, the epidemiologist first identifies an index group of subjects with disease and a second index group of subjects without disease (Figure 11–1). The epidemiologist then assembles an "exposed" cohort consisting of the initially unaffected relatives of the index persons with disease and an "unexposed" cohort consisting of the initially unaffected relatives of the persons without disease. To simplify interpretation, the cohorts often consist of first-degree relatives of those in the index groups. These two groups are then followed to determine subsequent occurrence of disease and to calculate incidence rates and rate ratios in the usual way. The (incidence) rate ratio estimates the extent to

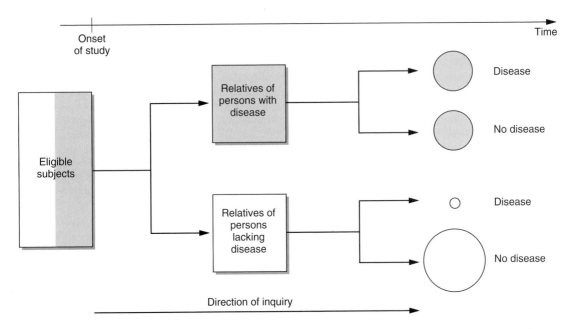

Figure 11–1. Schematic diagram of a cohort study to assess familial aggregation. Shaded areas represent "exposed" persons—those who are initially unaffected family members of index persons with the disease. Unshaded areas represent "unexposed" persons—those who are initially unaffected family members of persons without disease.

which people with an affected family member have a rate of disease that differs from those without an affected family member. Accordingly, a rate ratio greater than unity suggests familial aggregation, whereas the absence of familial aggregation is indicated by a rate ratio of unity or less.

This approach is illustrated by a study of Alzheimer's disease conducted by Huff and colleagues (1988): the exposed cohort consisted of siblings and parents of index cases who had Alzheimer's disease, and the unexposed cohort consisted of corresponding relatives of subjects without Alzheimer's disease (Figure 11–2). In this study, siblings and parents of patients with Alzheimer's disease had nearly a 50% lifetime risk of developing the illness, compared to a risk of about 10% among the corresponding relatives of comparison subjects. In other words, the lifetime risk of developing Alzheimer's disease was increased about fivefold (a risk ratio of about 5) for family members of patients with Alzheimer's disease. The authors noted that their results were consistent with an autosomal dominant pattern of transmission, but that other factors, such as a shared environment, could also explain the familial aggregation they found. Other investigators examining recurrence risk have suggested that the elevated risk among first-degree relatives does not follow an autosomal dom-

inant pattern of transmission, since female relatives of the index persons had a higher risk than male relatives. In that study, parents of index persons also had a higher risk than did siblings. Example 2 further illustrates use of the cohort design to study familial aggregation.

Example 2. As noted in Example 1, the incidence of Alzheimer's disease varies across ethnic and racial groups. To study familial risk factors for Alzheimer's disease, Payami and coworkers (1994) studied risk of developing this disease among three groups: parents and siblings of patients with Alzheimer's disease, parents and siblings of healthy elderly controls, and parents and siblings of randomly identified controls. The healthy elderly controls underwent neurologic examination and magnetic resonance imaging to ensure that they did not have dementia. The subjects and family members were interviewed to obtain histories of Alzheimer's disease and other dementia in relatives. The investigators found the risk of developing dementia by age 90 to be 0.44 for relatives of patients with Alzheimer's disease, 0.20 for relatives of randomly sampled controls, and 0.06 for relatives of healthy elderly controls. These observations demonstrate familial aggregation and are consistent with the presence in some families of genes that confer increased risk of developing Alzheimer's disease. The authors interpreted the

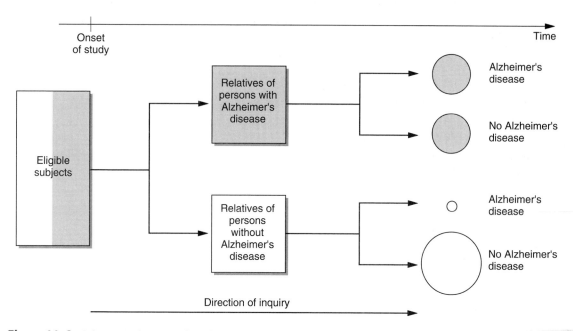

Figure 11–2. Schematic diagram of a cohort study of familial aggregation of Alzheimer's disease. Shaded areas represent "exposed" persons—those who are initially unaffected family members of patients with Alzheimer's disease. Unshaded areas represent "unexposed" persons—those who are initially unaffected family members of persons without Alzheimer's disease.

lower risk of aggregation in relatives of healthy controls as possibly suggesting the presence of "protective" genes whose presence reduces risk.

Epidemiologists also use the case–control study design to study familial aggregation. The design of this type of case–control study is analogous to that discussed in Chapter 9, except that exposure is determined by family history—the epidemiologist defines subjects who have one or more affected relatives to be "exposed" and subjects who do not have an affected relative to be "unexposed" (Figure 11–3). The odds ratio from this case–control study is calculated in the usual way. In this context, the odds ratio is the odds of having an affected family member among persons with the disease divided by the odds of having an affected family member among persons without the disease. Under appropriate circumstances, as outlined in Chapter 9, the odds ratio approximates the risk ratio—the risk of disease among those with an affected family member divided by the corresponding risk among those without an affected family member. Of course, odds ratios greater than one support familial aggregation. Interpretation can be difficult unless one specifies which relatives—and how many of them—to use in determining family history. For purposes of simplicity, limiting the relatives of interest to the parents of each subject avoids the problem

of any systematic differences in the average family sizes of cases and controls.

Case–control and cohort studies can provide useful information by documenting the presence and quantifying the degree of familial aggregation. These studies may also identify factors that create the aggregation by evaluating and assessing the roles of specific nongenetic risk factors. For example, in estimating recurrence risk for breast cancer among those with an affected relative, many other nongenetic exposures, such as diet and reproductive history, may be assessed.

Documentation and quantification of familial aggregation using the case–control or cohort study provide important information and may suggest a genetic etiology. Further studies of familial aggregation may assess the pattern of disease occurrence within the family to separate the relative roles of genetic and nongenetic factors. We consider two such studies—twin studies and inbreeding studies.

Twin studies can provide useful information about the role of possible genetic and environmental risk factors by comparing the pattern of risk among dizygotic (fraternal) twins with that among monozygotic (identical) twins. Monozygotic twins have identical genetic constitutions, whereas dizygotic twins have no more genetic similarity than do siblings.

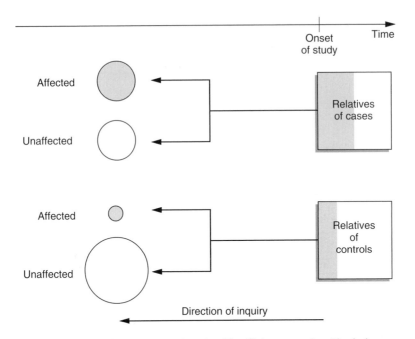

Figure 11–3. Schematic diagram of a case–control study of familial aggregation. Shaded areas represent "exposed" persons—those who are affected relatives of study subjects. Unshaded areas represent "unexposed" persons—those who are unaffected relatives of study subjects.

Accordingly, a pattern in which monozygotic twins have greater concordance for disease than dizygotic twins suggests genetically determined susceptibility. For example, twin studies of this type have provided evidence for genetic inheritance of Alzheimer's disease. In one such study, researchers identified 37 twin pairs in which at least one member had Alzheimer's disease. Among the 19 patients who had a monozygotic twin pairs, four (21.1%) were concordant for Alzheimer's disease, whereas among the 18 dizygotic twin pairs, only two (11.1%) were concordant for Alzheimer's disease (Figure 11–4). The greater concordance among monozygotic versus dizygotic twins suggests an underlying genetic predisposition to Alzheimer's disease.

In another type of twin study design, researchers study genetic and environmental factors by comparing disease concordance among twins reared together with that among twins reared apart. In this type of study, a pattern of risk of disease in which twins reared together have greater concordance for disease than twins reared apart suggests the importance of nongenetic factors, including social and environmental influences.

Studies of the association of inbreeding with risk of disease, so called **inbreeding studies,** also provide clues about the causes of familial aggregation. Because consanguineous marriages and

the resulting inbreeding increase the risk of autosomal recessive disorders, the epidemiologist can use these studies to assess whether familial aggregation reflects an autosomal recessive pattern of inheritance. Briefly, in these studies the exposure of interest is the degree of inbreeding that measures the likelihood that a subject has inherited two copies of the same allele from a single ancestor. If subjects with a higher degree of inbreeding also have higher risk of disease, autosomal recessive disease inheritance may be suggested.

EPIDEMIOLOGIC STUDIES OF SPECIFIC GENETIC FACTORS

The descriptive studies and the studies of familial aggregation considered so far can provide useful, but indirect, information about possible genetic and environmental causes of disease. If these studies suggest that the disease has, at least in part, a hereditary basis, further research can focus on the risks associated with specific genetic factors such as enzymes, receptors, or structural proteins. The following sections present a direct and an indirect approach to studying the association of disease with specific genetic factors.

To understand both the direct and indirect approach, as well as the more complex genetic linkage analyses, we must first understand genetic **linkage.**

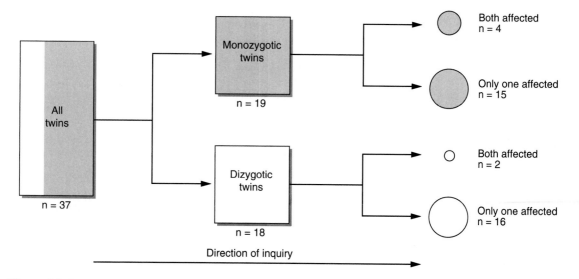

Figure 11–4. Schematic diagram of a study of concordance for Alzheimer's disease among monozygotic and dizygotic twins. (From Breitner JCS et al: Alzheimer's disease in the National Academy of Sciences-National Research Council Registry of Aging Twin Veterans. III. Detection of cases, longitudinal results, and observations of twin concordance. Arch Neurol 1995;**52**:763.)

Linkage between one gene and another arises because alleles that are closely situated on the same chromosome tend to be passed together as a group to offspring. Thus, if a subject inherits a particular allele, he or she will tend to also inherit other alleles present nearby on the same chromosome, a situation termed **cosegregation.**

At the population level, recombination or crossing over between genes tends to eliminate or reduce imbalances related to genetic linkage. This recombination tends to create an equilibrium in which the frequency with which two alleles (at different genes) occur together is simply the product of the frequencies with which each allele occurs in the population. Nevertheless, for some gene pairs an excess or deficiency of certain combinations of alleles occurs, a situation termed **linkage disequilibrium.** Such linkage disequilibrium can be present if a mutation (ie, a new allele) has recently arisen in a population, or if certain combinations of alleles at the two loci confer a survival advantage over other combinations.

The Direct Approach

With the direct approach, the researcher directly studies the possible increase in risk associated with a specific factor, such as an alteration in the DNA sequence or variations in enzyme activity. Using a cohort study, the researcher compares the risk among those with a specific variation in the DNA sequence or enzyme activity

with the risk among a similar group without that variant (Figure 11–5). Following the principles outlined in Chapter 8 for cohort studies and defining the "exposure" to be those with a particular genotype, the researcher follows two groups of subjects—one with the genetic variant and the other without the genetic variant—and then determines subsequent occurrence of disease. The investigator then calculates risks for each group, as well as the risk ratio that measures the increase (or decrease) in risk associated with the genetic variant. As in other cohort studies, subjects should be free of disease at the start of follow-up and should be comparable except for the genetic variant of interest.

Alternately, the researcher can use a case–control design to study the association between risk of disease and a specific genetic factor. In this type of case–control study, the "exposure" is the genetic factor of interest (Figure 11–6). As in other types of case–control studies (Chapter 9), cases consist of people with the disease of interest, and investigators select controls from the source population, that is, the population which gave rise to the cases. After assembling the case and control groups, the researcher compares the frequency of the genetic factor of interest among the cases to the corresponding frequency among the controls. The odds ratio—the odds of the genetic factor among cases divided by the odds of the genetic factor among controls—provides an approximation to the risk ratio, as described in Chapter 9. If cases have an elevated fre-

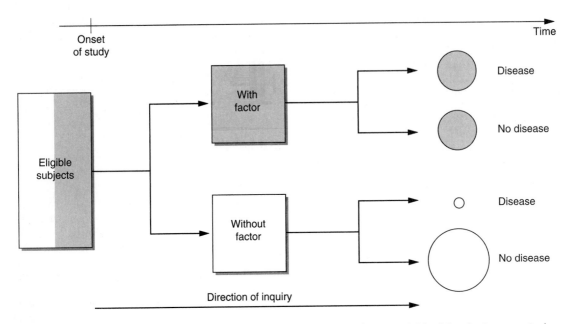

Figure 11–5. Schematic diagram of a cohort study of a specific genetic factor and risk of developing a particular disease. Shaded areas represent "exposed" persons—those with the specific genetic factor of interest. Unshaded areas represent "unexposed" persons—those who lack the specific genetic factor of interest.

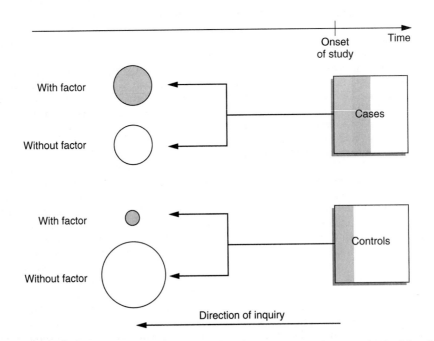

Figure 11–6. Schematic diagram of a case–control study of a specific genetic factor and risk of developing a particular disease. Shaded areas represent "exposed" persons—those with the specific genetic factor of interest. Unshaded areas represent "unexposed" persons—those lacking the specific genetic factor of interest.

quency of the genetic factor, the researcher must consider the possibility that this excess could be secondary to the disease itself or its treatment, rather than a cause of the disease. This possibility could occur, for example, in a study of the association between a particular mutation and risk of developing leukemia if the mutation was measured in blood obtained from cases after chemotherapy, since certain chemotherapeutic agents are known to be mutagens.

As with other types of epidemiologic studies, researchers must exercise care in interpreting results of genetic epidemiologic investigations. They must consider the possibility of selection bias, confounding, and misclassification in the interpretation of genetic epidemiologic findings, as those biases can affect genetic epidemiologic results just as they can affect other types of research. The possibility of selection bias must be considered, particularly in case–control studies, if controls are not selected from the source population that gave rise to the cases. The possibility of confounding must be considered, particularly by factors such as race and ethnicity, as these factors relate to risks for many types of disease and also can be linked with genetic markers.

Another important consideration arises in interpreting studies of the association between risk of disease and a specific DNA alteration, as measured by a marker allele. This kind of study is typified by studies of the association between insulin-dependent (type I) diabetes mellitus and certain human leukocyte antigens (HLAs). These studies have documented an increased risk of diabetes mellitus in association with the presence of the HLA DR3 allele. It is possible, however, that it is not the HLA DR3 allele per se, but rather some companion alteration at a nearby genetic locus, that is responsible for increasing the risk of developing diabetes mellitus. This phenomenon can arise if noncausal marker alleles at one genetic locus are in **linkage disequilibrium** with alleles at the causal genetic locus. If linkage disequilibrium is present, an association between risk of disease and the marker may reflect linkage disequilibrium between the marker and the gene that confers disease susceptibility—and not a causal association between the marker itself and risk of disease. Nevertheless, direct evidence of increased risk in association with a marker allele, if valid, suggests that the marker allele or another allele linked to it relates to susceptibility to disease.

With increasing frequency, researchers are now using single nucleotide polymorphisms or SNPs to measure alterations in the DNA sequence. The SNP reflects a change in a single base-pair at particular point in the DNA sequence. An advantage of SNPs is that they can be measured relatively easily in the laboratory, but a disadvantage is that many SNPs may be required to detect a relevant mutation in a particular gene since the SNP measures change only at a single point.

Finally, it should be noted that consideration of possible gene–environment interactions is important. For example, failure to account for important environmental factors in the design or the analysis of the study can lead to an underestimate of the influence of a genetic factor. The genetic characteristic of interest may contribute to risk of disease only in the presence of some environmental trigger. Accordingly, failure to account for a critical environmental trigger may obscure the role of an underlying genetic susceptibility.

The Indirect Approach

With the indirect approach, the researcher also looks for evidence of an association with a genetic factor. The indirect approach differs from the direct approach in that a marker is used for the genetic factor that may not be the same as the causal genetic factor itself. This approach depends on genetic **linkage** between the genetic marker and the disease susceptibility gene. Documentation of an association between the marker and risk of disease provides evidence that a gene near the marker allele affects risk of disease.

Linkage analysis (1) provides information about the magnitude of risk association with a genetic marker, (2) identifies the chromosome that bears the susceptibility gene locus, and (3) provides information about the site on the chromosome of a disease susceptibility gene.

A straightforward epidemiologic approach to the study of linkage involves estimating recurrence risks in siblings of index subjects with a specific disease. For a particular marker locus, a sibling can share by descent either zero, one, or two marker alleles with the case. If the marker locus is linked to a disease susceptibility locus, a sibling who shares two alleles with the index case should have the highest chance of having the same disease susceptibility allele as the case—and hence the highest risk of disease. A sibling who shares one allele with the case should have an intermediate chance of having the same disease as the case, and a sibling who shares no alleles with the case should have the lowest chance of having the same disease susceptibility allele and hence the lowest risk of disease. If risk of disease in siblings parallels the number of alleles shared with the case, the data suggest the presence of a disease susceptibility gene near the marker gene on the same chromosome. This type of study, sometimes called **sib-pair analysis,** is a simple example of genetic linkage analysis.

In more complex applications of genetic linkage analyses, the geneticist measures a genetic marker among a group of family members that is not restricted to siblings. If subjects who share the genetic marker, such as a particular allele, also tend to be concordant for occurrence of disease, the disease susceptibility gene may be located on the same chromosome near the marker allele. As with sib-pair analyses, these more complex linkage analyses rest on the rationale that if the measured genetic marker is located near the disease susceptibility allele, the marker allele and the susceptibility allele will tend to be passed together, that is, to cosegregate. Cosegregation of the marker allele and the disease susceptibility allele will then create concordance between occurrence of disease and presence of the genetic marker. Example 4 illustrates a linkage study.

Example 3. To study the role of apolipoprotein E (Apo E), a specific genetic factor suspected of playing a role in the causation of Alzheimer's disease, Tsai and coworkers (1994) conducted a case–control study. They obtained blood from 77 cases with Alzheimer's disease and 77 matched controls, then determined the presence of three isoforms of Apo E—denoted e2, e3, and e4. About 35% of the cases had the e4 allele, compared with 13% of controls. The results support the role of Apo E as a risk factor for Alzheimer's disease. Although the mechanism remains uncertain, results of other studies suggest that Apo E may bind to β-amyloid and change it to a neurotoxic form.

Example 4. To help in the search for possible genetic factors associated with Alzheimer's disease, Schellenberg and colleagues (1992) conducted linkage analyses in a series of 14 families, each of which had at least three members with Alzheimer's disease in at least two generations. Using several markers for loci on chromosome 14, the investigators found that within some families with early-onset Alzheimer's disease, members who shared the same markers tended to be concordant for Alzheimer's disease. The evidence suggested that a gene on chromosome 14 codes for susceptibility to early-onset Alzheimer's disease. If so, this would be a separate locus from the one coding for apolipoprotein E, as the Apo E gene is located on chromosome 19.

COMPLEX GENETIC ANALYSES

To study the possibility of genetic inheritance, the researcher also can apply methods from population genetics. In this section, a commonly used, powerful approach called **segregation analysis** is presented.

Briefly, segregation analysis is a complex statistical technique that geneticists use to study the pattern of occurrence of disease within pedigrees. The goal of segregation analyses is (1) to provide evidence that a particular disease has, at least in part, a genetic origin, and (2) to suggest the mode of inheritance. On the other hand, segregation analysis does not evaluate the role of specific genetic factors or markers. With segregation analyses, the geneticist attempts to identify which, if any, type of genetic inheritance

(eg, autosomal dominant, autosomal recessive, or multifactorial) is most consistent with the pattern of disease occurrence seen within families. Segregation analysis rests on the rationale that disease within a family will tend to occur in different patterns for different modes of inheritance. For example, an autosomal dominant pattern of inheritance is suggested when the following types of pedigrees predominate:

- One half of the offspring affected are from marriages in which only one parent has the disease
- Three fourths of the offspring affected are from marriages in which both parents have the disease
- None of the offspring affected is from a marriage in which neither parent has the disease.

In contrast, autosomal recessive or multifactorial patterns of inheritance will result in other characteristic patterns of disease occurrence within pedigrees.

In population studies, diseases do not tend to occur in such idealized patterns following the classical risks associated with the modes of inheritance. Segregation analysis provides a probabilistic method to assess the statistical consistency of the observed pattern of disease with the hypothesized mode of genetic inheritance.

SUMMARY

In this chapter, an overview of genetic epidemiology was presented. The field of genetic epidemiology uses the same basic principles of study design and analysis as are used in other areas of epidemiology. Researchers in genetic epidemiology conduct three basic types of studies: descriptive studies, studies of familial aggregation, and studies of specific genetic markers. Each type of study typically involves a case–control or cohort design and differs from other types of epidemiologic studies primarily in the "exposure" of primary interest being a genetic factor.

In the initial phase of studying the etiology of a disease, the researcher may use descriptive studies to look for characteristics that suggest genetic and nongenetic etiologies of disease, for example, person, place, and time. In a second phase, the researcher may study familial aggregation to look for evidence of increased risks of recurrence in relatives of cases and to look for further etiologic clues. Finally, the researcher may study specific genetic characteristics, such as gene markers or products, as well as gene–environment interactions. The researcher may also apply some of the more complex analytic methods derived from population genetics, such as segregation or linkage analyses, to study patterns of genetic inheritance.

STUDY QUESTIONS

Questions 1–5: For each numbered study of genetic factors in relation to the occurrence of a newly recognized disease, select the appropriate study design from the following lettered options. Each option can be used once, more than once, or not at all.

  A. Sib-pair (linkage) study

  B. Familial aggregation study

  C. Cohort study

  D. Migrant study

  E. Twin study

  F. Inbreeding study

  G. Segregation study

1. The recurrence risk among first-degree relatives of cases is compared with risk among first-degree relatives of people without the disease.

2. The number of alleles that each person with disease shares with their sibling without the disease is studied.

3. Concordance of the disease in monozygotic twins is compared with that among dizygotic twins.

4. The likelihood that cases inherited two copies of the same allele from a single ancestor is compared with the corresponding likelihood among controls.

5. During 5 years of follow-up, the risk of developing Alzheimer's disease among those with a particular allele versus among those without this allele.

Questions 6–10: The following statements refer to a case–control study designed to determine whether selected alleles at one locus are risk factors for coronary artery disease. For each numbered statement, select the most appropriate bias from the following lettered options. Each option can be used once, more than once, or not at all.

  A. Inbreeding

  B. Confounding

  C. Misclassification

  D. Linkage disequilibrium

  E. Selection bias

  F. None of these applies

6. The blood used to assess genotype was stored in a freezer, later determined to have a defective thermostat.

7. The cases are identified from those admitted to a cardiology ward and the controls are sampled from those hospitalized with a neurologic disease.

8. One of the alleles is found more frequently among those in a particular ethnic group; this group also has high rates of cardiac disease under study.

9. A laboratory technician incorrectly records a series of results for controls.

10. Identical twins are more likely to enroll in a twin study than are nonidentical twins.

FURTHER READING

Graff-Radford N, et al. Association between apolipoprotein E genotype and Alzheimer Disease in African American subjects. Arch Neurol 2002;**59**:594.

Nussbaum RL, Ellsi CE: Alzheimer's disease and Parkinson's disease. N Engl J Med 2003;**348**:1356.

Page GP et al: "Are we there yet?": deciding when one has demonstrated specific genetic causation in complex diseases and quantitative traits. Am J Hum Genet 2003;**73**:711.

Rocchi A et al: Causative and susceptibility genes for Alzheimer's disease: a review. Brain Res Bull 2003;**61**:1.

REFERENCES

Clinical Background

Clark CM, Karlawish JHT: Alzheimer disease: current concepts and emerging diagnostic and therapeutic strategies. Ann Intern Med 2003;**138**:400.

Ingram V: Alzheimer's disease. Am Scientist 2003;**91**:312.

Sloane PD et al: The public health impact of Alzheimer's disease, 2000–2050. Ann Rev Pub Health 2002;**23**:213.

Descriptive Epidemiologic Studies

Evans DA et al: Prevalence of Alzheimer's disease in a community population of older persons: Higher than previously reported. JAMA 1989;**262**:2551.

Epidemiologic Studies of Familial Aggregation

Breitner JCS et al: Alzheimer's disease in the National Academy of Sciences-National Research Council Registry of Aging Twin Veterans. III. Detection of cases, longitudinal results, and observations of twin concordance. Arch Neurol 1995;**52**:763.

Huff FJ et al: Risk of dementia in relatives of patients with Alzheimer's disease. Neurology 1988;**38:**786.

Lautenschlager NT et al: Risk of dementia among relatives of Alzheimer's disease patients in the MIRAGE study: What is in store for the oldest old? Neurology 1996;**46:**641.

Payami H et al: Evidence for familial factors that protect against dementia and outweigh the effect of increasing age. Am J Hum Genet 1994;**54:**650.

Epidemiologic Studies of Specific Genetic Factors

Beaty TH: Applications of the case–control method in genetic epidemiology. Epidemiol Rev 1994;**16:**134.

Ellsworth DL, Manolio TA: The emerging importance of genetics in epidemiologic research. II. Issues in study design and gene mapping. Ann Epidemiol 1999;**9:**75.

Khoury MJ et al: Epidemiologic approaches to the use of DNA markers in the search for disease susceptibility genes. Epidemiol Rev 1990;**12:**41.

Khoury MJ, Khoury MJ et al: Penetrance in the presence of genetic susceptibility to environmental factors. Am J Med Genet 1988;**29:**403.

Pericak-Vance MA et al: Complete genomic screen in late-onset familial Alzheimer's disease. Neurobiol Aging 1998;**19**(No. 1S):S39.

Risch N: Evolving methods in genetic epidemiology. II. Genetic linkage from an epidemiologic perspective. Epidemiol Rev 1997;**19:**24.

Tsai MS et al: Apolipoprotein E: Risk factor for Alzheimer's disease. Am J Hum Genet 1994;**54:**643.

Complex Genetic Analyses

Schellenberg GD et al: Genetic evidence for a familial Alzheimer's disease locus on chromosome 14. Science 1992;**258:**668.

e-PIDEMIOLOGY

Further Reading

http://www.pitt.edu/~super1/lecture/lec3301/index.htm

Clinical Background

http://www.pitt.edu/~super1/lecture/lec9341/index.htm

Epidemiologic Studies of Familial Aggregation

http://www.hhmi.org/GeneticTrail/searching/search.htm

Epidemiologic Studies of Specific Genetic Factors

http://www.journals.uchicago.edu/AJHG/journal/issues/v66n3/991345/991345.html

Complex Genetic Analyses

http://www.journals.uchicago.edu/AJHG/journal/issues/v63n4/980693/980693.html

Clinical Decision-Making

KEY CONCEPTS

1. Decision analysis is a formal process used to determine the preferred course of action from two or more potential approaches to clinical management.

2. Decision analysis is most appropriate when there is both some uncertainty about the preferred course of action and a meaningful trade-off of risks and benefits for the alternative management strategies.

3. A decision tree or decision diagram is the underlying structure of the clinical situation, including all uncertainties and choices, as well as all outcomes.

4. The expected utility is the estimated typical or average outcome for a population of patients managed with a particular strategy.

5. Substituting a range of values for a particular probability in a decision tree and determining the impact on the expected utility is referred to as a sensitivity analysis.

PATIENT PROFILE

A 50-year-old man presented to his physician with a high fever and severe abdominal pain. This patient occasionally worked as a house painter, and although he reported heavy use of alcohol, he had been in generally good health. There was no history of exposure to toxic substances or intravenous drug use. On physical examination, the patient was jaundiced, and he had severe tenderness to palpation in the right upper quadrant of his abdomen. Laboratory examination revealed leukocytosis accompanied by elevations in the serum levels of bilirubin, alkaline phosphatase, and serum glutamic oxaloacetic transaminase (SGOT, aspartate aminotransferase). It was considered that the patient had either alcoholic hepatitis or cholangitis (inflammation of a bile duct). It is nec-essary to differentiate cholangitis, which requires surgery, from alcoholic hepatitis, in which surgery is contraindicated. In fact, the postoperative mortality for alcoholic hepatitis is very high. The issue for the medical decision-maker is to choose the alternative that will carry the greatest benefit for the patient with the lowest achievable risk.

CLINICAL BACKGROUND

Cholangitis, an infection of the biliary ductal system, classically presents with a triad of fever, jaundice, and pain in the right upper quadrant of the abdomen. The clinical illness arises in the presence of bacterial colonization of the bile, most commonly because of obstruction of biliary tract flow. Historically, the most common underlying cause of obstruction was blockage

189

of the biliary tract by stones, although malignant strictures have become increasingly important contributors in recent years. The increased pressure within the bile ducts resulting from obstruction produces bacterial reflux into the hepatic veins and perihepatic lymphatics, with subsequent bacterial spread into the circulating bloodstream. The bacteria associated with cholangitis include *Escherichia coli, Klebsiella* species, and the enterococci, with a shift more recently to include *Enterobacter* and *Pseudomonas* species. Infections typically involve multiple species of organisms.

The clinical manifestations of cholangitis range from asymptomatic illness to severe toxic symptoms, including septic shock. Fever is present in almost all patients, typically accompanied by chills. Jaundice and abdominal pain in the right upper quadrant of the abdomen are part of the classical description of presenting symptoms, although they may not be present in the absence of obstructive stones. Complications of advanced disease can include confusion, liver abscess, low blood pressure, and kidney failure. Laboratory examination usually reveals an elevation of leukocytes in the blood, with moderate elevation of bilirubin and liver enzymes.

The clinical management of patients with cholangitis is adapted to the severity of the illness, with severely ill patients requiring intensive care and monitoring. General supportive care typically includes stopping oral intake, starting intravenous fluids, and after taking appropriate cultures, initiating antibiotics for a broad range of potential pathogens. Relieving the elevated pressure within the biliary tract also is important, particularly for patients with severe symptoms. This can be accomplished through a variety of means, including using an endoscope to drain the tract. If there is an obstructing stone, this can be removed with an endoscope, or if an obstruction cannot be removed, a stent can be inserted to maintain flow of bile. Surgical drainage is associated with a high risk of morbidity and mortality, and therefore generally is a choice of last resort.

Alcoholic hepatitis is an inflammatory process that occurs in persons with long-term heavy consumption of alcohol, although only a minority of heavy consumers will develop this problem. As with cholangitis, the clinical severity of alcoholic hepatitis ranges widely from asymptomatic illness at one extreme to severe incapacitating disease at the other extreme. Patients often experience loss of appetite, nausea and vomiting, weight loss, and malaise. Fever is present in about half of all patients. The physical examination typically reveals jaundice, enlargement of the liver, and tenderness in the right upper quadrant of the abdomen. With advanced disease, patients may present with abnormal fluid collections in the soft tissues (edema) or abdominal cavity (ascites), bleeding, or impaired central nervous system functioning.

The laboratory evaluation of patients with alcoholic hepatitis often reveals an elevated level of leukocytes in the blood. Bilirubin levels can be elevated to varying extents, typically accompanied by abnormal levels of liver enzymes. To the extent that hepatic function is disordered, prolonged prothrombin time, depressed levels of serum albumin, or elevated blood ammonia may also be observed. Microscopic examination of the liver reveals infiltration with leukocytes, accompanied by degeneration and necrosis of liver cells. The damaged liver cells often include material that stains with eosin dye and that are referred to as Mallory bodies.

The clinical management of patients with alcoholic hepatitis involves initial supportive therapy. The recommended regimen typically includes abstinence from further consumption of alcohol, rest, and nutritional therapy. In addition, patients who present with severe complications, such as bleeding, ascites, or central nervous system dysfunction, may require specific therapy directed at these disorders. Other therapeutic approaches have an uncertain benefit. Some patients may benefit from corticosteroid treatment. The role of liver transplantation for patients with end-stage alcoholic liver disease is still a matter of debate.

CLINICAL DECISION-MAKING

The practicing physician is a problem solver whose clinical task is to maximize benefit to the patient by correctly diagnosing illness and instituting appropriate treatment. The problem-solving process in medicine involves

1. Collection and evaluation of diagnostic information
2. Formulation of diagnostic hypotheses
3. Consideration of alternative hypotheses
4. Appropriate use of an efficacious therapy or procedure.

This process is made difficult, in part, because of inherent uncertainty in the information both for diagnosis and for treatment. For example, information elicited from patients may be false, inconclusive, and of uncertain validity; signs often are not perfect indicators of the presence of specific diseases; and even laboratory and other diagnostic tests can yield misleading information—either false-negative or false-positive results. In addition, treatment modalities are far from perfect, and there is always uncertainty about how efficacious a therapy may be in an individual patient. This uncertainty that bedevils the practice of medicine may be ameliorated, in part, by effective use and measurement of probabilities to assess the validity of diagnostic data and the efficacy of therapies, thus demonstrating that the practice of medicine is probabilistic—not deterministic—in nature.

An understanding of the derivation, calculation, and use of probabilities is important in making clinical decisions, and thus is an important topic in clinical education. The subjects presented in this book have direct applicability to clinical decision-making. Although developed in populations, the concepts and measurements of disease frequency (incidence, prevalence, risk, and probability) have direct applicability to probability of disease in single patients. The sensitivity and specificity of information collected from the patient's history, the physical examination, and laboratory tests are probability measures that play a significant role in determining the diagnostic utility of the work-up. In addition, the clinical trial assesses the efficacy of a therapy in terms of proportions of patients who benefit, so this probability of benefit derived from a population of patients can be used to predict the outcome of treatment in a single patient.

Formal decision analysis is an explicit process that utilizes information from epidemiologic and clinical studies to determine the preferred course of action. Not all clinical decisions are amenable to a formal decision analysis. Two important criteria should be borne in mind in deciding whether a formal decision analysis is appropriate.

The first criterion is whether there is some reasonable uncertainty about what the optimal treatment strategy is. In some instances, there is clear and compelling evidence about what diagnostic or therapeutic approach is the best course of action. Unfortunately, in spite of considerable effort to generate and synthesize such clear and compelling evidence for medical practice, it is not available for the vast majority of clinical decisions. The second criterion is that there must be a meaningful trade-off between the options under consideration. A formal decision analysis always involves a comparison of two or more alternative strategies. If one strategy always offers higher potential benefits and lower potential risks, there is no need to conduct a formal decision analysis. The challenge comes in sorting out the potential trade-off between risks and benefits of alternative strategies. One approach may offer greater potential benefits than another approach, but those benefits may come at the price of greater risks. Formal decision analysis is a tool to help the clinician weigh the relative advantages and disadvantages of these management alternatives.

FORMAL DECISION ANALYSIS

Decision analysis is an explicit process that considers medical choices, medical outcomes, and the uncertainty in the clinical and test data used to make decisions. The process is explicit in that the medical alternatives present and the choices available in the management of a patient's care may be clearly specified and demonstrated to others: physicians, students, and with care, the patient. The elements in a formal decision analysis include the following:

1. An underlying structure termed the decision tree (or decision diagram)
2. The probabilities for uncertain events
3. The incorporation of test results
4. The medical outcomes of the alternative choices to be made.

Table 12–1 summarizes the considerations: the decision problem must be explicitly stated, the problem must be structured over time, the information about uncertainties and the value of outcomes must be characterized, and a preferred course of action must be demonstrated.

The important underlying structure of the process is the **decision diagram** or **decision "tree"** (Table 12–2). The diagram flows from left to right with choices (**decision nodes**) represented by boxes and probabilities (**chance nodes**) represented by circles; outcomes (often termed **terminal nodes**) are inserted at the far right of the appropriate branches (Figures 12–1 and 12–2). The tree should contain all appropriate outcomes and all uncertainties and choices. Appropriate numeric values for probabilities and values of outcomes are included in the dia-

Table 12–1. Considerations for the analytic approach to decision-making.

I. Identify and set bounds for the decision problem:
   A. Identify alternative actions
   B. Identify clinical information needed
   C. Determine clinical status of the patient including possible outcomes of morbidity and mortality
II. Structure the problem over time:
   A. Identify choices to be made
   B. Identify uncertainties to be encountered
   C. Identify possible outcomes
   D. Draw a decision tree
III. Characterize the information needed for the decision tree:
   A. Indicate probabilities for uncertain outcomes including risks and test characteristics
   B. Assign values to outcomes
IV. Choose a preferred course of action:
   a. Quantify uncertainties and values to determine expected values
   b. Perform sensitivity analysis

Table 12–2. Characteristics of decision trees.

I. Decision trees are based on models that incorporate the following features of clinical practice:
   A. It is necessary to choose between alternative management strategies
   B. The natural history of disease and effects of intervention for individual patients are uncertain, and can be represented in terms of likelihoods of outcomes
   C. Trade-offs often must be considered, which involves weighing the relative desirability of the outcomes under consideration
II. Decision trees allow the systemic evaluation of components of a complex situation. On the other hand, all relevant features of a clinical situation may not always be adequately represented
III. As a quantified display of clinical reasoning, decision trees allow consideration of both beliefs (about probabilities) and preferences (among the outcomes)
IV. Decision trees are tools to help in selecting a strategy for patient care that maximizes the expected value for the patient

gram. Several types of outcome measures may be considered:

1. **Clinical measures:** a variety of patient outcomes might be considered, including, among others, functional status, probability of survival (or death), risk of complications, and years of life expectancy.
2. **Economic measures:** models that include the costs of management alternatives are useful for assessing the cost effectiveness of treatment alternatives; these models typically take the societal perspective of costs, but other perspectives are possible.
3. **Utility measures:** quality-of-life measures, termed utilities, represent how patients value life in a particular health state. Utilities typically are placed on a relative scale, with the extremes being zero, corresponding to death, and one, corresponding to perfect health.

The process of assigning values to the elements of a decision tree can be challenging. For clinical events, probabilities may be obtained from systematic reviews of the medical literature. For many situations, however, published information may be limited or nonexistent. In the absence of published data, the parameters of interest may be estimated by the collection of new information, or by reference to existing databases, such as disease registries, electronic medical record systems, or reimbursement claims. Under certain circumstances, clinical opinion may be used, particularly if the analysis reveals that the conclusions are not highly sensitive to these estimates.

A variety of approaches can be used to estimate utilities, including surveys in which subjects rate health states, or to make judgments about willingness to trade risk for benefit in moving from one health state to another. For example, persons may be asked to determine whether they are willing to accept a more aggressive treatment regimen by weighing the risk of death against the gain of additional functional status.

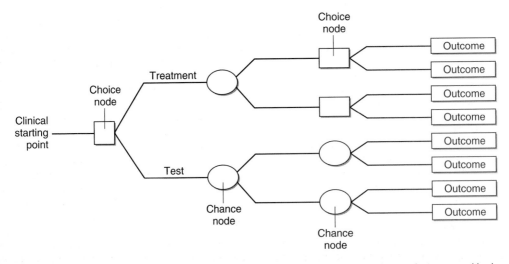

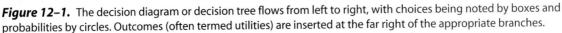

Figure 12–1. The decision diagram or decision tree flows from left to right, with choices being noted by boxes and probabilities by circles. Outcomes (often termed utilities) are inserted at the far right of the appropriate branches.

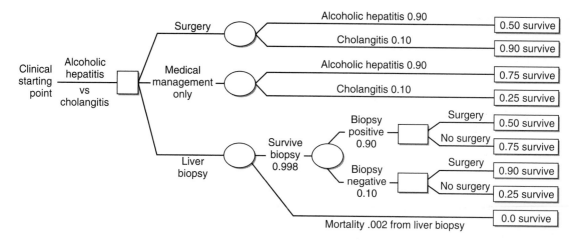

Figure 12–2. Decision tree applied to a patient presenting with alcoholism, jaundice, fever, leukocytosis, and an elevated alkaline phosphatase level. Initial options are to (1) go to surgery, (2) manage medically with supportive care, or (3) do a liver biopsy. For each of these potential decisions, probabilities are generated (arms of the respective chance nodes). The outcome of each probability is given in terms of probability of survival. Note that the value for the limb of a chance node is the probability that outcome or clinical state will occur, that is, there is a 0.9 (90%) chance that the patient has alcoholic hepatitis and only a 0.1 (10%) chance that the patient has cholangitis. Note also that the sum of the probabilities about a chance node always equals 1.0 (100%).

In constructing a decision tree, it is useful to bear in mind two competing considerations. On the one hand, the tree must be complex enough to represent the key events and probabilities in the decision-making process. On the other hand, the tree must be simple enough to be able to be understood. Inevitably, the tree is a model of reality, and as such cannot capture all of the complexities of a particular clinical situation. To reach a valid conclusion, however, the model must include the key elements needed to determine relative risks and benefits.

Alternative paths that may be chosen are termed clinical scenarios. For each path, an **Expected Utility** (expected outcome) is a numeric value that may be calculated as described below. The Expected Utility is interpreted as the average, or the expected result, if the decision-maker follows a specific path (clinical scenario). The Expected Utility can combine medical data in the form of probabilities with human values in the form of utilities. The integration of evidence-based medicine, with both patient preferences and economic considerations, allows for a holistic approach to health care decision-making.

The purpose of a decision analysis is to identify a preferred path among two or more clinical scenarios. The preferred path may be selected as the best outcome on the basis of clinical response, utility, or cost effectiveness.

It should be emphasized that the expected outcome is a "typical" or average result for a population of patients who are all managed in the same way. Variation in outcomes across patients is to be expected, but the Expected Utility represents the best estimate of the overall risks and benefits for a particular management decision.

The numeric calculations used to derive the Expected Utility are simple in concept. At each chance node, the probabilities and numeric outcomes of each branch of the path are multiplied, and the results from separate branches are summed. This process is termed *averaging out*. In this manner, calculations are performed from *right to left* to obtain the Expected Utility, which is always presented in the same numeric terms as the outcome. When certain pathways clearly will not, for medical reasons, be considered, the branch is folded back using double slash lines to indicate a path that is not considered appropriate. The calculations of Expected Utilities, which may become tedious to perform, are easily handled by available computer programs.

One of the challenges of a formal decision analysis is deciding how many pathways should be included. In many clinical situations, a large number of combinations of tests and interventions is possible. Rather than considering all possible options, it is advisable to limit the number of pathways considered to a subset that is clearly different from other subsets and covers the full range of options that might be pursued.

The element of time also is fundamental to the conduct of a decision analysis. It is common practice to emphasize current events more than future ones. Assigning greater value to near-term events is referred to as *discounting* or *valuing* time. For example, if an intervention will save money many years down the road, the present value of those savings is less because of inflation. Similarly, near-term clinical benefits may be valued more highly than clinical benefits that will be experienced in the future. Many of the aspects of a formal decision analysis are best illustrated by considering a specific clinical problem. The situation introduced in the Patient Profile affords us an opportunity to examine a decision analysis in detail.

THE DECISION EXAMPLE

The patient had a history of heavy use of alcohol and presented with fever, jaundice, and abdominal pain. The clinical presentation—along with laboratory findings of leukocytosis and elevated levels of bilirubin and liver enzymes—suggested a diagnosis of either cholangitis or alcoholic hepatitis. Beyond initial supportive care, endoscopic or surgical intervention would be warranted to relieve the biliary obstruction precipitating cholangitis, but these procedures, particularly surgery, would be contraindicated for a patient with alcoholic hepatitis. This decision problem can be examined using the process of decision analysis. The various probabilities of uncertainty and outcome are presented in Table 12–3.

The structure of the tree (Figure 12–2) indicates the outcomes in terms of probabilities of survival for each alternative, as well as probabilities of each clinical state or test result (the branches of the chance nodes). Note that if a biopsy is done, the decision for surgery or no surgery awaits the biopsy result, exactly as it would in the clinical setting. Note also that the summation of all probabilities at any chance node always equals 1 (100%). Once constructed, the tree is *solved* by multiplying the outcome values (survivals in this case) by their respective probabilities. Around each chance node, the products of the branches are added to give the value at that chance node. After all the chance nodes from a single decision arm are summed, the Expected Value (expected utility) of that decision is achieved. This can be compared with the values of the other branches of the choice node; then the best numeric choice may be selected as the most favorable option. The other potential choices are excluded or folded back (by convention with double slash lines). Values of each chance node are shown in that node.

Table 12–3. The elements to be included in the clinical decision analysis problem.

I. A 50-year-old man with a history of heavy alcohol use, presenting with fever, jaundice, abdominal pain, leukocytosis, and abnormal liver functions.

II. Choices in initial clinical management:
   A. Surgery
   B. Medical therapy
   C. Further diagnostic testing with a liver biopsy

III. Probabilistic events:
   A. 90% of patients who present with this clinical picture will have alcoholic hepatitis and 10% will have ascending cholangitis
   B. 0.2% of patients undergoing diagnostic liver biopsy will have a fatal complication

IV. Outcomes:
   A. 75% of patients with alcoholic hepatitis who do not have surgery survive
   B. 50% of patients with alcoholic hepatitis who have surgery survive
   C. 25% of patients with cholangitis who do not have surgery survive
   D. 90% of patients with cholangitis who have surgery survive

The calculations are straightforward. For example, the Expected Utility at the surgery node, expressed as the probability of survival, is calculated as

Expected
Utility = (likelihood of alcoholic hepatitis)
   × (survival probability if alcoholic hepatitis)
   + (likelihood of cholangitis)
   × (survival probability if cholangitis)
   = $(.9 \times .5) + (.1 \times .9) = .54$

In this model, although there is a small risk of mortality associated with performing a diagnostic liver biopsy, the information gained from the biopsy helps to optimize the subsequent treatment decision (Figure 12–3). On the basis of this probabilistic argument, the clinical preference would be to perform a diagnostic liver biopsy. Note, however, that using this approach does not *ensure* the best outcome for the patient, as there is a small (0.2%) but real risk of a fatal complication from the biopsy. Nevertheless, after weighing the relative risks and benefits of performing the diagnostic biopsy, the most favorable outcome is likely to be achieved if a liver biopsy is performed first. This is reflected in Figure 12–3 by the Expected Utility for liver biopsy (0.76), which is somewhat more favorable than

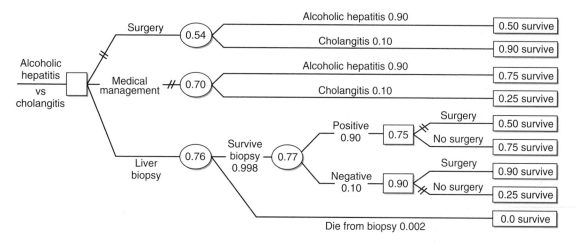

Figure 12–3. Completed decision tree with values shown. Each outcome is multiplied by the value (probability) of its respective chance node arm, and the sum of the two products about each chance node is obtained. For example, on the top or surgical decision limb, the value for the chance node is equal to $(0.5 \times 0.9) + (0.9 \times 0.1) = 0.54$. A value is likewise obtained for the other two decision limbs in similar fashion. Note that in doing the liver biopsy, it is necessary to take into account the possibility of a fatal complication of the biopsy itself (outcome value = 0.0). After biopsy is obtained, it is necessary to decide whether to do surgery. Note that at a choice node, only the highest value limb is taken for the value of that choice node. The remainder of the lower value limbs at that choice node are folded back (by convention with double slash lines) and discarded. A positive biopsy indicates the presence of alcoholic hepatitis, in which case surgery would not be indicated. A negative biopsy indicates cholangitis, and surgery is indicated.

medical management alone (0.70), and clearly better than surgical intervention.

This probabilistic approach contrasts with the traditional method of decision-making, in which the outcome is frequently the only criterion for assessing the method, so that good results may positively reinforce bad decision methods, and bad results may negatively reinforce good decision methods. It should also be noted that other outcomes could have been used, such as surgical morbidity, biopsy morbidity, and others. To the extent that morbidity parallels mortality, the optimal approach will remain the same. However, circumstances can be envisioned in which there may be discrepancies in Expected Utilities depending on the choice of outcome. For this reason, it may be useful to consider different choices of outcome.

A criticism of formal decision analysis has been that the input data (probabilities) may not be verifiable, and the values may be subject to doubt. Data obtained through the conduct of large and well-designed studies typically are the most reliable, and hence when available, are preferred for use in decision analysis. For many clinical scenarios, however, carefully designed studies have not been conducted, so it is necessary to rely on data of less certain reliability and validity. The latter type of information can be collected by retrospective review of outcomes for a series of patients treated at a particular facility, and in the absence of any observational data, on clinical impression based on prior experience with treated patients.

The use of data that are little more than a "best guess" is subject to question. A method for handling this problem in decision analysis is called **sensitivity analysis.** The term sensitivity analysis should not be confused with the sensitivity of a diagnostic test. It also should not be confused with the use of the same term in the context of meta-analysis. In meta-analysis (Chapter 7), we referred to sensitivity analysis in the context of examining the pattern of results across subgroups of studies to understand possible sources of heterogeneity in results.

In the context of decision analysis, we use the term sensitivity analysis to describe the process of substituting the reasonable maximum and minimum values of a particular probability in question into the decision tree. An upper and lower bound is then calculated on the outcome in question. If the preferred clinical scenario remains unchanged, the analysis and results may be considered robust. That is to say, the preferred management does not change for a broad range of estimated underlying probabilities.

In applying sensitivity analysis to the problem illustrated above, for example, among patients with alcoholic hepatitis the impact of allowing the probabilities of death following surgery can be considered to range between 50% and 75%. When these values are inserted into the tree and the problem is solved, performing a diagnostic liver biopsy remains the preferred clinical scenario. It can be concluded, therefore, that the inferences from the decision analysis are invariant to at least this range of postsurgical mortality probabilities for patients with alcoholic hepatitis.

Any of the variables (probabilities) may be subjected to sensitivity analysis, and if a reasonable maximum or minimum value changes the inference from the analysis, this circumstance should be considered in choosing the preferred clinical scenario. Sensitivity analysis can be performed easily with a personal computer and appropriate software. The analysis may be done using either a spreadsheet program or a more specific program, of which there are several (see references). The computer allows rapid calculations over a wide range of probabilities, so that the answers are quickly available, often in easily understood graphs.

It is also necessary to consider that any test is less than 100% sensitive and specific in classifying disease. If the liver biopsy misses 5% of alcoholic hepatitis and incorrectly labels other diseases as alcoholic hepatitis 2% of the time, then these considerations must be included in the decision tree. The new tree will be slightly more complicated, but it can easily accommodate these differences. For this particular problem, sensitivity analysis of the possibility of alcoholic hepatitis using values for sensitivity and specificity of the biopsy ranging from 50% to 100% does not change the preference for performing the diagnostic test. The likelihood that the biopsy is positive has little influence on the decision to test over a wide range of probabilities.

In contrast, it can be shown that the preferred clinical scenario will vary somewhat with the probability of alcoholic hepatitis versus cholangitis. The results of a sensitivity analysis for alcoholic hepatitis over a range of probabilities from 0% to 100% is given in Table 12–4. Over most of the range of values (10–90%), there is clear benefit to obtaining the diagnostic liver biopsy. Only at the extremes of probability of alcoholic hepatitis is there any question about the value of the diagnostic biopsy. When it is certain that the patient has cholangitis, proceeding directly to decompression of the biliary obstruction offers an Expected Utility comparable with that of obtaining the diagnostic liver biopsy first. On the other extreme, when it is virtually certain that the patient has alcoholic hepatitis, proceeding directly to medical management offers an Expected Utility comparable with that of obtaining the diagnostic liver biopsy first.

As might be suspected, the estimated probability that the liver biopsy itself will produce a fatal complication also influences the decision of whether or not to test. The results of a sensitivity analysis of surviving a liver biopsy using estimated probabilities ranging from 90% to 94% are shown in Table 12–5. In this problem, the sensitivity analysis indicates that the preferred alternative is liver biopsy *unless* the risk of a fatal complication is greater than 8%.

SUMMARY

Reaching optimal decisions in clinical practice is complex, in part because the decision may involve the use of information that is imperfect or of uncertain validity. The estimation of the degree of uncertainty in clinical information, based on the concept of probability esti-

Table 12–4. Sensitivity analysis varying the baseline probability of alcoholic hepatitis.

Probability (%) of Alcoholic Hepatitis	Expected Utilities			Preferred Decision
	Surgery	Medical	Biopsy	
0	.900	.250	.898	Surgery
10	.860	.300	.883	Biopsy
20	.820	.350	.868	Biopsy
30	.780	.400	.853	Biopsy
40	.740	.450	.838	Biopsy
50	.700	.500	.823	Biopsy
60	.660	.550	.808	Biopsy
70	.620	.600	.793	Biopsy
80	.580	.650	.778	Biopsy
90	.540	.700	.764	Biopsy
100	.500	.750	.749	Medical

Table 12–5. Sensitivity analysis varying the probability of surviving the liver biopsy.

Probability (%) of Surviving Biopsy	Expected Utilities			Preferred Decision
	Surgery	Medical	Biopsy	
94	.540	.700	.719	Biopsy
93	.540	.700	.712	Biopsy
92	.540	.700	.704	Biopsy
91	.540	.700	.696	Medical
90	.540	.700	.689	Medical

mates, and the use of these estimates in a logical structure are useful tools for making objective decisions in medicine. Formal decision analysis requires the specification of alternative management strategies and provides an explicit probabilistic method for choosing the most favorable anticipated course of action.

The elements of a formal decision analysis include the following: (1) identification of an underlying set of management options, (2) application of probabilities to uncertain events, (3) incorporation of test results, and (4) inclusion of anticipated clinical outcomes for alternative management options. Within the formal structure of the process, referred to as a decision diagram or tree, numerical values are inserted for the anticipated likelihoods of diagnoses, test results, and treatment outcomes. The clinical end points can be assessed in a variety of different ways, such as morbidity, mortality, or quality of life. The alternative management options within the decision diagram are referred to as clinical scenarios, each of which is associated with an Expected Utility (or outcome). The Expected Utilities of different scenarios are compared to arrive at the most favorable approach to management. In many circumstances, precise estimates of alternative diagnoses, test performance, or clinical outcomes are unavailable. In these situations, the impact of assuming different values for the unknown parameters can be explored through sensitivity analysis.

Some clinicians may object to the use of probability estimates, arguing that their use may imply more precision than is warranted by the clinical information, that it dehumanizes the doctor–patient relationship, that it may somehow increase liability, and so on. Although these concerns may limit the widespread use of formal decision analysis, this technique can serve as a useful tool to aid in appropriate patient management. As the stethoscope aids an experienced clinician in making a diagnosis, decision analysis provides insight into alternative management strategies, taking advantage of clinical and epidemiologic methods, many of which are outlined in this book.

For the situation described in the Patient Profile, the clinical presentation suggested a diagnosis of either cholangitis or alcoholic hepatitis. Cholangitis requires surgery to relieve biliary obstruction, whereas surgery is contraindicated in alcoholic hepatitis. By framing this management problem in a formal decision analysis, performing a liver biopsy to reduce uncertainty about the diagnosis was shown to result in a more favorable outcome (in terms of mortality) than proceeding directly to either surgical or medical management.

Sensitivity analysis further demonstrated that the decision to perform an initial liver biopsy would be preferred under a fairly wide range of expected mortality probabilities for alcoholic hepatitis and test accuracy. There were only two circumstances in which an initial liver biopsy did not appear warranted: when there was minimal baseline uncertainty about the diagnosis, and when the anticipated likelihood of a fatal complication of the biopsy reached an appreciable level. Using the available information, the physician in the Patient Profile would be justified in opting for a diagnostic liver biopsy before proceeding further in patient management.

STUDY QUESTIONS

Questions 1–4: For each numbered question below, select the most appropriate answer based on the decision diagram in Figure 12–4.

The diagram represents the decision to use medical therapy or bypass surgery in a 50-year-old patient with severe angina. The utilities are hypothetical outcomes scored from 0 to 100. Respective probabilities are also shown on the diagram. The preferred outcome is to survive as long as possible without angina.

1. In Figure 12–4, the expected utility for medical therapy is

    A. 57 + 62 = 119.0

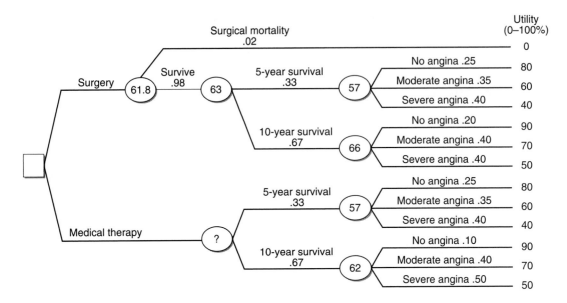

Figure 12–4. Decision tree for coronary bypass surgery.

B. $(57 + 62) \times (.67) = 79.73$

C. $(57 \times .67) + (62 \times .33) = 58.65$

D. $(57 \times .33) + (62 \times .67) = 60.35$

E. $(57 \times .33) + (5\ years) = (62 \times .67) + (10\ years)$
= 75.35

2. If you were to base your decision on the Estimated Utility (EU) in Figure 12–4, what would your preferred choice be?

A. Bypass surgery

B. Medical therapy

C. Observe the patient and consider bypass surgery in 6 months

D. Observe the patient and consider bypass surgery in 9 months

E. No rational therapeutic choice can be made based on the available data

3. Because the survival at 5 and 10 years is the same for surgery and medical therapy, what outcome event has led to the preferred choice in question 2?

A. A greater proportion of surgery patients has no angina at 10 years

B. A greater proportion of surgery patients has no angina at 5 and 10 years

C. A greater proportion of medical patients has no angina at 10 years

D. A greater proportion of medical patients has no angina at 5 and 10 years

E. An equal proportion of surgery and medical patients has no angina at 10 years

4. What is the mortality threshold, that is, the probability of death associated with surgery that would necessitate a decision to change to medical therapy for the 50-year-old patient described above?

A. .03

B. .04

C. .05

D. .06

E. .07

Questions 5–6: For each numbered question below, select the most appropriate answer based on the decision diagram in Figure 12–5, which represents the portion of a decision tree that depicts the use of a test to make a medical decision.

The probability that the test is positive is represented by p(Pos), and the probability that the test is negative is indicated by p(Neg). If the test is positive, the patient may have disease (ie, a true-positive) or the patient may not have disease (ie, a false-positive) with probabilities represented by p(Dis) and p(No Dis), respectively.

The same disease outcomes are possible with a negative test. If the test is negative, the probability of disease is represented by p(Dis–N) and the probability of no disease is represented by p(No

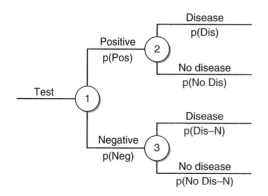

Figure 12–5. Portion of a decision tree that illustrates the use of a test to formulate a medical decision

Dis–N). N indicates that the test is scored as negative.

5. The probability that the test is positive can be easily determined based on the concept of predictive values discussed in Chapter 6. In Figure 12–5, consider true-positives, true-negatives, false-positives, and false-negatives (TP, TN, FP, and FN) as proportions, and Prev. as the pretest prevalence, which is occasionally termed the pretest probability. Which of the following calculations can be used to determine the probability p(Pos) at the chance node 1?

   A. $TP \times Prev. + FN \times Prev.$

   B. $TP \times Prev. + TN \times (1 - Prev.)$

   C. $TP \times Prev. + FP \times (1 - Prev.)$

   D. $TP \times (1 - Prev.) + FP \times Prev.$

   E. $TP \times (1 - Prev.) + FN \times (1 - Prev.)$

6. In Figure 12–5, consider PVP as the predictive value positive and PVN as the predictive value negative. At the chance node labeled 2, the probability of disease is given by which of the following?

   A. The PVP

   B. The 1 – PVP

   C. The PVN

   D. The 1 – PVN

   E. The $TP \times FP$

FURTHER READING

Elwyn G et al: Decision analysis in patient care. Lancet 2001; **358:**571.

REFERENCES

Clinical Background

Cholangitis

Carpenter HA: Bacterial and parasitic cholangitis. Mayo Clin Proc 1998;**73:**473.

Westphal J-F, Brogard J-M: Biliary tract infections. Drugs 1999; **57:**81.

Alcoholic Hepatitis

Morgan MY: The treatment of alcoholic hepatitis. Alcohol 1996; **31:**177.

Formal Decision Analysis

Detsky AS et al: Primer on medical decision analysis: Part 1—Getting started. Med Decis Making 1997;**17:**123.

Detsky AS et al: Primer on medical decision analysis: Part 2—Building a tree. Med Decis Making 1997;**17:**126.

Hollenberg JP: SMLTREE. Version 2.9. Roslyn, NY.

Krahn MD et al: Primer on medical decision analysis: Part 4—Analyzing the model and interpreting the results. Med Decis Making 1997;**17:**142.

Naglie D et al: Primer on medical decision analysis: Part 3—Estimating probabilities and utilities. Med Decis Making 1997; **17:**136.

Sonnenberg FA, Parker SG: *Decision Maker,* Version 6.2. New England Medical Center, 1988.

e-PIDEMIOLOGY

Further Reading

http://www.bmj.com/cgi/content/full/317/7155/405

Formal Decision Analysis

http://www.usd.edu/~dstevens/ctrial.htm

Interpretation of Epidemiologic Literature

13

KEY CONCEPTS

1. The literature on a topic of clinical interest often includes conflicting or inconclusive studies, thereby requiring the development of critical skills for interpreting the results.

2. A systematic approach to evaluating the features of individual studies can provide thoroughness and consistency to a review of the literature.

3. The evaluation of an individual study should include the research hypothesis, the study design, the predictor and outcome variables, the methods of analysis, possible sources of bias, and interpretation of results.

4. In considering whether a statistical association is likely to represent a causal relationship, one should consider the strength of the association, the presence of a dose-response trend, correct timing of events, consistency across studies, and biological plausibility.

5. A meta-analysis is a quantitative systematic review in which the results of multiple studies are combined to obtain a precise, and hopefully unbiased, estimate of the association under study.

PATIENT PROFILE

A 40-year-old accountant visited her family physician for a routine checkup. The patient's mother had been diagnosed with breast cancer in the past year, and the patient wanted advice about what she could do to reduce her own risk of developing this disease. The patient had two children aged 6 and 8 years. She was in good health, with regular menstrual cycles, and she had a recent normal Papanicolaou smear and mammogram.

In responding to the patient's questions about breast cancer, the physician confirmed that a positive family history increases the risk of developing this disease. A number of other characteristics are associated with a reduced risk of developing breast cancer, such as early age at first full-term

pregnancy and increasing number of pregnancies. Unfortunately, these factors are not easily susceptible to intervention, and the patient already had completed her childbearing. The physician was also aware of a controversy regarding the relationship between the intake of dietary fat and the occurrence of breast cancer. Before recommending that the patient reduce her fat intake, however, the physician wished to review the pertinent medical literature.

INTRODUCTION

The recommendations that physicians make to patients depend on the current state of knowledge available about diseases, the underlying pathophysiology of diseases, and the most effective treatment for diseases. The knowledge base of clinical medicine is continuously expanding, and physicians must therefore develop methods to seek out and apply new information.

This process is complicated when inconclusive or conflicting results are found in the medical literature. The publication of articles, even in the most respected journals, does not guarantee that the investigators' conclusions are valid, or even if valid, relevant to the daily practice of a particular physician. The history of medicine includes countless examples of therapies that were once widely accepted but later were shown to be ineffective or even harmful to patients. Clinicians must develop skills that will allow them to update and reevaluate their knowledge, enabling them to provide optimal patient care.

SEARCHING THE LITERATURE

The first step in acquiring new medical knowledge is to locate the appropriate literature. This is an increasingly difficult task as the number of medical journals increases each year. It is not possible for any physician to read, as it is published, everything relevant to his or her practice. Fortunately, help of various kinds is available to assist with literature searching when necessary.

With the advent of computer technology, it has become possible to search the medical literature in an automated manner. For example, a search through a standard database, such as *Medline,* could be performed to assemble lists of articles that might be of interest. *Medline* is a database of articles published in any one of 4600 biomedical journals. The earliest citations in this database are indexed from 1966, with coverage up through the present time. Although journals published from around the world are included in *Medline,* the vast majority are English language publications. The National Library of Medicine has made the *Medline* database available through the Internet at the following address: http://www.ncbi.nlm.nih.gov/entrez/query .fcgi

The search process is based on a few key words chosen to recover articles on relevant subjects. The search can be limited to a specific time period, which is helpful if you want to focus on the most recently published information. For example, a recent *Medline* search for the title words "breast cancer and dietary fat" retrieved about 70 journal articles over the previous 2-year period. These articles included a range of investigations, including laboratory animal studies, descriptive studies, case–control studies, cohort studies, randomized controlled clinical trials, and reviews, including meta-analyses. Most computer databases include abstracts of articles from major journals, and some even include the entire text of articles from selected publications.

REVIEWING INDIVIDUAL STUDIES

Once the appropriate literature is identified, it is useful to apply a uniform and thorough approach to evaluating the articles. This process will encourage the reader to consider all aspects of a study before passing judgment on its validity and utility. The following sections provide one such approach to evaluating individual published studies. The steps in the review are presented in Figure 13–1 in the general sequence in which they should be considered. However, each component of a review is dependent on the others to some extent, so that they are often considered collectively. The details of the review process for an individual paper are outlined in Table 13–1.

Research Hypothesis

It is important to consider the research hypothesis that is addressed by the study. In practice, this may be a difficult task. Authors often do not state

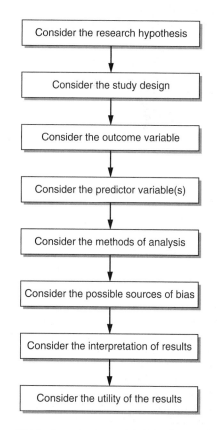

Figure 13–1. Steps in the evaluation of an epidemiologic study.

Table 13–1. Stepwise approach to critical appraisal of published medical research.

Step 1. Consider the research hypothesis
  Is there a clear statement of the research hypothesis?
  Does the study address a question that has clinical relevance?
Step 2. Consider the study design
  Is the study design appropriate for the hypothesis?
  Does the design represent an advance over prior approaches?
  Does the study use an experimental or an observational design?
Step 3. Consider the outcome variable
  Is the outcome being studied relevant to clinical practice?
  What criteria are used to define the presence of disease?
  Is the determination of the presence or absence of disease accurate?
Step 4. Consider the predictor variable(s)
  How many exposures or risk factors are being studied?
  How is the presence or absence of exposure determined?
  Is the assessment of exposure likely to be precise and accurate?
  Is there an attempt to quantify the amount or duration of exposure?
  Are biological markers of exposure used in the study?
Step 5. Consider the methods of analysis
  Are the statistical methods employed suitable for the types of variables (nominal versus ordinal versus continuous) in the study?
  Have the levels of type I and type II errors been discussed appropriately?
  Is the sample size adequate to answer the research question?
  Have the assumptions underlying the statistical tests been met?
  Has chance been evaluated as a potential explanation of the results?
Step 6. Consider possible sources of bias (systemic at errors)
  Is the method of selection of subjects likely to have biased results?
  Is the measurement of either the exposure or the disease likely to be biased?
  Have the investigators considered whether confounders could account for the observed results?
  In what direction would each potential bias influence the results?
Step 7. Consider the interpretation of results
  How large is the observed effect?
  Is there evidence of a dose-response relationship?
  Are the findings consistent with laboratory models?
  Are the effects biologically plausible?
  If the findings are negative, was there sufficient statistical power to detect an effect?
Step 8. Consider how the results of the study can be used in practice
  Are the findings consistent with other studies of the same questions?
  Can the findings be generalized to other human populations?
  Do the findings warrant a change in current clinical practice?

the hypotheses they wish to test. Sometimes the goal of the study is stated as a research question, but occasionally a reader is left to infer the purpose of the study from a set of complicated analyses.

Once the purpose of the study is discerned, the reader should attempt to determine if the study addresses a question that has clinical importance. If the study does not, the results may have little relevance to clinical practice. For the physician who needs information to counsel a patient about the relationship of dietary fat and risk of breast cancer, it is necessary to identify articles that address that topic. A number of

different kinds of hypotheses, however, may be relevant to the general topic. For example, a study of the effects of varying dietary fat composition on the occurrence of mammary tumors in mice may be useful, because studies conducted in laboratory animals can be more tightly controlled than studies conducted in humans. It may be useful to read a study on the effect of a high-fat diet on circulating estrogen levels in women, as this may have relevance to the biologic plausibility of a potential relationship between dietary fat and breast cancer. This type of research may yield information about the mechanism of disease development and prevention.

The various types of **significance** that may be ascribed to a research finding should be distinguished (Table 13–2). It is common to refer to results as significant if a statistical test indicates that the findings are unlikely to be attributable to chance alone. The evaluation of statistical significance—and therefore the likelihood of committing a type I (false-positive) error—is useful in the interpretation of results.

Even if a finding is statistically significant, however, it may not be biologically or clinically important. For instance, a small difference in the risk of developing breast cancer with increasing levels of dietary fat could be judged to be statistically significant if the finding were based on a large number of observations. Nevertheless, this elevation in risk may be so small that an individual woman's risk of developing breast cancer would not be appreciably altered by changing her diet. As a result, a clinical recommendation to reduce dietary fat might not be supportable on the basis of the evidence. The biological significance of a finding addresses yet another issue: Do the epidemiologic observations help to clarify the causal mechanism? This type of insight is most likely to be gained if the epidemiologic study involves biological markers of exposure, susceptibility, and outcome.

Study Design

If the study question is of interest, the reader should then determine what type of study design was employed. As noted in Chapters 7–9, certain designs may be more or less useful in answering specific kinds of questions. Another factor that may have determined the type of study design used by the investigator is the current state of knowledge. Early studies of a particular hypothesis may have a simple design, such as a descriptive study. As the hypothesis is refined, more definitive study designs can be utilized.

The appropriateness of the study design to the research question should be assessed. The incidence rate of the disease in question may be a determining factor. For example, although breast cancer is the most common form of cancer among women in the United States, this disease is diagnosed among only a small pro-

portion of women during a short period of time. Accordingly, a case–control study would offer an efficient approach to studying this disease, since the sampling scheme for this type of study identifies affected women once they are diagnosed. In fact, studies of dietary fat intake and occurrence of breast cancer have utilized several different designs, including descriptive, case–control, and cohort studies. The descriptive studies are useful for hypothesis generation, but not for hypothesis testing. The case–control and cohort designs provide more compelling evidence to test specific hypotheses. To date, all of the published studies of dietary fat and risk of developing breast cancer in humans have employed observational designs. A large, multicenter experimental study in which women are randomly assigned to groups receiving different levels of dietary fat and followed for the occurrence of breast cancer is underway in the United States, but this is a long-term study and results have not yet been published.

Outcome Variable

The outcome of interest in the Patient Profile is the development of breast cancer. In investigations of the relationship between dietary fat intake and risk of developing breast cancer, it is important to specify how the presence or absence of breast cancer was determined. There are several possibilities.

1. Death certificates limit information to deceased subjects. In addition, a variety of studies have shown that information on death certificates may be incomplete or inaccurate, as discussed in Chapter 4.

2. Self-reports require that subjects be alive or have relatives who can provide information on breast cancer. If the subjects are not medically sophisticated, they may mistake benign forms of breast disease for breast cancer.

3. Medical records may provide more accurate information. However, it is possible that diagnostic criteria differ from physician to physician, over time, or across geographic regions or countries.

Table 13–2. Types of significance in clinical research.

Type	Meaning	Assessment
Statistical	Exclusion of chance as an explanation for findings	Statistical test
Clinical	Importance of findings for changing current clinical practice	Magnitude of clinical response to an intervention
Biological	Findings help to clarify mechanism of action	Compare findings to information from in vitro and in vivo laboratory experimentation

4. Histopathologic diagnoses provide the most definitive information, but adequate tissue must be available for pathologic examination.

It is desirable to have the most definitive information possible on the presence of disease. This will tend to minimize the likelihood of misclassification of subjects. For breast cancer, it is possible that a small proportion of apparently healthy women may actually have occult (undiscovered) breast cancer. This could be evaluated by performing a screening test, such as mammography, on all apparently unaffected subjects. However, because so few asymptomatic cancers are likely to be detected, study findings probably would not be affected greatly by limiting detection to routine histopathologic diagnosis.

It is also important to judge how precisely the investigator defines the outcome. In general, it is useful to specify a single disease entity when searching for causes. For example, a study of dietary fat and the risk of all cancers combined may produce misleading results, as different cancers have different causes, and only some causes may involve dietary fat. Restricting the study to breast cancer improves the likelihood of obtaining a definitive result for this disease of primary interest.

Predictor Variables

The predictor variable is the risk factor or exposure under investigation. Studies may involve a single risk factor of interest or several different predictor variables. If a number of exposure variables are included, they may or may not be closely linked.

In a study of the cause of breast cancer, an investigator might choose to examine a variety of exposure variables, including reproductive factors such as age at first full-term pregnancy, hormone levels, exposure to radiation, and dietary fat intake. Although this sort of study may provide a more comprehensive picture of the causes of breast cancer, it may limit the ability to collect detailed information on each exposure of interest. Even if a study is focused on the question of dietary fat and the risk of developing breast cancer, it is necessary to collect some basic information on other possible determinants of breast cancer that could act as confounders.

The reader must determine whether the methods used to characterize the presence or absence of exposure are reliable and accurate. Possible methods of ascertainment include subject or surrogate respondent reports, direct observation, or measurement of a biological marker. The reader should ask whether there are better ways to define the exposure levels of subjects.

The assessment of a dietary exposure can be particularly difficult. In one method, asking subjects about their past dietary habits, the subjects must remember the kinds and the amounts of foods that they ate. Various studies have indicated that such recall, although imperfect, may suffice to determine whether a subject consumed a relatively high, moderate, or low amount of dietary fat. Generally, it is desirable to have several levels of exposure defined, so that a dose–response relationship can be evaluated.

Another approach to determining dietary fat intake is to have subjects record what they currently eat. This can be done by keeping a diary or by using a list of commonly eaten foods to check off the meals and snacks being ingested. There are problems with this approach, however. Subjects may forget to record what they eat, or they may incorrectly estimate the size of portions. To help offset such problems, plastic models of different portion sizes are available to provide visual cues and reminders. It is important to remember that a subject's current diet may not accurately reflect their past diet. In a case–control design based only on current diet information, it is crucial to know if subjects with breast cancer changed their diets because of (1) the disease, (2) the side effects of treatment, or (3) the hope of influencing prognosis.

Another approach to collecting information on diet is to measure what subjects eat. This could be useful for a prospective cohort study in which subjects are followed to determine whether they develop breast cancer. However, this approach to measuring dietary intake would be extremely difficult in practice, as it would require a tightly controlled environment in which the investigator could observe the foods eaten by subjects.

Epidemiologists occasionally take advantage of a situation in which people maintain certain dietary habits for religious or other reasons. Thus, an epidemiologist may identify a group of people (eg, vegetarians) who consume very little fat in their diets. The frequency of occurrence of breast cancer in this group could be compared with the experience of another group whose members consume large amounts of fat. However, the problem of determining the precise intake of fat for subjects in both groups still remains. Furthermore, it is likely that the groups will differ in life-style factors other than intake of dietary fat, giving rise to potential confounding.

The use of biological markers of exposure has become more common in clinical research (see Chapter 10). Biological markers are important because they can provide quantitative documentation of exposure in certain circumstances. No biological markers of fat intake are currently available, but to assess long-term intake of dietary fat, the fatty acid content of adipose tissue could be measured in biopsies. Obviously, the utility of such a measure depends on the extent to which it accurately reflects consumption patterns. The willingness of study participants to undergo a tissue biopsy must also be considered.

Methods of Analysis

The emphasis placed on a particular research finding often depends on the ability of the investigator to exclude chance as an explanation for the observed results. This is accomplished by the use of statistical tests. Readers should have a basic understanding of which statistical tests are appropriate for which types of analysis. The type of statistical test that should be used is determined by the goal of the analysis (eg, to compare groups, to explore an association, or to predict an outcome) and the types of variables used in the analysis (eg, categorical, ordinal, or continuous variables).

By convention, the 5% level of statistical significance is used as a standard in many biomedical studies. That is, the investigator is willing to accept a 1 in 20 risk that the observed effect is a result of chance variation alone. However, care must be taken to avoid oversimplistic interpretations of p values. One common mistake is to assume that a statistically significant result is biologically or clinically important. As discussed above, the clinical importance and biological plausibility of results are not assessed by hypothesis tests.

A second common mistake is to dismiss a finding because it has not reached the predetermined level for statistical significance. A p value of 0.08, for example, although not statistically significant in common practice, still represents a finding that is relatively unlikely to be attributable to chance. It would be unwise, therefore, to conclude on the basis of such a p value that there is no relationship between dietary fat intake and development of breast cancer in a particular study. The heavy reliance on p values is particularly dangerous when the sample size of a study is small and the statistical power is therefore low as well. In such situations, even moderate differences between groups may fail to reach a conventional level of statistical significance, and the ability to reach a definitive conclusion is limited.

Possible Sources of Bias

A result must also be examined to determine whether it could be due to systematic errors related to the sampling strategy or to data collection procedures. A statistical test cannot address whether biases of any sort are responsible for the observed results. As discussed in Chapter 10, the consideration of potential bias often cannot be assessed in precise quantitative terms. Bias can occur in any study, although certain designs are more susceptible to specific types of bias. Regardless of the study design, the potential for three distinct types of bias should be considered (Table 13–3).

The first concern is whether the selection of subjects is likely to have distorted the results (**selection bias**). Because few studies (if any) can examine an entire population, the investigator must draw a sample to make inferences about the population. The reader must determine if the samples are likely to be representative of the population to which extrapolations are made.

Table 13–3. Types of bias in clinical research.

Bias	Source of Error
Selection bias	Sample distorted by selection process
Information bias	Misclassification of the variables
Confounding	An extraneous variable that accounts for the observed result rather than the risk factor of interest

The methods section of any published medical research paper should include details of how subjects were selected for the study. In a case–control study, selection bias could arise from the approach used to select cases, controls, or both. In the context of a case–control study of dietary fat and occurrence of breast cancer, selection bias might occur if prevalent (surviving) cases are used rather than newly diagnosed (incident) cases. This distortion would occur if prediagnostic nutritional status were related to disease prognosis. For example, if women who consumed high-fat diets before developing breast cancer survived longer than women who consumed low-fat diets, prevalent cases would overrepresent high-fat consumption, and the observed risk ratio may be biased toward larger values. The bias is presented schematically in Figure 13–2.

In a case–control study, the sampling of controls can be as great a source of selection bias as the sampling of cases. Consider a hospital-based sample of control subjects with diagnoses other than breast cancer. If the diseases of the control subjects are caused by dietary factors (eg, atherosclerotic heart disease) or, conversely, if the diseases influence dietary intake (eg, gastrointestinal disease) a biased case–control comparison may result. Sampling from the general population typically results in control subjects who better reflect the exposure patterns of persons without the disease of interest. However, even general population sampling schemes can result in a distorted control group. For example, a telephone sampling technique might preferentially include higher income women, because they are more likely to have telephones than lower income women. Also, if higher income women are less likely to work outside of the home, they would be more available when the sampling is performed. Because the diets of higher income women may differ from those of other women, a biased case–control comparison may occur. To determine whether a telephone sampling scheme is likely to yield an unbiased sample of control subjects, it is necessary to know the completeness of telephone coverage of the

Incident cases

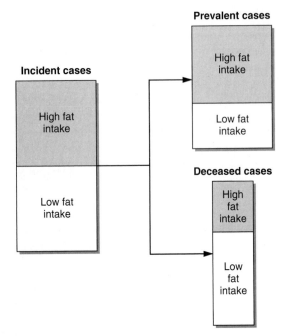

Prevalent cases

Deceased cases

Figure 13–2. Schematic diagram of bias introduced by study of prevalent cases when the risk factor (high fat intake) is related to prognosis. Shaded areas represent cases with high fat intake and unshaded areas represent cases with low fat intake. Note that the deceased cases included a relatively large proportion of persons with diets low in fat, resulting in overrepresentation of high-fat consumers among the prevalent cases.

target population. Also, multiple calls should be made to sampled residences, at varying times of the day and days of the week, to reach persons who work outside the home.

Cohort studies of the association between dietary factors and occurrence of breast cancer are also subject to potential selection bias. The major source of selection bias in such studies is loss to follow-up during the study. If women who eat a high-fat diet and develop breast cancer tend to discontinue participation in the study for some reason prior to the diagnosis of cancer, the investigator will underestimate the risk of developing breast cancer in women whose diets are high in fat. To date, cohort studies of this question have yielded conflicting results. An important consideration in such a situation is the extent to which bias due to loss to follow-up could explain the discrepancy.

Another source of bias can arise from systematic errors in measuring either the independent variable (exposure) or the dependent variable (disease). This type of bias is often referred to as **information bias** or **mis-**

classification bias. For example, in a case–control study, the validity of information on exposure may be questioned because the data are gathered retrospectively. Because the cases are aware of their disease and have undergone treatment for it, their reporting of past exposures may differ systematically from the reporting of control subjects. This is referred to as **recall bias.** Studies of dietary risk factors may be susceptible to recall bias. For example, if patients with breast cancer have wondered why they developed their cancer, they may tend to overestimate past exposure to dietary fat, particularly when the potential relationship has been widely publicized. Control subjects may be less concerned about past diet or may be worried about other problems such as obesity, which would tend to make them underreport exposure to dietary fat.

If recall bias occurred in a study, the investigator might overestimate the relationship between dietary fat intake and the risk of developing breast cancer. In fact, a number of studies have demonstrated problems of imperfect recall of dietary history. Only a few studies, however, have examined differential (biased) recall in cases versus controls by comparing prospectively collected dietary data with subsequent data collected retrospectively from the same subjects. In general, these investigations have not demonstrated differential recall of food intake in cases of breast cancer compared with controls. This would suggest that recall bias is an unlikely explanation for inconsistent results reported from case–control studies of the association of dietary fat intake and occurrence of breast cancer.

It should be remembered, however, that even if cases and controls do not differ in the ability to recall dietary exposure, misclassification bias still could occur. Errors in reporting that are comparable between cases and controls give rise to nondifferential misclassification. If nondifferential misclassification occurs, it may reduce the estimated risk ratio. In other words, such misclassification tends to make it more difficult to detect any true differences between cases and controls.

The final consideration of bias is to determine whether **confounding** could account for the observed result. A confounder is an extraneous correlate of disease that, because of its association with the risk factor of interest, accounts for some or all of the observed association between the risk factor and the disease. In studies of dietary fat intake and occurrence of breast cancer, it is important to determine if the investigator has accounted for the effects of known risk factors for breast cancer. These factors include age, race, reproductive characteristics (eg, age at first full-term pregnancy, number of pregnancies, duration of lactation), obesity among postmenopausal women, alcohol intake, and exposure to radiation. A schematic diagram for confounding of the relationship between dietary fat intake and

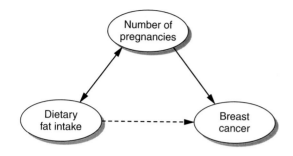

Figure 13–3. Schematic diagram of confounding of the dietary fat–breast cancer relationship by number of pregnancies.

occurrence of breast cancer by number of pregnancies is presented in Figure 13–3. If women who eat a high-fat diet have fewer pregnancies than those who eat a low-fat diet, an apparent association between consumption of dietary fat and occurrence of breast cancer could be attributable to the effects of reproductive history rather than to diet per se.

In an observational study, confounding can be controlled either in the design of the study (by restricting subject inclusion to persons with a narrow range of the confounder values or by matching study groups on confounders) or in the analysis of the results (through stratification by confounders or by regression techniques). All of these adjustment methods, however, are contingent on knowing which variables are confounders. Because the known risk factors for developing breast cancer do not account for all occurrences of the disease, other unknown risk factors must exist. Any observed association between dietary fat intake and occurrence of breast cancer could be explained, at least in part, in that way.

When the reader detects the potential for bias, it is important to try to estimate both the magnitude and the direction of the effect the bias could have on the results. In this way, the reader can determine if the bias is likely to have inflated the results or to have diminished the exposure's effect. In a case–control study, for example, if it is suspected that women with breast cancer are more likely than control subjects to remember and report fat intake, the risk ratio could be overestimated. In contrast, if it seems likely that patients with breast cancer underreport their dietary fat intake in comparison with control subjects, the observed results may underestimate the true impact of dietary fat intake on the occurrence of breast cancer. In discussing the results, an investigator may attempt to convince the reader that the magnitude of bias would not be sufficient to skew the results, or that the true relationship is as strong as or stronger than that observed.

Interpretation of Results

If the investigator reports a statistically significant result that cannot be explained by bias, the reader must then decide whether the result is clinically important. Consider, for example, a study concluding that a 50% decrease in dietary fat intake is associated with a 5% decrease in risk of developing breast cancer. Even if this result is statistically significant, the magnitude of the reduction in risk is so slight in exchange for the major change required in diet that individual patients may be poorly motivated to make the dietary change. On the other hand, the benefit to society in eliminating 5% of all breast cancer cases may well justify a mass public education effort to reduce consumption of dietary fat.

Conversely, results that are not statistically significant need not be considered useless. In particular, when there is a small sample size or when the relationship between the exposure and the disease is weak, the possibility of a false-negative conclusion must be considered. The statistical power of the study to detect the observed effect may be too low to allow a definitive conclusion from the study.

Practical Utility of Results

When reviewing a published study, the reader must determine the practical utility of the results. The usefulness of a study finding depends on various factors, including the purpose of the study, the limitations of the study population, the clinical and biologic importance of the results, and consistency with findings from other published studies. Clinical and epidemiologic research has various purposes. The clinical utility of a particular research finding must be viewed in the context of the type of question posed. As indicated in Table 13–4, a particular study may lead to findings relevant to disease causation, early detection of disease, the prediction of prognosis, or improved treatment. Studies of the rela-

Table 13–4. Clinical applications of various types of studies.

Type of Study	Application to Clinical Practice
Etiologic	Can risk be reduced among susceptible persons?
Diagnostic	Can accuracy and timeliness of diagnosis be improved?
Prognostic	Can prognosis be determined more definitively?
Therapeutic	Can treatment be improved?

tionship between dietary fat intake and occurrence of breast cancer relate to disease causation. Unfortunately, there is no standard by which to judge whether an association between a risk factor and a disease is clinically important. Clearly, the stronger the association (ie, the farther the risk ratio is from the null value), the greater the potential impact of eliminating the exposure. In assessing clinical utility, consideration must be given to how difficult it is to change the risk factor (in this case, to reduce dietary fat intake) and to the amount of morbidity and mortality associated with the disease.

The ability to generalize the findings beyond the study population should be taken into account. For this purpose, the definition and limitations of the study sample must be understood. For example, some studies of risk factors for developing breast cancer have focused on postmenopausal women. This may limit the applicability of such studies to the premenopausal patient in the Patient Profile. Investigators are often forced to restrict the sample by age, race, or other factors. The reader must decide what effect these restrictions may have on the broader applicability of results.

In determining whether the findings of a particular study can be generalized to other populations, it is useful to assess whether similar results have been obtained in other studies. It often happens that the first evaluation of a risk factor, diagnostic test, or therapeutic regimen is favorable, whereas subsequent reports demonstrate more limited utility. One reason for this pattern is that initial assessments often involve selected populations that offer a best-case scenario. Subsequent attempts to broaden the applicability may prove less successful.

ESTABLISHING A CAUSAL RELATIONSHIP

Ultimately, the reader may question whether a causal relationship between a risk factor and occurrence of a disease has been supported by the results of a study. Table 13–5 presents selected criteria that can be used to evaluate suspected causal relationships. The consideration of causality is based on the findings of a particular study, within the context of what is already known about a disease process.

Table 13–5. Selected criteria for evaluating a suspected causal relationship.

Strength
Presence of a dose–response relationship
Correct temporal sequence
Consistency of results across studies
Biological plausibility

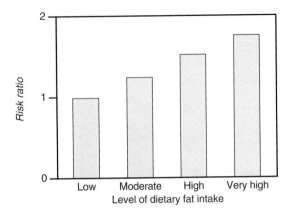

Figure 13–4. Hypothetical dose–response relationship between level of dietary fat intake and risk ratio of developing breast cancer. The reference category of exposure is low dietary fat intake.

The **strength of the observed association** is a primary criterion in evaluating whether a risk factor causes a disease. The strength of the association is indicated by the distance of the risk ratio or odds ratio from the null value. When the association is very strong, it is less likely that the association can be explained by chance or bias. Weak associations also may be causal, indicating only a lower risk of disease development. With a weak association, however, it is more difficult to exclude other factors and biases that may account for the relationship.

It is useful to examine whether there is a **dose–response relationship** between the proposed risk factor and the disease. If there is, increased levels of the risk factor will be associated with a greater risk of developing the disease (or with protection in the case of a beneficial factor). For example, as the level of dietary fat intake increases, the risk of developing breast cancer would be expected to increase if a causal relationship exists (Figure 13–4). However, the absence of a progressive, graded dose–response relationship does not preclude a causal relationship. For example, there may be a threshold above which the level of the risk factor confers increased risk. In this case, risk of disease will not be affected by changes in exposure below a certain level, but risk does vary with exposure at higher levels.

With any association, it is helpful to compare the findings with the results of other studies. If other investigators studying different populations in differing settings find similar results, a causal explanation is supported. However, the reader must be careful when judging consistency of results, because it is possible that the same flaw could lead to incorrect conclusions in several studies.

The proposed causal relationship should be consistent with what is currently known about biology and the disease process. This is often referred to as **biological plausibility.** If the proposed cause-and-effect relationship is not in accordance with current knowledge, causality may be questioned. The assessment of biological plausibility often requires a review of research on other human populations, as well as a review of research that involves laboratory animal models.

The **temporal relationship** between a suspected cause and an effect is important. That is, *a cause must always precede an effect in time.* This seems intuitive, but in reality, factors that are suspected to be causes sometimes turn out to be effects of the disease. For example, a person with an early undiagnosed cancer may make a change in food choices because of unrecognized systemic effects of the cancer. Consequently, the dietary change may appear to be the cause of, rather than an effect of, the later diagnosed cancer. Case–control studies of chronic diseases with long latent periods are particularly susceptible to this problem. For a factor to be considered the cause of a disease, it is theoretically important that removal or modification of that factor will prevent the disease from occurring or will ameliorate the disease once it has occurred. This criterion may have been met for the example cited in Chapter 9, as the incidence of eosinophilia-myalgia syndrome appears to have declined with the removal of L-tryptophan from the market. However, surveillance for eosinophilia-myalgia syndrome is not as active as it was when the syndrome was first reported, so unreported cases of eosinophilia-myalgia syndrome may still be occurring. For example, cases of eosinophilia-myalgia syndrome continue to occur in Canada, where L-tryptophan is available only by prescription (Spitzer et al, 1995). This means that the true incidence of eosinophilia-myalgia syndrome is not currently known; nor do epidemiologists know the extent to which the incidence may have changed.

In practice, the criterion of removal or modification of a suspected causal factor may not always be satisfied. There are some instances in which a causal factor may set off a protracted chain of events. Once established, this sequence may no longer depend on the presence of the causal agent for progression. For example, many cancers are thought to develop in response to an initiating event, followed by promotional effects that occur for many years. If the risk factor of interest contributes to initiation only, removal of the exposure during the promotional phase will not affect the subsequent risk of developing cancer. Thus eliminating an initiating risk factor for cancer may not affect the incidence of this disease for many years into the future.

DIETARY FAT AND BREAST CANCER

As mentioned previously, the relationship between dietary fat intake and the risk of developing breast cancer was investigated in a variety of epidemiologic studies. These studies included case series reports, ecologic analyses, case–control studies, and cohort studies. To date, no randomized controlled clinical trial of the relationship between consumption of a low-fat diet and prevention of breast cancer has been published.

Ecologic or correlation studies have demonstrated a consistently strong relationship between dietary habits, as estimated by per-capita consumption of dietary fat, and breast cancer occurrence in different countries. Plots of these data have yielded a linear relationship, with increasing fat consumption associated with higher breast cancer occurrence. The problem with such studies is that they do not demonstrate that increased dietary fat in *individuals* is associated with breast cancer occurrence in the same individuals (ie, the **ecologic fallacy** may be involved). For example, in industrialized countries in which fat consumption and breast cancer mortality tend to be higher than in developing countries, it may not be the high fat consumers who are developing breast cancer. The comparatively high mortality rates of breast cancer in industrialized countries may be attributable to other factors, such as earlier menarche, delayed childbearing, or other reproductive factors.

Case–control studies have yielded conflicting results on the question of diet and breast cancer. The reasons for these conflicting results are not clear. One criticism is that dietary data collected retrospectively are inaccurate (ie, dietary exposure is misclassified). General difficulties in recalling diet could contribute to nondifferential misclassification, and case–control differences in ability or motivation to recall dietary fat could result in differential misclassification. Another potential explanation is that the influence of dietary fat could have been exerted many years prior to the diagnosis of breast cancer. Most case–control studies have included diet information from the recent but not from the remote past. Some reviewers have concluded that none of the studies, when viewed individually, had a large enough sample size to provide adequate statistical power. In other words, a true relationship between dietary fat intake and risk of developing breast cancer might be missed because of inadequate discriminatory ability (ie, a type II error may be involved).

Some of these problems can be avoided with the cohort study design. Prospective cohort studies eliminate the potential for distortion of results from differential recall of dietary history. This type of study was used to investigate the question of fat in the diet and the risk of developing breast cancer. Again, the published results of cohort studies of this question have yielded conflicting results. Some studies have produced evidence of a relatively weak association, with risk ratios in the range of 1.2 to 1.7. Other cohort studies, however, have indicated little or no association. In general, the dose–response relationship suggested by the ecologic studies has not been borne out in the case–control and cohort studies. Some reviewers have argued that the range of dietary fat intake in the analytic studies is smaller than in the international ecologic studies. Within a single country, there may be too little variation in fat intake to demonstrate a dose–response relationship in case–control and cohort studies. Others have argued that factors other than diet (ie, confounders) that could not be controlled easily in ecologic studies were the real explanation for the association between fat intake and development of breast cancer observed in correlation analyses.

Was there biological plausibility to the relationship? What pathophysiologic mechanism might be involved? Were there animal models that showed the relationship between fat in the diet and development of breast cancer? In fact, animal studies have found an association between fat intake and the development of mammary cancers in mice bearing the mammary tumor virus. Similar findings have been reported in other animal models. The pathophysiology involved in this process is less clear, but potential mechanisms have been discussed. It has been speculated that mammary neoplasms are controlled by endocrine balance, which in turn is affected by dietary factors, including fat intake. For example, women consuming high-fat diets have been shown to have more circulating estrogen than women on low-fat diets. In postmenopausal women, adipose tissue has been demonstrated to be a contributor to the production of estrogen. Dietary fat intake may also have modified DNA synthesis and cell duplication. If this were found to be true for breast tissue, this could be relevant to breast carcinogenesis. In animal studies, certain types of fatty acid in the diet modulate mammary tumor growth and metastasis. The evidence is strongest for a promotional effect of polyunsaturated fat. The potential differential effect of various types of fatty acid on development and progression of cancer might explain some of the variation observed in studies of fat intake and breast cancer risk in humans. Most epidemiologic studies have evaluated total fat intake. Some studies have used adipose tissue levels of fat as a surrogate measure of fat intake. Adipose tissue levels, however, do not provide an indication of dietary intake of fatty acids that can be synthesized internally. The Nurses Health Study did include a prospective evaluation of different types of fatty acid intake. In this study, none of the various types of dietary fat was associated with the risk of developing breast cancer.

Systematic Reviews

In Chapter 7, we introduced the concept of a **meta-analysis**. A meta-analysis is a type of quantitative systematic review in which the results of multiple studies that are considered combinable are aggregated together to obtain a precise, and hopefully unbiased, estimate of the relationship in question. As already illustrated in the dietary fat–breast cancer question, single studies rarely provide the definitive answer on a topic. A systematic review helps in two specific ways:

1. By combining a series of smaller studies, each with a statistically imprecise estimate of effect, a larger sample size is obtained, with a corresponding increase in statistical precision.
2. By identifying the differences in findings across different studies, sensitivity analyses can be conducted that may lead to greater insight into the sources of heterogeneity.

The steps in a systematic review should follow a clear sequence. The first step is to formulate a clear and meaningful question to be addressed. Elements to be considered in the formulation of this question are (1) the type of person(s) involved, (2) the type of exposure that the person(s) experiences (eg, a risk factor, a prognostic factor, a diagnostic procedure, or a therapeutic intervention), (3) the type of control with which the exposure is compared, and (4) the outcomes to be addressed. In the context of the patient profile, we might specify the question in the following way: *For premenopausal women with a family history of breast cancer, is reduction of dietary fat consumption substantially below levels typical of the American diet likely to reduce the risk of developing breast cancer?*

Note that even with this level of specification, there is some ambiguity. The characteristics of the population could have been delimited further, by noting other characteristics of the patient, such as her age of 40, a history of having her first child after age 30, and a recent normal mammogram. The precise level of dietary fat reduction was characterized as substantial, but not quantified further. Although greater specificity is desirable in formulating the question, if the question becomes too specific, there may be an insufficient amount of pertinent literature available to address it. With insufficient data, it may be impossible to answer the question. As a general rule, features of the patient or the intervention that are thought in advance to affect the answer should be considered.

Once the question is formulated, the next step is to decide what studies to include. A pragmatic approach is to limit the source studies to those published in the English language. There is a possibility that this will introduce some bias, as studies with positive findings may be submitted preferentially to journals with wider circulation, which tend to be the English language journals. A further consideration is whether to limit the review to published studies, as these are peer reviewed and presumably of higher quality. As noted in Chapter 7, however, a **publication bias** might result, as studies with positive findings may be more likely to be submitted and accepted for publication. Of course, the identification of unpublished work may be incomplete.

The next step is to search for the studies of interest. As suggested earlier in this chapter, an automated search of an electronic database, such as *Medline,* is an efficient way to identify the relevant published literature. Such a search, however, is limited to the articles contained in the database, which will tend to exclude the proceedings of meetings that are not published in journals, doctoral dissertations, and journals that are not indexed.

Once the articles for potential inclusion are identified, they must be reviewed one at a time. Specific eligibility criteria for inclusion must be specified. The included studies should be directly relevant to the question under consideration. In the present context, they must include, at a minimum, a study sample including healthy premenopausal women, information on dietary consumption of fats, comparison of higher and lower fat intakes, and estimation of breast cancer risk. If a qualitative review is under consideration, a wide range of studies, including those involving laboratory animals, human case series, cross-sectional, case–control, and cohort studies, as well as clinical trials might be included. If there is interest in a statistical integration of data from the various studies, the analysis may be limited to studies in which the data are combinable (eg, case–control and cohort studies and clinical trials). The next step is to extract the key data elements from the included studies. A pretested standard abstract form should be used to collect the relevant information from each source paper. To ensure reliability, it is advisable to have two independent reviewers collect information from each paper.

The actual analysis of the data begins with an estimation of the effect of interest in each of the included studies. It is useful to display the individual study results as shown in Figure 13–5. In this graph, the results of five separate hypothetical studies of the relationship between reduced dietary fat intake and risk of developing breast cancer are presented. The findings of each investigation are summarized with a point estimate of effect and a corresponding confidence interval around that estimate. The point estimate is represented as a solid circle, with a horizontal line stretching in both directions to the upper and lower bounds of the confidence interval. By convention, the effect typically is

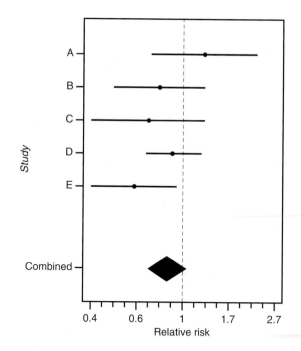

Figure 13–5. Meta-analysis of five hypothetical epidemiologic studies (A–E) of the relationship between reduced dietary fat intake and the risk of developing breast cancer.

measured in terms of either an odds ratio or a relative risk (risk ratio).

In Figure 13–5, the results are displayed in terms of estimated relative risk of developing breast cancer associated with a reduced level of dietary fat intake. If reducing fat in the diet decreases the risk of developing breast cancer, a relative risk less than 1 would be expected. The point estimates for the relative risks in these hypothetical studies ranged from a low of 0.6 (Study E) to a high of 1.3 (Study A). Four of the five studies (Studies B through E) had point estimates lower than 1, consistent with the possibility of a reduction in breast cancer risk. On the other hand, most of these estimates are close to the null value of 1 (no association between dietary fat intake and risk of developing breast cancer). It is possible, therefore, that these small benefits suggested by a reduction in fat consumption may have arisen by chance.

Examination of the corresponding confidence intervals for the individual studies provides some insight into the statistical precision of the results and whether they are statistically significant. By convention, 95% confidence limits typically are calculated. The odds or risk ratio often is displayed on a logarithmic scale as in

Figure 13–5, so as to make the confidence intervals symmetrical around the point estimate.

It can be seen from Figure 13–5 that the precision of the five study results varied, with the narrowest confidence intervals (greatest precision) for Study D and the widest confidence intervals (least precision) for Study A. Only one of the five studies had a result that was statistically significant at the 5% level, as indicated by the fact that its confidence interval did not cross the dashed vertical line corresponding to the null value of one.

Statistical integration of the results of the individual studies allows calculation of a summary estimate of effect. On the bottom of Figure 13–5, the combined point estimate for the five hypothetical studies is shown as a diamond. The vertical points of the diamond are located at the point estimate of the summary effect, and the horizontal points are located at the upper and lower bounds of the 95% confidence interval, respectively. In this example, the combined point estimate was 0.86, with a corresponding 95% confidence interval from 0.70 to 1.05. The summary estimate is based on a larger sample size than any of the individual study results. Accordingly, the combined estimate is more precise, which is reflected in the figure by comparatively narrow confidence intervals. In this example, it can be seen that the combined effect is consistent with a small reduction in risk of developing breast cancer, but even with the large sample size of the five studies combined, chance cannot be excluded as a possible cause of the findings.

Once the individual and combined estimates are obtained, it is useful to consider the level of heterogeneity across the individual results. A graphic display of the data, as in Figure 13–5, provides some insight into this question. Although there is some variation in the individual results, the impression is that there is considerable overlap in the values of the relative risk that are consistent with each result. This would suggest that heterogeneity of findings is not a problem in summarizing these data. A formal test of heterogeneity can be performed to address this issue from a statistical perspective.

Sensitivity analysis can be performed to identify patterns of results across the individual study results and potentially provide insight into any heterogeneity that exists. For example, two questions may be examined: do studies of a particular design (eg, case–control studies) tend to yield results that differ from studies of other designs (eg, cohort studies), and do investigations with younger study populations tend to have results that differ from investigations with older populations?

In the present hypothetical example, it is unclear that a sensitivity analysis would yield great insights for two reasons. First, there are a relatively modest number of studies involved, which limits the ability to explore findings across subgroups. Any differences that were observed might arise on the basis of chance, leading to false-positive interpretations. Second, the results across studies are reasonably consistent, further limiting the ability to find different underlying patterns. From a descriptive point of view, it might be useful to consider possible reasons (other than chance) for an apparently different result in Study A.

Meta-analysis can be useful in achieving greater statistical power, but it cannot overcome the limitations and potential biases of individual studies. The investigator performing a meta-analysis must also be careful that selection of some studies and exclusion of others do not lead to a distorted conclusion.

A meta-analysis published in 2003 explored the relationship between dietary fat intake and risk of breast cancer. This systematic review included 45 studies (31 case–control and 14 cohort), with a combined total of over 25,000 breast cancer patients and 580,000 control or comparison subjects. An overall small increase in risk of breast cancer was associated with elevated total fat intake in both the case–control (OR = 1.14) and cohort studies (RR = 1.11). The combined association was statistically significant and was higher in the studies judged to be of better quality. Similar findings were observed in analyses of saturated fat and meat intake.

In the Patient Profile, the physician wanted to determine whether dietary fat intake is causally related to the development of breast cancer. The findings of studies were inconsistent, and the strength of association was weak at best, without clear evidence of a dose–response relationship. The temporal sequence of dietary fat intake and development of breast cancer appeared to be reasonable.

The physician in the Patient Profile, however, is left without a firm answer to the question about the relationship between consumption of dietary fat and risk of developing breast cancer. Even if research has demonstrated a small increase in risk with high-fat diets, it is unclear whether the patient can meaningfully reduce her risk of breast cancer by changing her diet. The physician may believe, however, that a low-fat diet is justifiable for other reasons, including reduction of risk for cardiovascular disease. In addition, there are other cancers, such as colon cancer, for which the protective effect of a low-fat diet may be beneficial.

This type of uncertainty is common in clinical medicine. Physicians often must weigh potential risks and benefits of an intervention and make decisions without complete information. The goal of medical research is to continue to provide better answers to important clinical questions. The best way to resolve the issue of the relationship between dietary fat intake and risk of developing breast cancer is through large randomized controlled trials comparing occurrence of breast cancer in women randomized to a low-fat diet with women randomized to a high-fat diet. Clearly, this type of study would provide the most definitive evidence about a causal relationship between consumption of dietary fat and risk of developing breast cancer. Such a study is underway, but until the results are available, the best evidence is that which has been obtained through observational studies. Much of the satisfaction derived from patient care relates to the ability to incorporate new knowledge into the practice of medicine. It is imperative to develop the skills required for a critical review of the medical literature to keep current on the state of information. This is a difficult task, but the reward is enormous when it results in improved patient care.

SUMMARY

In this chapter, a structured approach to reviewing published epidemiologic studies was presented. The ultimate goal of this approach is to help integrate epidemiologic information into clinical practice. As a focus for discussion, the literature on dietary fat intake and risk of developing breast cancer is used to illustrate the evaluation process.

The initial step in reviewing the medical literature is to conduct a thorough search for relevant recent publications. Screening for appropriate articles can be accomplished through a manual or a computer-assisted approach. In either case, a correct choice of key words calculated to retrieve pertinent articles is essential. Computer searches can save time and consequently are extremely popular.

The actual review of a publication begins with the stated purpose of the investigation. For the medical practitioner, a primary consideration is whether a particular study addresses a clinically important question. Are the results likely to influence the delivery of patient care? In the present context, clinical importance might be assessed in terms of whether the findings support a recommendation to lower dietary fat intake so as to reduce the risk of developing breast cancer.

The design of an investigation determines the types of inferences that can be drawn from it. The most compelling evidence for cause-and-effect relationships is derived from randomized controlled clinical trials. Among observational investigations, prospective cohort studies generally are least susceptible to bias, followed by retrospective cohort and case–control studies. Descriptive studies are useful for generating research questions but not for testing hypotheses.

The measurement of outcome (ie, development of disease) as well as the documentation of exposure to risk factors can be complicated in observational research. Emphasis must be placed on obtaining the most accurate information possible, recognizing that the ideal often cannot be achieved. Whenever possible, assessment should be performed in a blinded manner and should be based on objective, standard criteria.

A distinction must be made between the concept of statistical significance, which can be evaluated by a hypothesis test, and clinical or biological significance. p values should not be used to indicate the importance of a finding, but rather the likelihood that sampling variability can explain the results. Clinical importance relates to whether a difference in outcomes observed between study groups is large enough to warrant a change in clinical practice. Biological significance refers to the extent to which findings help to elucidate the underlying biological processes.

Systematic errors may arise in observational research from the approach to sample selection, information collection, or confounding. It is usually impossible to determine whether a particular bias actually has occurred. Attention, therefore, is focused on strategies to minimize the likelihood that systematic errors will affect the study conclusions. When bias is suspected in an investigation, the exact level of distortion generally is unknown. However, the direction of the systematic error (ie, a tendency to either overestimate or underestimate the strength of association) may be clear. The assessment of whether an observed association is likely to be one of cause and effect is based on specific criteria, including strength of association, presence of a dose–response relationship, appropriateness of the temporal sequence of exposure and outcome, consistency of results across studies, and biological plausibility.

When applied to the literature on dietary fat and breast cancer, this process of reasoning leads to an inconclusive assessment. The most consistent supporting evidence comes from the least compelling types of study. In situations in which an association has been observed, the magnitude generally has been weak. Results have been somewhat inconsistent across studies, perhaps due in part to limitations of the study design and in part to the weakness of the relationship, even if it does exist. The ultimate test of this hypothesis—a randomized controlled clinical trial—has not yet been published.

As with many issues in medicine, the dietary fat–breast cancer hypothesis remains unresolved. Because little harm probably results from restriction of dietary fat intake and because other benefits may accrue (ie, a reduction in risk of cardiovascular disease), it may be reasonable for the clinician in the Patient Profile to recommend this change in dietary habits to the patient. Until more definitive information is available, however, the patient should be counseled that the effect of restricting dietary fat intake on the risk of developing breast cancer is uncertain.

☑ STUDY QUESTIONS

Questions 1–5: For each research study described in the numbered questions, select the most likely form of bias or error from the lettered options.

1. A study is performed that examines the prevalence of hypertension and the per capita intake of sodium in the diet. It is found that the countries with higher sodium consumption have a higher prevalence of hypertension.
   A second study is performed in an individual country that examines the intake of sodium in the diet and the level of blood pressure. In this study subjects with higher sodium intake in the diet do not have higher blood pressure.
   A. Selection bias
   B. Random error
   C. Information bias
   D. Ecologic fallacy
   E. Confounding
   F. Birth cohort effect

2. In a cohort study of cigarette smoking and prostate cancer, 42% of the subjects are lost to follow-up after 5 years.
   A. Selection bias
   B. Random error
   C. Information bias
   D. Ecologic fallacy
   E. Confounding
   F. Birth cohort effect

3. In a case–control study of rheumatoid arthritis and alcohol intake, the cases tend to overreport drinking alcohol, whereas the controls who were hospitalized with gastrointestinal illnesses tend to underreport drinking alcohol.
   A. Selection bias
   B. Random error
   C. Information bias
   D. Ecologic fallacy
   E. Confounding
   F. Birth cohort effect

4. In a cohort study of the relationship of intake of fruits and vegetables and protection against coronary artery disease, blood pressure is associated positively with coronary artery disease and is inversely associated with dietary intake of fruits and vegetables. The investigators report that fruit and vegetable intake protects against the development of coronary artery disease, but does not control for the effects of blood pressure.
   A. Selection bias
   B. Random error
   C. Information bias
   D. Ecologic fallacy
   E. Confounding
   F. Birth cohort effect

5. In a case–control study of dietary intake and the development of colon cancer, the food frequency questionnaires yield imprecise estimates of actual food consumption for all respondents.
   A. Selection bias
   B. Random error
   C. Information bias
   D. Ecologic fallacy
   E. Confounding
   F. Birth cohort effect

Questions 6–10: For each study described in the numbered questions, select the most appropriate study design from the lettered options.

6. A study is conducted in a country to evaluate the prevalence of type 2 diabetes.
   A. Case–control study
   B. Cohort study
   C. Clinical trial
   D. Cross-sectional study
   E. Meta-analysis
   F. Ecologic study

7. Patients with newly developed breast cancer are asked about previous dietary intake of fat. Their responses are compared to patients admitted to the hospital for plastic surgery procedures.
   A. Case–control study
   B. Cohort study
   C. Clinical trial
   D. Cross-sectional study
   E. Meta-analysis
   F. Ecologic study

8. Two hundred patients with rheumatoid arthritis are randomly assigned to 6 months of a new anti-inflammatory drug or standard care.
   A. Case–control study
   B. Cohort study
   C. Clinical trial

D. Cross-sectional study

E. Meta-analysis

F. Ecologic study

9. A study evaluates the per-capita intake of calcium and the prevalence of hypertension in 8 different countries.

A. Case–control study

B. Cohort study

C. Clinical trial

D. Cross-sectional study

E. Meta-analysis

F. Ecologic study

10. The results of several case–control studies of the association between exposure to rug shampoo and the development of Kawasaki disease are examined to produce a summary conclusion.

A. Case–control study

B. Cohort study

C. Clinical trial

D. Cross-sectional study

E. Meta-analysis

F. Ecologic study

Questions 11–13: For each numbered situation below, choose the most appropriate criterion for establishing a causal relationship from the lettered options.

11. Five published case–control studies of the association between exposure to lead and diminished cognitive function in children yield the following odds ratios: 1.4 (95% CI 0.9–2.5), 1.7 (95% CI 1.3–2.5), 2.4 (95% CI 1.1–4.5), 1.9 (95% CI 1.4–2.4), and 1.2 (95% CI 1.05–1.6).

A. Strength of the association

B. Dose–response relationship

C. Correct temporal sequence

D. Consistency of results

E. Biologic plausibility

12. In a study of risk factors for the development of coronary artery disease and coronary heart disease mortality as depicted in Figure 13–6, the following relationship is found.

A. Strength of the association

B. Dose–response relationship

C. Correct temporal sequence

D. Consistency of results

E. Biologic plausibility

13. A case–control study shows an association between exposure to aluminum and Alzheimer's disease. At autopsy the pathologic lesions in the brains of patients who have died with Alzheimer's disease are found to contain elevated amounts of aluminum.

A. Strength of the association

B. Dose–response relationship

C. Correct temporal sequence

D. Consistency of results

E. Biologic plausibility

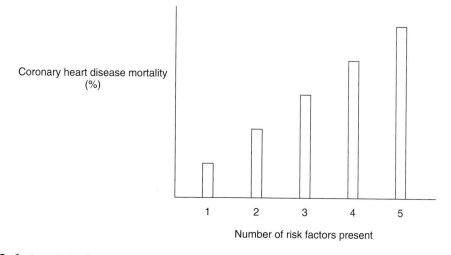

Figure 13–6. Association between the number of risk factors and coronary heart disease mortality.

FURTHER READING

Kushi L, Giovannucci E: Dietary fat and cancer. Am J Med 2002; **113**(9B):63S.

REFERENCES

Critical Review

Bingham SA et al: Are imprecise methods obscuring a relation between fat and breast cancer? Lancet 2003;**362**:212.

Greenhalgh T: How to read a paper: Getting your bearings (deciding what the paper is about). BMJ 1997;**315**:243.

Grimes DA, Schulz KF: Clinical research in obstetrics and gynecology: a Baedeker for busy clinicians. Obstet Gynecol Surv 2002;**57**(Suppl 3):S35.

Spitzer WO et al: Continuing occurrence of eosinophilia-myalgia syndrome in Canada. Br J Rheumatol 1995;**34**:246.

Dietary Fat and Breast Cancer

Boyd NF et al: Dietary fat and breast cancer risk revisited: a meta-analysis of the published literature. Br J Cancer 2003;**89**:1672.

Greenwald P, Sherwood K, McDonald SS: Fat, caloric intake, and obesity: Lifestyle risk factors for breast cancer. J Am Diet Assoc 1997;**97**(Suppl):S24.

Holmes MD et al: Association of dietary intake of fat and fatty acids with risk of breast cancer. JAMA 1999;**281**:914.

Hunter DJ et al: Cohort studies of fat intake and the risk of breast cancer—a pooled analysis. N Engl J Med 1996;**334**:356.

Wu AH, Pike MC, Stram DO: Meta-analysis: Dietary fat intake, estrogen levels, and the risk of breast cancer. J Natl Cancer Inst 1999;**91**:529.

e-PIDEMIOLOGY

Further Reading

http://www.bmj.com/epidem/epid.c.shtml

Searching the Literature

http://www.bmj.com/archive/7101/7101ed.htm

Critical Review

http://www.bmj.com/archive/7103/7103ed.htm
http://www.bmj.com/archive/7102/7102ed.htm

Methods of Analysis

http://www.pitt.edu/~super1/lecture/lec10401/index.htm

Possible Sources of Bias

http://www.pitt.edu/~super1/lecture/lec10391/index.htm

Establishing a Causal Relationship

http://www.bmj.com/archive/7105/7105ed.htm

Dietary Fat and Breast Cancer

http://envirocancer.cornell.edu/FactSheet/Diet/fs27.fat.cfm

Appendix A: Answers to Study Questions

CHAPTER 1

1. G
2. C
3. A
4. E
5. J
6. B
7. H
8. L
9. N
10. M

CHAPTER 2

1. B
2. C
3. A
4. F
5. D
6. E
7. C
8. D
9. A
10. D
11. C
12. D
13. C
14. A
15. B

CHAPTER 3

1. B
2. C
3. A
4. E

5. D
6. C
7. B
8. E
9. D
10. E
11. A
12. B

CHAPTER 4

1. B
2. D
3. A
4. C
5. E
6. A
7. C
8. D
9. E
10. A
11. C
12. D

CHAPTER 5

1. A
2. C
3. D
4. E
5. E
6. C
7. B
8. C
9. C
10. A

CHAPTER 6

1. E
2. K
3. L
4. G
5. F
6. H
7. M
8. I
9. J
10. B
11. A
12. D
13. C

CHAPTER 7

1. C
2. B
3. D
4. C
5. E
6. D
7. C
8. A
9. A
10. E

CHAPTER 8

1. C
2. A
3. D
4. B
5. A
6. D
7. A
8. D
9. C
10. D

CHAPTER 9

1. D
2. F
3. D

4. C
5. F
6. B
7. A
8. E
9. A
10. F
11. G
12. B
13. E
14. C

CHAPTER 10

1. A
2. B
3. C
4. B
5. C
6. D
7. A
8. B
9. C
10. C

CHAPTER 11

1. B
2. A
3. E
4. F
5. C
6. C
7. E
8. B
9. C
10. F

CHAPTER 12

1. D
2. A
3. A
4. C
5. C
6. A

CHAPTER 13

1. D
2. A
3. C
4. E
5. B
6. D
7. A
8. C
9. F
10. E
11. D
12. B
13. E

Appendix B: Estimation of Sample Size Requirements for Randomized Controlled Clinical Trials

The formulas used to estimate sample size requirements are provided in this appendix. Also provided are illustrative calculations relative to the Diabetes Control and Complications Trial described in Chapter 7.

Prior to undertaking this study, the investigators specified an alpha level (0.05, or 5%), statistical power (90%, and thus a beta level of 10%), and the outcome difference that should be detected by the trial (a reduction in the proportion of patients diagnosed with diabetic retinopathy from 20% to 10%). The baseline proportion of subjects who would develop retinopathy is derived from previous literature. The amount of reduction in retinopathy is based on clinical judgment; the following question was posed: "What would be a clinically important difference in the proportion of patients who would suffer this complication?"

The equation for sample size for a comparison of two proportions is as follows:

$$n = \left[\frac{z_a \sqrt{2\pi_c(1-\pi_c)} = z_\beta \sqrt{\pi_t(1-\pi_t) + \pi_c(1-\pi_c)}}{\pi_t - \pi_c} \right]^2$$

where n is the number of subjects for each treatment group, π_c and π_t are the proportion of patients that develops retinopathy within 5 years in the control group (standard therapy) and treatment group (intensive therapy), respectively, and z_α and z_β are the values that include alpha in the two tails and beta in the lower tail of the standard normal distribution. These values can be determined from tables available in most statistical texts (see Dawson and Trapp, 2004; complete publication data can be found at the end of Chapter 7). The value for a type I error of 5% is 1.96, and the z_β value for a type II error of 10% is −1.28. As the acceptable level of error decreases, z_α and z_β increase.

Note that in equation (1), the larger the z_α and z_β— that is, the smaller the acceptable type I and type II er-

rors—the larger the sample size required; also the smaller the difference in π_c and π_t, the larger the sample size required. What may not be so intuitively obvious is the relation of sample size to the distance of π_c from 0.5. The part of the equation $\pi_c(1 - \pi_c)$ is maximized, and therefore the numerator is greater when $\pi_c = 0.5$. Movement of π_c away from 0.5 reduces the required sample size.

If we expected the proportion of patients on standard insulin therapy for diabetes that would develop retinopathy by year 5 to be 0.20, and we wanted this trial to be able to detect a reduction in retinopathy at 5 years from 0.20 to 0.10, then the sample size would be calculated as follows:

$$n = \left[\frac{1.96\sqrt{2 \times 0.2 \times 0.8} - (-1.28)\sqrt{(0.1 \times 0.9) + (0.2 \times 0.8)}}{0.1 - 0.2} \right]^2$$

and $n = 305$. Therefore, a total of 610 subjects equally divided between groups would be required to answer the following question: "Is there a reduction in the rate of retinopathy at 5 years from 20% to 10% using intensive rather than standard insulin therapy?" This can be restated as follows: If the true difference in rate of retinopathy at 5 years is 10% versus 20%, then the probability that the researchers will find no difference between the proportion of subjects developing retinopathy during the first 5 years of therapy with an equally divided sample size of 610 would be only 10%.

Because the diabetes trial had over 305 subjects in each group, the likelihood of not finding a true difference of this magnitude was actually less than 10%.

If average glucose levels 5 years after beginning therapy had been the measure chosen to compare the two treatment groups, the required sample size could have been determined using the following equation:

$$n = 2 \left[\frac{(z_\alpha - z_\beta)\sigma}{\mu_1 - \mu_2} \right]^2$$

where n is the number of subjects for each treatment group, $\mu_1 - \mu_2$ is the detectable difference between the means of the two groups, σ is the common standard deviation of each group, and z_α and z_β have the same meaning as in equation (1).

Again, without memorizing this formula, we can intuitively understand how its various components contribute to sample size. The greater the absolute values of z_α, z_β, and σ, and the smaller the difference in the means, $\mu_1 - \mu_2$, the larger the n, or sample size, required (see Table 7–3). This makes sense, as smaller differences in means between groups would be harder to detect, and greater variability within the groups would tend to blur intergroup differences. As in all sample size calculations, the larger the values of z_α and z_β—that is, the smaller the acceptable type I and type II errors—the larger the sample size required.

Suppose the investigators estimated that the mean glucose levels at 5 years after the start of therapy would be 200 mg/dL for patients on standard insulin therapy and 175 mg/dL for those on intensive therapy, and the pooled standard deviation would be 45 mg/dL. The sample size for each group would be calculated using equation (3):

$$n = 2 \left[\frac{(1.96 + 1.28)45}{175 - 200} \right]^2$$

and $n = 68$. This end point would have required far fewer patients to be enrolled in the trial. At the conclusion of the trial, treating physicians may not have considered a reduction in glucose levels to be a sufficiently important outcome to warrant a change to the more intensive therapy; however, if the trial found that intensive therapy reduced the onset of retinopathy, intensive therapy would be judged to be a superior treatment regimen.

Appendix C: Method for Determining the Confidence Interval Around the Risk Ratio

An approximate 95% confidence interval (*CI*) around the point estimate of the risk ratio (*RR*) can be calculated using the following formula:

95% *CI*

$$= (RR) \exp\left[\pm 1.96\sqrt{\mathrm{VAR(lnRR)}}\right]$$

where

$$\sqrt{\mathrm{VAR(lnRR)}}$$
$$= \sqrt{\frac{1-A/(A+C)}{A} + \frac{1-B/(B+D)}{B}}$$

where exp is the base of the natural logarithm raised to the quantity within the brackets and *A, B, C,* and *D* represent the numerical entries in the summary format in Table 8–6, and VAR(ln*RR*) is the estimated variance of the natural logarithm of the *RR*. This confidence interval is approximate because it is based on a computa-

tional short-cut for estimating the variance of the natural logarithm of the *RR*. For relatively large samples, this approximation yields confidence limits that are quite close to the exact values, which are much more difficult to calculate.

The 95% *CI* for the 10-minute Apgar score (0–3 versus 4–6) relationship to infant mortality described in Chapter 8 is

95% *CI*

$$= (2.8) \exp\left[\pm 1.96\sqrt{\frac{1-0.344}{42} + \frac{1-0.125}{43}}\right]$$

$$= (2.8) \exp\left[\pm 1.96\sqrt{0.0156 + 0.0203}\right]$$

$$= (2.8) \exp\left(\pm 0.37\right)$$

Lower bound $= (2.8) \exp(-0.37) = 1.9$

Upper bound $= (2.8) \exp(+0.37) = 4.1$

Appendix D: The Odds Ratio as an Estimator of the Incidence Rate Ratio

To understand further the design of a case–control study, and why the odds ratio from a case–control study estimates the incidence rate ratio, consider first the occurrence of a particular disease within an underlying population that gives rise to the cases. This underlying cohort is sometimes called the source population. At the start of follow-up, all subjects are disease-free; P people are exposed and Q are not. After following the cohort for t years, A of the P exposed and B of the Q unexposed subjects develop disease (Table D–1).

To calculate incidence rates for this cohort, as discussed in Chapter 2, first calculate the person-years of observation (py), which is given by

$$py = \text{average size of source population} \times \text{length of follow-up}$$

This equation simplifies if few people develop disease during the follow-up period and the population undergoes no major demographic shifts, a situation termed the "**steady state.**" If the steady state holds, the size of the source population is nearly constant and the equation above simplifies to

$$py = \text{size of source population} \times \text{length of follow-up}$$

Application of the latter equation to the hypothetical cohort yields $P \times t$ and $Q \times t$ person-years of observation for the exposed and unexposed subjects, respec-

tively (Table D–1). Thus, the incidence rate in the exposed subjects is $A/(P \times t)$ and in the unexposed subjects is $B/(Q \times t)$, and the incidence rate ratio (IRR) is

$$IRR = (A/P \times t)/(B/Q \times t) = (A \times Q)/(B \times P)$$

Now, turning to the case–control study design, cases arise from a clearly defined source population and the investigator then chooses controls from this same population. Thus, to conduct a case–control study using the source population described in Table D–1, subjects with disease (cases) and subjects without disease (controls) are sampled and their respective exposure histories are then determined. Excluded from both the case and control groups are potential subjects known to have had disease when the study began—only newly diagnosed or "**incident**" cases are included. In practice, it is possible to contact newly diagnosed cases and a sample from the general population, ask each subject about prior disease, and exclude those who were diagnosed prior to the study period. The data can be summarized as in Table D–2.

Cases and controls are selected without regard to exposure. For example, it is possible to randomly sample cases from all those in the population who develop disease during the study period and randomly select controls from all those without disease. Sampling is "blind" to exposure, so that the proportion of cases in the study that was exposed should, on average, equal the proportion of cases in the full cohort. Similarly, the propor-

Table D–1. Disease occurrence in a cohort by exposure status.

	Exposed	Unexposed
Number of new cases during follow-up	A	B
Person-years of observation	$P \times t$	$Q \times t$
Incidence rate	$A/(P \times t)$	$B/(Q \times t)$

Table D–2. Data from a hypothetical case-control study of a disease and a dichotomous exposure.

	Exposed	Unexposed	Total
Diseased	a	b	M_1
Not diseased	c	d	M_2
Total	N_1	N_2	T

tion of controls in the study that was exposed should, on average, equal the proportion of those without disease in the full cohort. Thus, the exposure odds among cases, *a/b,* is an estimate of *A/B,* the corresponding odds among new cases arising from the full cohort. In a parallel manner, the exposure odds among controls, *c/d,* is an estimate of *P/Q,* the corresponding odds among persons without disease in the full cohort. The cross-product or **odds ratio** (*OR*) is the odds that a case is exposed, *a/b,* divided by the odds that a control is exposed, *c/d:*

$$OR = (a \times d) / (b \times c)$$

The odds ratio from the case–control study is therefore an estimate of the incidence rate ratio in the full cohort, which was shown above to equal $(A \times Q)/(B \times P)$.

If exposure increases risk, more cases than controls will be exposed, so that *a/b > c/d,* or *OR* > 1. On the other hand, if exposure decreases risk, fewer cases than controls will be exposed, so that *a/b < c/d,* or *OR* < 1. Thus, an *OR* greater than one suggests that exposure is associated with higher incidence rates or risk, an *OR* less than one suggests that exposure is associated with lower incidence rates or risk, and an *OR* near one suggests that exposure is not associated with higher or lower than average risk.

Appendix E: Method for Determining the Confidence Interval Around the Odds Ratio

An approximate 95% confidence interval (CI) around the point estimate of the odds ratio (OR) for an unmatched case–control study can be calculated using the following formula:

$$95\% \; CI = (OR) \; \exp\left[\pm 1.96 \sqrt{\frac{1}{A} + \frac{1}{B} + \frac{1}{C} + \frac{1}{D}}\right]$$

where exp is the base of the natural logarithm raised to the quantity in the brackets, and A, B, C, and D represent the numerical entries into the summary format in Table 9–4. This confidence interval is approximate because it is based on a computational short-cut to estimating the variance of the natural logarithm of the OR. For relatively large sample sizes, this approximation yields confidence bounds that are quite close to the exact values, which are much more difficult to calculate.

For the data in Table 9–5 relating L-tryptophan brand use to eosinophilia-myalgia syndrome in an unmatched case–control study, the 95% CI was calculated as follows:

$$95\% \; CI = (7.5) \; \exp\left[\pm 1.96 \sqrt{\frac{1}{22} + \frac{1}{36} + \frac{1}{7} + \frac{1}{86}}\right]$$

$$= (7.5) \; \exp[\pm 0.94]$$

Lower bound $= (7.5) \; \exp[-0.94] = 2.9$

Upper bound $= (7.5) \; \exp[+0.94] = 19.1$

Similarly, an approximate 95% CI around the point estimate of an OR from a pair-matched case–control study can be calculated using the following formula:

$$95\% \; CI = (OR) \; \exp\left[\pm 1.96 \sqrt{\frac{1}{X} + \frac{1}{Y}}\right]$$

where exp is the base of the natural logarithm raised to the quantity in the brackets, and X and Y represent the numerical entries in the summary format in Table 9–6.

For the data in Table 9–7 relating L-tryptophan use to eosinophilia-myalgia syndrome in a hypothetical pair-matched case–control study, the 95% CI was calculated as follows:

$$95\% \; CI = (11.4) \; \exp\left[\pm 1.96 \sqrt{\frac{1}{57} + \frac{1}{5}}\right]$$

$$= (11.4) \; \exp[\pm 0.91]$$

Lower bound $= (11.4) \; \exp[-0.91] = 4.6$

Upper bound $= (11.4) \; \exp[+0.91] = 28.3$

Glossary

Accuracy: the extent to which a measurement or study result correctly represents the characteristic or relationship that is being assessed.

Acquired immunodeficiency syndrome (AIDS): a disease characterized by a marked reduction in CD4$^+$ T lymphocytes and associated defects in immune response caused by the human immunodeficiency virus (HIV).

Active surveillance: a system of data collection in which those responsible for collecting the information go into the community under observation (typically defined by geographic boundaries) to gather data from various sources.

Acute: a disease of short duration.

Acute myelogenous leukemia (AML): a heterogeneous group of disorders, also known as acute nonlymphocytic leukemia, each of which involves the uncontrolled proliferation of primitive blood-forming cells.

Adjustment: a procedure for overall comparison of two or more populations in which background differences in the distribution of covariables are removed. (See also **Standardization.**)

Age adjustment: a procedure used to calculate summary rates for different populations in which underlying differences in the age distributions are removed. (See also **Age standardization.**)

Age-specific rate: a rate (usually incidence or mortality) for a particular age group.

Age standardization (direct): a procedure for obtaining a weighted average of age-specific rates in which the weights are selected on the basis of a standard age distribution (eg, the population of the United States in 1940).

Allele: an alternate form of a gene or a genetic locus that differs from other forms in its specific sequence of nucleotides; certain alleles may affect the structure and function of the corresponding protein coded for by that gene, in turn affecting the susceptibility to a particular condition.

Alpha error: see **Type I error.**

Alzheimer's disease: the most common form of dementia in many populations, first described in 1907 by Alois Alzheimer; affected individuals have characteristic abnormalities in their brains, including neurofibrillary tangles and plaques with a protein fragment, β-amyloid, at their core.

Analytic epidemiology: activities related to the identification of possible determinants of disease occurrence.

Analytic study: a research investigation designed to test a hypothesis, often used in reference to a study of an exposure–disease association.

Anthrax: an infectious disease caused by a spore-forming bacterium *Bacillus anthracis*. The natural occurrence of this illness typically involves inhalation of spores from animal products. This agent was used as a weapon of bioterror in 2001 in the United States, resulting in 22 cases and 5 deaths.

Antibody: a protein, often produced in response to exposure to an antigen, that binds to the antigen and thereby stimulates its inactivation by the immune system.

Antigen: a protein, usually foreign in origin, that is capable of generating an immune response in a host animal.

Antigenic drift: mutation of a pathogen (eg, influenza A), such that the surface antigens differ from those of previously existing strains.

Apgar score: a system of evaluating the health status of a newborn using five indicators, each assigned a maximum of two points; the score is named after its originator, Dr. Virginia Apgar.

Arithmetic mean: see **Mean.**

Arteriosclerosis: hardening of the arteries.

Association: the extent to which the occurrence of two or more characteristics is linked either through a causal or noncausal relationship.

Asymptomatic persons: individuals who have a particular disease but do not manifest abnormalities of function, appearance, or sensation typically associated with that disease.

Atrophy: abnormal wasting of tissues, organs, or the entire body.

Attack rate: the proportion of persons within a population who develop a particular outcome within a specified period of time.

Attributable risk percent: the percentage of the overall risk of a disease outcome within exposed persons, related to the exposure of interest.

Autoimmune disorder: a disease state in which affected individuals produce antibodies against their own cells or tissues.

Benign: a mild illness; when applied to an abnormal growth of cells (viz, a neoplasm), it connotes a slowly progressing defect that is not invading adjacent tissues (in contrast to the rapid growth and invasive behavior of a malignant neoplasm).

Beta error: see **Type II error.**

Bias: a nonrandom error in a study that leads to a distorted result.

Biological marker: a measurable characteristic that helps to classify either level of exposure to a risk factor or susceptibility to (or presence of) a disease.

Bioterrorism: the threat of use of biological agents by individuals or groups in order to create fear or cause illness or death.

Birth cohort effect: an unusual age-specific rate (either incidence or mortality) within cross-sectional data that reflects the shared experience of persons born in specific years (birth cohort).

Blinding: assignment of treatment to individual subjects in a way such that subjects only (**single blinding**) or both subjects and treating physicians (**double blinding**) do not know the actual treatment allocation.

Borrelia burgdorferi: a spirochete that is borne by a particular deer tick that when transmitted to humans can cause Lyme disease (a systemic illness characterized by a skin rash, joint pains, and in advanced cases, cardiac and neurologic manifestations).

Botulism: a muscle-paralyzing disease caused by a toxin produced by the bacterium *Clostridium botulinum.* Natural occurrence typically results from consumption of contaminated food, but the toxin is now considered a potential agent of bioterrorism.

Bronchoscopic examination: the insertion of an instrument (viz, bronchoscope) to help visualize the trachea and bronchi and to facilitate the collection of specimens from these tissues.

Campylobacter jejuni: a species of the bacterial genus *Campylobacter* that is a leading cause of food-borne illness, most often arising in isolated events (rather than outbreaks), and characterized by fever, abdominal cramping, and diarrhea (occasionally bloody).

Cancer: a heterogeneous group of diseases characterized by the abnormal, uncontrolled growth of cells, which are capable of crossing normal anatomic boundaries to invade other tissues and even spread to remote anatomic sites.

Candidate region: a physical location on a chromosome believed to contain a potential disease susceptibility gene and identified by a genomewide scan and subsequent linkage analysis.

Case: a person who has a disease of interest. (See also **Incident case** and **Prevalent case.**)

Case–control study: an observational study in which subjects are sampled based on the presence (cases) or absence (controls) of the disease of interest. Information is collected about earlier exposure to risk factors of interest.

Case fatality: the proportion of persons with a particular disease who die from that disease within a specified period of time.

Causality: the extent to which the occurrence of a risk factor is responsible for the subsequent occurrence of a disease outcome.

Cerebral palsy: a disorder manifested by speech disturbances and lack of muscular coordination that arises from damage to the brain of a newborn before, during, or shortly after birth.

Cerebrovascular accident: a deficit in the delivery of oxygenated blood to the brain that may occur because of a blood clot or a hemorrhage; a synonym for a stroke.

Chance node: an element in a decision analysis that represents a point at which specified outcomes are determined on the basis of probability.

Cholesterol: a steroid that is abundant in animal tissues and is necessary for normal function; elevated levels of total cholesterol circulating in the blood of a host are associated with increased risks of cardiovascular disease.

Chronic: a disease of long duration.

Chronic obstructive pulmonary disease (COPD): an abnormal and long-standing reduction in airflow into and out of the lungs, typically caused either by chronic bronchitis or emphysema.

Clinical scenario: one of two or more alternative paths of management available in a decision analysis.

Clinical trial: an experimental study that is designed to compare the therapeutic benefits of two or more treatments.

Clostridium botulinum: the bacterium that produces a toxin responsible for causing botulism. Natural occurrence typically results from consumption of contaminated food, but the toxin is considered a potential agent of bioterrorism.

Clostridium perfringens: the bacterium responsible for a food-borne illness that often occurs in outbreaks and is characterized by diarrhea and abdominal cramping.

Cluster: a group of cases of a disease closely linked in time, place of occurrence, or both.

Cochrane Collaboration: an international organization dedicated to promoting well-informed health care decisions by preparing, maintaining, and ensuring accessibility to current, rigorous, systematic reviews of the benefits and risks of health care interventions. The organization is named in memory of Archie Cochrane, a physician epidemiologist who advocated using the best available evidence to guide health care decisions.

Coefficient of determination: the square of the correlation coefficient; it represents the proportion of total variability in an outcome that can be explained by the predictors in a regression model.

Cohort: a group of persons that shares a common attribute, such as birth in a particular year or residence in a particular town, and is followed over time.

Cohort study: an observational study in which subjects are sampled based on the presence (exposed) or absence (unexposed) of a risk factor of interest. These subjects are followed over time for the development of a disease outcome of interest. (See also **Prospective cohort study** and **Retrospective cohort study**.)

Common-source exposure: contact with a risk factor that originates in the shared environment of multiple persons.

Concordant results: the same outcome status for two or more individuals, as in a pair-matched case–control study in which both the case and the control are exposed (or unexposed).

Confidence interval: a range of values for a measure that is believed to contain the true value within a specified level (eg, 95%) of certainty.

Confounder: a variable that distorts the apparent relationship between an exposure and a disease of interest.

Confounding: a systematic error in a study that arises from mixing of the effect of the exposure of interest with other associated correlates of the disease outcome.

Control: in a case–control study, a subject without the disease of interest. (See also **Adjustment**.)

Control group: a population of comparison subjects in an analytic investigation.

Coronary artery disease: complete or partial blockage of the blood vessels that bring oxygenated blood to the heart muscle (myocardium), usually arising from atherosclerosis; if the reduction in blood flow is severe, a myocardial infarction may result.

Coronavirus: a family of viruses characterized by the appearance of a corona (crown) on electron microscopic imaging. These viruses are frequent causes of the common cold, and in the winter of 2002–2003, a new member of the family emerged as the cause of severe acute respiratory syndrome (SARS).

Correlation coefficient: a statistical measure of the relatedness of two variables; it can range from −1 (perfectly related inversely to each other) to +1 (perfectly related in the same direction to each other). When the variables are unrelated to each other, the correlation coefficient has a value of zero.

Correlation study: a hypothesis-generating investigation in which the values of two or more summary characteristics are associated across different population groups.

Cosegregation: the tendency of alleles on the same chromosome to be inherited together.

Cross-sectional study: an analytic investigation in which subjects are sampled at a fixed point or period of time, and the associations between the concurrent presence or absence of risk factors and diseases are then investigated.

Crude mortality rate: the rapidity with which persons within a given population die from a particular disease, without adjustment for the underlying age distribution of the population.

Cumulative incidence: the risk of developing a particular disease within a specified period of time.

Cutoff point: a value on an ordinal or a continuous scale of measurement used to distinguish categories. For example, values above this threshold may be classified as "abnormal" and values below this point may be classified as "normal."

Death rate: see **Mortality rate**.

Decision analysis: a formal probabilistic process for making clinical decisions that incorporates information on medical options, anticipated likelihoods of various outcomes, and the uncertainty associated with clinical information.

Decision diagram: a flow chart used in decision analysis that identifies the clinical management choices, probabilities of events, and likelihoods of outcomes.

Decision node: an element of a decision tree that represents a choice between two or more competing alternative management approaches.

Decision tree: see **Decision diagram**.

Dementia: a condition characterized by impaired short- and long-term memory, along with disturbances of other cognitive functions, such as speech and the perception of spatial relationships.

Dependent variable: see **Outcome variable**.

Descriptive epidemiology: activities related to characterizing patterns of disease occurrence.

Diabetes mellitus: a disorder of carbohydrate regulation caused by either a markedly reduced or absent production of insulin by the pancreas (**type I**) or a decreased sensitivity to the effects of insulin in the peripheral tissues (**type II**).

Differential misclassification: incorrect categorization of the status of subjects with regard to one variable (eg, exposure) that is influenced by other characteristics of interest (eg, disease status).

Discordant results: different outcome status for two or more individuals, as in a pair-matched case–control study, when one subject in a pair is exposed and the other individual is unexposed to the risk factor of interest.

Disease outbreak: a sudden, unexpected increase in the occurrence of a disease within a relatively limited geographic area.

Diuresis: an abnormally elevated volume of urine production.

Dizygotic twin: fraternal twins resulting from the fertilization of two separate ova by two separate spermatozoa; the members of this pair are no more similar genetically than are two nontwin siblings.

Dose–response relationship: an exposure–disease association in which the risk of developing a disease varies with respect to the intensity or duration of exposure.

Ebola virus: a filovirus named after a river in the Democratic Republic of the Congo where it was first identified. It is responsible for a life-threatening illness characterized by fever, headache, joint and muscle pains, diarrhea, vomiting, and in some patients, external bleeding.

Eclampsia: the occurrence of one or more seizures that cannot be attributed to an underlying neurologic condition (such as epilepsy or a cerebral hemorrhage) in a patient with preeclampsia.

Ecologic fallacy: an association between summary characteristics across populations without actual linkage of the characteristics within individual persons.

Ecologic study: see **Correlation study.**

ELISA: enzyme-linked immunosorbent assay; it can be used to test for antibodies to an infectious agent.

Emerging infectious disease: an infection that has newly appeared within a population or has existed but is rapidly increasing in incidence or geographic range.

Empiric treatment: in the context of infectious illness, the initiation of an antibiotic treatment against a spectrum of suspected potential pathogens, in the absence of a documented specific pathogen(s).

Endemic rate: the usual rate of occurrence of particular events within a population.

Eosinophilia-myalgia syndrome: a condition characterized by muscle pains, and in some patients joint pains, skin thickening, hair loss, or intestinal disease, accompanied by an abnormally elevated level of eosinophil cells in the blood.

Epidemic: a dramatic increase above the usual or expected rate of occurrence of particular events within a population.

Epidemiology: the study of the distribution and determinants of disease within human populations.

***Escherichia coli* O157:H7:** a strain of bacteria that is a cause of the hemolytic uremic syndrome, which occurs in humans who consume food products contaminated with this pathogen.

Etiology: the cause(s) of a disease or the study of disease causation.

Evidence-based medicine: the integration of current best evidence from research with clinical expertise, pathophysiologic knowledge, and patient preferences, used to make health care decisions.

Excess risk: the extra risk of the occurrence of a particular disease among persons exposed to a risk factor of interest. (See also **Risk difference.**)

Exclusions: persons who are eliminated from an analytic study because they do not satisfy the eligibility (inclusion) criteria.

Expected utility: a numerical value that represents the average result if the decision maker follows a particular path in a decision analysis.

Exposure: contact with or possession of a characteristic that is suspected to influence the risk of developing a particular disease.

External validity: the extent to which the conclusions of a study can be correctly applied to persons beyond those who were investigated. (See also **Generalize.**)

False-negative: a test result that is normal (negative) despite the true presence of the disease of interest or a study result that incorrectly fails to identify a true effect. (See also **Type II error.**)

False-positive: a test result that is abnormal (positive) despite the true absence of the disease of interest or a study result that incorrectly suggests an effect, when in truth, the purported effect does not exist. (See also **Type I error.**)

Familial aggregation: the extent to which the occurrence of a particular disease tends to cluster within families.

Fixed effects model: a statistical approach to combining information from multiple sources in which it is assumed that the investigated relationship is constant across sources and any differences in individual results are attributable entirely to random variation.

Follow-up study: see **Cohort study.**

Food-borne disease: an illness that is caused by the ingestion of food or food products, often arising from contamination of the food with microbes or other toxic materials.

Framingham Heart Study: a landmark prospective cohort study of risk factors for cardiovascular disease initiated in 1950 among residents of Framingham, Massachusetts.

Generalize: the ability to extrapolate study results from the study subjects to other persons who were not investigated.

Genetic epidemiology: the use of epidemiologic techniques to study hereditary determinants of disease in human populations.

Genetic (linkage) map: a type of map of the genome in which markers are identified on the chromosomes and the relative distances between these markers are estimated by the frequency with which the markers are inherited together.

Genome: the full complement of genes on all chromosomes.

Genomewide scan: an approach to localizing candidate regions for genes contributing to the susceptibility for a specific disease by analyzing the extent to which the disease occurs in members of affected families in association with markers at known locations throughout the genome.

Genotype: the genetic constitution of an individual; may be used in reference to the particular allele(s) present at one or more gene loci.

Glucosuria: an abnormally elevated level of glucose in the urine, as my occur in diabetes mellitus.

Granulocyte: a mature granular white blood cell, which includes neutrophils as well as other types of cells.

Granulocytopenia: a condition marked by an abnormally low number of granulocytes in the blood, and which may predispose the host to infection.

Hantavirus: a virus named for a river in South Korea, where human infection was first recognized; this pathogen is capable of causing a hemorrhagic fever and a separate pulmonary syndrome in infected human hosts.

Hematologic: of or relating to the blood or blood-forming tissues.

Heterogeneity: the statistical property of variation in an investigated relationship across individual studies or across subgroups within a particular study.

Historical cohort study: see **Retrospective cohort study.**

Historical controls: subjects in a clinical study who were previously treated with the standard therapy before the new experimental treatment was introduced.

HIV: see **Human immunodeficiency virus.**

Homogeneity: the statistical property of lack of variation of an investigated relationship across individual studies or across individual subgroups within a particular study.

Human immunodeficiency virus: the cause of the acquired immunodeficiency syndrome (AIDS) and other HIV-related disorders.

Hyperglycemia: an abnormally high level of glucose in the blood, as may occur in untreated patients with diabetes mellitus.

Hypertension: an abnormal elevation in blood pressure.

Hypoglycemia: an abnormally low level of glucose in the blood, as may result from an overly aggressive administration of insulin in patients with diabetes mellitus.

Hypothesis-generating study: an exploratory investigation designed to formulate questions that are evaluated in subsequent analytic studies.

Hypothesis-testing study: an analytic investigation in which one or more specific refutable suppositions are evaluated.

Hypoxia: an abnormally low level of oxygen in the arterial blood.

Immunity: a state in which a host is not susceptible to a particular infection or disease.

Inbreeding study: a study in which the degree of selective breeding among members of a particular group is assessed with respect to risk of developing a particular disease.

Incidence density: see **Incidence rate.**

Incidence rate: the rapidity with which new cases of a particular disease arise within a given population.

Incident case: a person who is newly diagnosed with a disease of interest.

Incubation period: the time interval between contact with a risk factor (often an infectious agent) and the first clinical evidence of the resulting illness.

Independent variable: a factor that is suspected to influence the outcome of an analytic study.

Index case: in a disease outbreak, the first affected individual to be identified; in genetics, see **Proband.**

Information (or observation) bias: a systematic error in a study that arises from the manner in which data are collected from participants.

Informed consent: the process of providing a patient with information about the risks and benefits of a proposed treatment plan and then securing the patient's (or if the patient is a child, the guardian's) agreement to undergo the planned intervention recognizing the risks and benefits.

Insulin: a peptide hormone produced in the pancreas and secreted into the blood, which delivers it to target organs to help regulate glucose utilization, protein synthesis, and formation and storage of lipids.

Intention to treat: analysis of the results of a clinical trial based on initial treatment assignment regardless of whether the subjects completed the full course of treatment.

Internal validity: the extent to which the conclusions of a study are correct for the subjects under investigation.

Ketosis: a condition characterized by the enhanced production of ketone bodies, as may occur in the metabolic abnormalities associated with diabetes mellitus.

Latent period: time between exposure to a risk factor and subsequent development of clinical manifestations of a particular disease.

Lead-time bias: apparent increase in the length of survival of patients with a disease as a result of earlier detection of the disease through the use of a screening procedure.

Length-biased sampling: preferential detection of less aggressive forms of a disease through the use of a screening procedure.

Life expectancy: the expected, or average, duration of life for persons in a particular population, under the assumption that current age-specific mortality patterns continue to apply.

Likelihood: the probability of the occurrence of a specified event.

Likelihood ratio: the probability of a particular test result for a person with the disease of interest divided by the probability of that test result for a person without the disease of interest.

Likelihood ratio for a negative test result: the probability of a negative test result for a person with the disease of interest divided by the probability of a negative test result for a person without the disease of interest.

Likelihood ratio for a positive test result: the probability of a positive test result for a person with the disease of interest divided by the probability of a positive test result for a person without the disease of interest.

Linkage: the proximity of multiple genes or genetic markers on the same chromosome, which is related to the probability that a certain combination of alleles at these sites will be inherited as a linkage group or haplotype.

Linkage analysis: a statistical technique used to identify candidate regions for genes based on the examination of the closeness of association between the inheritance within affected families of the condition of interest and markers at known locations throughout the genome.

Linkage disequilibrium: an excess or deficiency of certain combinations of alleles from genes or markers that are located on the same chromosome; alleles at tightly linked sites often are inherited together, and therefore linkage disequilibrium may help to identify the location of a particular susceptibility gene that is inherited as part of a linkage group with genes or markers at known locations within the genome.

Longitudinal study: see **Cohort study.**

Malignancy: the property of being malignant, often used interchangeably with the term cancer.

Malignant: a severe disease that is resistant to treatment (eg, severe hypertension); the term often is used in relation to the behavior of cancers.

Marker: in genetics, an identifiable physical location on a chromosome or DNA segment useful in mapping genes and in performing linkage analysis.

Matching: a procedure for sampling comparison subjects based on whether key attributes (ie, **matching factors**) are similar to those of subjects in the index group.

Mean: the arithmetic average of a distribution of values; calculated as the sum of the individual values divided by the number of observations.

Meconium: the first intestinal discharges of a newborn; if passed prior to delivery, it may serve as a sign of fetal distress, and if aspirated by the newborn, may give rise to acute pulmonary distress.

Median: a measure of central tendency of a distribution; calculated as the mid-point of the distribution when individual values are ordered from the smallest to the largest.

Median survival time: the duration of time from diagnosis to death that is exceeded by exactly 50% of subjects with a particular disease.

Medical outcome: see **Outcome.**

Meta-analysis: a statistical combination or integration of the results of several independent research studies that are considered to be combinable.

Metabolic acidosis: an abnormally high level of acid and low level of bicarbonate in the blood and other tissues resulting either from an accumulation of acids from metabolic processes (as in diabetes mellitus) or from an abnormally high loss of bases from the body (as in diarrhea or renal disease).

Misclassification bias: incorrect characterization of the status of subjects with regard to a study variable, leading to a distorted conclusion. (See also **Information bias.**)

Mode: a measure of central tendency of a distribution; it is the value that occurs most frequently within the distribution.

Monozygotic twin: genetically identical individuals arising from the division of a single fertilized ovum.

Morbidity: a state of illness produced by a disease.

Mortality: death, usually in reference to death caused by a particular disease (viz, **cause-specific mortality**).

Mortality rate: the rapidity with which persons within a given population die from a particular disease.

Mycobacterium: a genus of bacteria, a member of which is *M tuberculosis,* also known as tubercle bacillus, the pathogen responsible for tuberculosis in humans.

Myocardial infarction: a sudden diminution in the delivery of oxygenated blood to the heart muscle (viz, **myocardium**), most commonly caused by partial or complete blockage of one or more of the coronary arteries.

Natural history: the progression of a disease through successive stages, often used to describe the course of an illness for which no effective treatment is available.

Negative predictive value: the probability that a person with a negative (normal) test result actually does not have the disease of interest.

Neoplasm: a new growth that arises from the abnormal proliferation of cells; the proliferation may be benign or malignant (viz, **cancer**).

Nephropathy: a disorder of the kidney; among diabetics, the disorder arises because of damage to the small blood vessels of the kidney, which can lead to failure of the kidneys in an advanced stage.

Neutropenia: the presence of an abnormally low level of neutrophils in the blood, placing the host at increased susceptibility to infection.

Neutrophil: a mature white blood cell in the granulocyte series necessary for normal host defense responses.

Nondifferential misclassification: incorrect categorization of the status of subjects with regard to one variable (eg, exposure) that is unrelated to another characteristic of interest (eg, disease status).

Nosocomial infection: an illness caused by exposure to a pathogen during hospitalization of the host.

Notifiable disease: a disease for which regular, frequent, and timely information on individual cases is considered necessary for the prevention and control of the disease.

Null value: the point on the scale of a measure of association that corresponds to no association (eg, 1 for the risk ratio and the odds ratio and 0 for the risk difference and the attributable risk percent).

Observation bias: see **Information bias.**

Observational study: a nonexperimental analytic study in which the investigator monitors, but does not influence, the exposure status of individual subjects and their subsequent disease status.

Odds: the probability that a particular event will occur divided by the probability that the event will not occur.

Odds ratio: the odds of a particular exposure among persons with a specific disease divided by the corresponding odds of exposure among persons without the disease of interest.

Opportunistic infection: an illness caused by a microorganism that is capable of causing disease only in a host whose resistance is lowered below normal levels.

Outbreak: see **Disease outbreak.**

Outcome: clinical events that result from patient management decisions (eg, morbidity, complications, quality of life, or mortality).

Outcome variable: in an analytic study, the response of interest (eg, development of disease).

Pandemic: an elevated occurrence of a disease across a wide geographic area, affecting a substantial proportion of the population.

Passive surveillance: a system of data collection in which those responsible for collecting information rely upon voluntary reporting by other individuals or groups without entering the community to gather data.

Pathogen: an agent responsible for the development of a particular disease.

Pathophysiology: derangement of function associated with a disease process.

Pedigree: the family members of a proband, identified with respect to their biological relationship to the proband and whether they are known to have the disease of interest.

Penetrance: the proportion of individuals with a particular genotype that exhibits the same phenotype under similar environmental conditions.

Perinatal asphyxia: an abnormally reduced level of oxygenation of a fetus during labor and delivery, or shortly thereafter.

Person-time: a unit of measurement used in the estimation of rates that reflects the amount of time observed for persons at risk of a particular event.

Person-to-person spread: propagation of a disease within a population by transfer from an affected person to susceptible persons.

Person-years: a common unit for measuring person-time; one person-year corresponds to one person being followed for one year, or alternatively, two persons each followed for one half year, and so forth.

Person-years of life lost: a measure of total life expectancy lost within a particular population because of premature death.

Phenotype: a category or group to which an individual may be assigned on the basis of one or more characteristics observable clinically or by laboratory assessment that reflect genetic variation or gene–environment interactions.

Placebo: an inert substance.

Placebo effect: occurs when persons affected with a specific illness demonstrate clinical improvement when treated with an inert substance.

Plague: an infectious disease caused by the bacterium *Yersinia pestis.* It is naturally transmitted to humans by the bite of a rodent flea and is a potential agent for bioterrorism.

Polymerase chain reaction: a laboratory technique for rapidly synthesizing large quantities of a particular portion of genetic material.

Population at risk: persons who are susceptible to a particular disease but who are not yet affected.

Population-based study: an analytic study in which subjects are sampled from the general population.

Positive predictive value: the probability that a person with a positive (abnormal) test result actually has the disease of interest.

Posttest odds of disease: the estimated probability, after the administration of a diagnostic test, that a patient has the disease of interest divided by the probability that the patient does not have the disease of interest.

Posttest probability of disease: the estimated likelihood, after the administration of a diagnostic test, that a patient has the disease of interest.

Power: see **Statistical power.**

Precision: the extent to which a measurement is narrowly characterized. **Statistical precision** is inversely related to the variance of the measurement.

Predictor variable: see **Independent variable.**

Preeclampsia: the abnormal occurrence of hypertension accompanied by either an abnormal collection of fluid in body tissues or abnormally increased levels of protein in the urine, or both, due to pregnancy.

Premature death: a death that occurs earlier than would be expected in the absence of a particular disease.

Pretest odds of disease: the estimated probability, prior to the administration of a diagnostic test, that a patient has the disease of interest divided by the probability that the patient does not have the disease of interest.

Pretest probability of disease: the estimated likelihood, prior to the administration of a diagnostic test, that a patient has the disease of interest.

Prevalence: the proportion of persons in a given population that has a particular disease at a point or interval of time.

Prevalent case: a person who has a disease of interest that was diagnosed in the past.

Proband: the first affected individual who brings his or her family to the attention of a researcher or clinician for the purposes of medical care or investigation.

Prognosis: the predicted rate of progression of a disease process and its likely outcome(s).

Prognostic factor: an attribute anticipated to be related to the progression and outcome of a disease process.

Proportion: one quantity divided by another quantity in which the population in the numerator is a subset of the population in the denominator. The possible values of a proportion range from zero to one.

Prospective cohort study: a cohort study in which exposure status and subsequent occurrence of disease both occur after the onset of the investigation.

Publication bias: a distortion in conclusions derived from published studies because of the selective factors associated with the likelihood of publication, including whether the findings were positive and statistically significant, and the potential proprietary interests of sponsors.

Random effects model: a statistical approach to combining information from multiple sources in which it is assumed that the investigated relationship varies across individual sources, in addition to the influences of random variation in estimates.

Randomization: procedure for assigning treatments to patients by chance.

Rate: the rapidity with which health events such as new diagnoses or deaths occur. (See also **Incidence rate** and **Mortality rate.**)

Rate ratio: the rate of occurrence of a specified health event among persons exposed to a particular risk factor divided by the corresponding rate among unexposed persons.

Ratio: one quantity divided by another quantity, in which the population in the numerator is not a part of the population in the denominator. The possible values of a ratio range from zero to positive infinity.

Recurrence risk: in genetic epidemiology, the risk of developing a particular disease experienced by relatives of a subject with that disease.

Relapse: the return of the manifestations of a disease after a period of diminished manifestations.

Relative risk: see **Risk ratio.**

Reliability: the extent to which multiple measurements of a characteristic are in agreement.

Remission: elimination or reduction in the number or severity of the manifestations of a disease, which may be transient or permanent.

Response variable: see **Outcome variable.**

Retinopathy: a disorder of the retina of the eye; among diabetics the disorder arises from damage to the small blood vessels of the retina and can lead to blindness.

Retrospective cohort study: a cohort study in which exposure status and subsequent development of disease both occur prior to the onset of the investigation.

Risk: the probability that an event (eg, development of disease) will occur within a specific period of time.

Risk difference: the risk of the occurrence of a particular disease among persons exposed to a given risk factor minus the corresponding risk among unexposed persons.

Risk factor: an attribute or agent suspected to be related to the occurrence of a particular disease.

Risk ratio: the likelihood of the occurrence of a particular disease among persons exposed to a given risk factor divided by the corresponding likelihood among unexposed persons.

Salmonella enteritidis: one of two serotypes of the bacterium *Salmonella* that is a common cause of salmonellosis, a food-borne illness characterized by fever, abdominal cramping, and diarrhea (sometimes bloody).

Salmonella typhimurium: one of two serotypes of the bacterium *Salmonella* that is a common cause of salmonellosis, a food-borne illness characterized by fever, abdominal cramping, and diarrhea (sometimes bloody).

Sample: a subset of a target population that is chosen for investigation.

SARS: see severe acute respiratory syndrome.

SARS-associated coronavirus (SARS-CoV): the agent which first emerged in the winter of 2002–2003 and is responsible for causing severe acute respiratory syndrome (SARS).

Screening: the use of tests to detect the presence of a particular disease among asymptomatic persons prior to the time that the disease would be recognized through routine clinical methods.

SEER Program: The Surveillance, Epidemiology and End Results Program of the National Cancer Institute; it consists of 11 population-based cancer registries in various locations within the United States.

Segregation analysis: a complex statistical technique used to assess whether a particular disease has, at least in part, a genetic origin, and if so the most likely mode of inheritance.

Selection bias: a systematic error in a study that arises from the manner in which subjects are sampled.

Sensitivity: the probability that a person who actually has the disease of interest will have a positive (abnormal) test result.

Sensitivity analysis: (1) in systematic reviews, including meta-analyses, the evaluation of the pattern of results across subgroups of studies to characterize possible sources of heterogeneity and their respective influences on the overall summary effect; (2) in decision analysis, use of different values for an uncertain likelihood to determine whether the preferred course of action remains unchanged.

Sentinel case(s): the initial person(s) affected by a particular illness during an outbreak.

Seroconversion: change in a person's status from not having evidence of infection (such as antibodies) in the serum to having such evidence.

Seronegative: absence of evidence of infection in a person's serum (synonym: antibody negative).

Seropositive: presence of evidence of infection in a person's serum (synonym: antibody positive).

Severe acute respiratory syndrome (SARS): a highly contagious and life-threatening respiratory illness that first emerged in the winter of 2002–2003 in China and rapidly spread throughout the world.

Shigella sonnei: one of four species of the bacterium *Shigella* and the most common cause of shigellosis, a food-borne illness characterized by diarrhea (often bloody), abdominal cramping, and fever.

Sib-pair analysis: statistical analysis for many genetic linkage studies attempting to locate susceptibility genes for a particular disease in which the fundamental unit of analysis is a pair of siblings.

Smallpox: an infectious disease caused by variola virus that was eradicated in 1977. The illness had a high case fatality and variola now is considered to be a potential agent for bioterrorism.

Specificity: the probability that a person who actually does not have the disease of interest will have a negative (normal) test result.

Squamous cell carcinoma: a malignant neoplasm (cancer) arising from stratified squamous epithelium, but that may also occur in sites in which glandular or columnar epithelium normally occur.

Standardization: an analytic procedure for obtaining a summary measure for a population by applying standard weights to the measures within subgroups of the population.

Statistical power: the ability of a study to detect a true effect of a specified magnitude. The statistical power corresponds to 1 (Type II error).

Statistical significance: the likelihood that a difference as large as or larger than that observed between study groups could have occurred by chance alone in a sample of the size investigated. Usually, the level of statistical significance is stated as a p value (eg, $p < 0.05$).

Stroke: a sudden derangement in function, as in sunstroke or heat stroke; often used in relation to a sudden neurologic deficit that occurs because of insufficient delivery of oxygenated blood to the brain, as may occur following a blood clot or hemorrhage.

Subacute: a rate of progression of a condition that is intermediate between acute and chronic.

Surveillance: ongoing observation of a population for rapid and accurate detection of changes in the occurrence of particular diseases.

Survival: the likelihood of remaining alive for a specified period of time after the diagnosis of a particular disease.

Systematic error: see **Bias.**

Systematic review: a synthesis of medical evidence on a topic, in which the synthesis has been prepared using strategies to minimize errors.

Terminal node: in a decision tree, an element that represents the outcome for a particular clinical scenario.

T lymphocyte: a white blood cell that is responsible for cell-mediated immunity in the host.

Transmission: the process by which a pathogen passes from one source of infection to a new host.

True-negative: a test result that is normal (negative) when the disease of interest is actually absent.

True-positive: a test result that is abnormal (positive) when the disease of interest is actually present.

Tuberculosis: an infectious illness caused by *Mycobacterium tuberculosis,* characterized by a brief initial illness; in a minority of cases, a chronic active illness, primarily affecting the lungs, will occur months to years following infection.

Tularemia: an infectious disease caused by the bacterium *Francisella tularensis.* Natural infection results from the bite of an infected tick, deerfly, or insect, but the bacterium also is now considered a potential agent of bioterrorism.

Tumor: a swelling that may occur from an inflammatory process or a benign or malignant neoplasm.

Twin study: a study of genetic susceptibility in which concordance for occurrence of a particular disease is compared between dizygotic (fraternal) twins and monozygotic (identical) twins, or between twins reared together versus apart.

Type I error: rejection of the null hypothesis when it is actually correct.

Type II error: failure to reject the null hypothesis when it is actually incorrect.

Underlying cause of death: (1) the disease or injury that initiated the train of morbid events leading directly to death, or (2) the circumstances of the accident or violence that resulted in fatal injury.

Utility: in decision analysis, a patient's preference for one outcome over another, usually graded on a scale of zero, representing death, to one, representing perfect health.

Validity: the extent to which a measurement or a study result correctly represents the characteristics or relationship of interest.

Variability: the property of having a spread of values, which may arise from random sources (viz, the operation of chance) or from systematic influences (viz, bias).

Viral hemorrhagic fevers: a group of life-threatening illnesses caused by the filoviruses (eg, Ebola and Marburg) and arenaviruses (eg, Lassa and Machupo). Natural occurrence is geographically limited, but these viruses now are considered potential agents of bioterrorism.

Viremia: the presence of virus particles in the blood of a host.

Vital statistics: information concerning patterns of registered life events, such as births, marriages, divorces, and deaths.

Weighted average: a summary measure in which some of the component data values are assigned greater influence than others. For example, precision-based weighting is the calculation of a summary measure in which the relative influence of individual results is based on statistical confidence in the respective results.

West Nile virus: a member of the Flavivirus genus first identified in 1937 in the West Nile district of Uganda. The virus is passed between birds by mosquitoes, which in turn can infect humans through bites. The illness first appeared in the Western Hemisphere in 1999 and is characterized by fever, nausea, vomiting, headache, myalgia, and in rare instances leads to a severe neurologic disease.

Withdrawals: subjects who are initially included in a study but later voluntarily or involuntarily terminate participation.

Years of potential life lost (YPLL): a measure of total life lost to a particular age (eg, 75 years) within a population because of premature deaths.

e-PIDEMIOLOGY

http://www.kings.cam.ac.uk/~js229/glossary.html

http://www.facsnet.org/report_tools/guides_primers/epidemiology/glossary.html

INDEX

NOTE: Page numbers in **bold face** type indicate a major discussion. A *t* following a page number indicates tabular material and an *f* following a page number indicates a figure.

Framingham Heart Study, as cohort study example, 135–136

Francisella tularensis, in bioterrorism, 86*t*

Fraternal (dizygotic) twins, genetic and environmental risk factors studied in, 181–182, 183*f*

G

Gastroenteritis
  as disease outbreak, 69–91
    attack rate and, 71–73, 71*t*, 72*t*
    common-source exposure in, 70, 73, 74*t*, 75
    incubation period and, 73–74, 74*t*, 75–77, 75*f*
    risk ratio and, 71–72, 73, 74
    profile of patient with, 69

Gender
  attack rate and, 71*t*, 72
  genetic and environmental risk factors and, 179
  matching and, 154, 154*f*
  mortality patterns affected by, 57, 58–59, 58*f*, 60*f*
  occurrence patterns affected by, 36, 36*f*

Gene–environment interactions, 185

Generalization of results, validity and. *See* External validity

Genetic epidemiology, **176–188**
  complex genetic analyses in, 178*t*, **186**
  descriptive studies for, **178–179**, 178*t*
  environmental interaction and, 185
  familial aggregation studies and, 178*t*, **179–182**, 180*f*, 181*f*, 182*f*, 183*f*

interpretation of studies in, 185
  specific genetic factors studied in, 178*t*, **182–186**, 184*f*
  types of studies in, 178, 178*t*

Genetic linkage, 182–183
  indirect approach to genetic epidemiology studies and, 185–186

Genetic markers
  linkage analysis in study of, 185–186
  linkage disequilibrium influencing studies of, 185

Genotype, as "exposure" for cohort study, 183

Geographic area, disease occurrence patterns and. *See* Place

Growth factors, for infection in neutropenic patients, 18

H

Hantavirus pulmonary syndrome, ecologic changes and, 80

Health Insurance Plan (HIP) study, 102–103, 102*f*

"Healthy worker" effect, 168

Hemorrhagic fevers, viral, in bioterrorism, 86, 86*t*, 87*t*

Hepatitis, alcoholic
  clinical background of, 190
  differentiation of from cholangitis, 189
  decision analysis and, 193*f*, 194–196, 194*t*, 195*f*
  sensitivity analysis and, 195–196, 196*t*, 197, 197*t*
  profile of patient with, 189

Heterogeneous results, of clinical trial, meta-analysis and, 125–126, 128

HIP (Health Insurance Plan) study, 102–103, 102*f*

Historical (nonconcurrent) controls, 113–114, 114*f*

Historical (retrospective) cohort study, 136–137, 136*f*, 137*t*, 144

HIV infection/AIDS
  epidemiologic contribution to understanding of, **1–16**
    approach to research and, 3–4
    causes of disease and, 7–8, 7*f*, 8*f*
    diagnostic testing and, 8–10, 9*f*
    disease surveillance and, 4–7, 5*f*, 6*f*
    effect of treatment and, 12–14, 13*f*
    natural history of disease and, 10–11, 11*f*
    person/place/time and, 2–3
    prognostic factors and, 11–12, 12*f*, 13*t*
    risk factor identification and, 3–4, 7–8, 7*f*, 8*f*
    sentinel cases and, 2–3, 3*t*
  incidence rates of, 6–7, 6*f*
  as pandemic, 2
  profile of patient with, 1
  surveillance definition of, 4
  transmission of, cohort studies in evaluation of, 7–8, 8*f*
  tuberculosis coexistence and, 42–43, 42*f*, 43*f*, 45

HLAs. *See* Human leukocyte antigens

Homosexuality, identification of as HIV infection/AIDS risk factor, 3

Hospital-based case–control study, **151–152**, 152*t*, 153*t*, 158
  selection bias and, 169